ALLE ZEIT WACH

1842

K. Yabe · K. Kusano · H. Nakata (Eds.)

Adapted Physical Activity

Health and Fitness

With 67 Figures

Springer Japan KK

Kyonosuke Yabe, ph.d.
Professor, Research Center of Health, Physical Fitness and Sports, Nagoya University, Furo-cho, Chikusa-ku, Nagoya, 464-01 Japan

Katsuhiko Kusano
Professor, Department of Education, Miyazaki University, 1-1 Gakuen Kibanadai Nishi, Miyazaki, 889-32 Japan

Hideo Nakata
Associate Professor, Institute of Special Education, University of Tsukuba, 1-1-1 Tennoudai, Tsukuba, 305 Japan

ISBN 978-4-431-68274-5 ISBN 978-4-431-68272-1 (eBook)
DOI 10.1007/978-4-431-68272-1

Printed on acid-free paper.

Library of Congress Cataloging-in-Publication Data
Adapted physical activity: health and fitness/K. Yabe, K. Kusano, H. Nakata (eds.). p. cm. Includes papers presented at the 9th International Symposium on Adapted Physical Activity (9th ISAPA), held in Yokohama, Japan, August 4–7, 1993. Includes bibliographical references and index. 1. Physical education for handicapped persons—Congresses. 2. Physical fitness for the physically handicapped—Congresses. 3. Physical fitness for the aged—Congresses. 4. Physical education for handicapped persons—Physiological aspects—Congresses. 5. Physical fitness for the physically handicapped—Physiological aspects—Congresses. 6. Physical fitness for the aged—Physiological aspects—Congresses. I. Yabe, K (Kyonosuke), 1937- . II. Kusano, K. (Katsuhiko), 1942- . III. Nakata, H. (Hideo), 1948- . IV. International Symposium on Adapted Physical Activity (9th: 1993: Yokohama-shi, Japan) GV445.A29 1994 796′.087—dc20, 94-31606

Originally published by Springer-Verlag Tokyo Berlin Heidelberg New York in 1994
Softcover reprint of the hardcover 1st edition 1994

Foreword

During the last decade, societal perception of disability has been changing; there has been a gradual shift in focus from the disabled person's limitations to the potential for maximizing his or her individual abilities. In the 1980s, numerous innovative educational and rehabilitation models were developed and implemented. The emphasis today is on psychological and physical health, fitness, and well-being rather than on sickness, disability, and pathology. The concept of adapted physical activity (APA) refers to the theory and practice of adaptation of physical activities to the specific needs of disabled persons.

In a nutshell, APA means *movement*: it is the comprehensive term for physical activities and sports in which the interests and capabilities of individuals with limiting conditions have been taken into special consideration. APA is an interdisciplinary field that includes education, rehabilitation, and sports sciences for the benefit not just of persons labelled as handicapped but also for anyone in need of pedagogic, therapeutic, or technical adaptations.

The adapted physical activity movement was launched with the founding of the International Federation in 1973, and the concept of APA rapidly gained momentum through international symposia held every two years in various cities around the world (Quebec City, Brussels, New Orleans, London, Toronto, Brisbane, Berlin, and Miami). The *Adapted Physical Activity Quarterly* was the first professional journal to disseminate the results of APA research; it was recently named as the official journal of the International Federation.

The purpose of APA symposia is to stimulate the development and implementation of research; to facilitate the interaction between theory and practice as well as among scientists and other APA professionals; and to improve the dissemination of knowledge and research findings. The Ninth International Symposium, held in Yokohama, Japan, in August, 1993, marked a new step in the simultaneous progress of science and practical work in the field of APA.

Both disability research in general and the field of physical activity and sports for the disabled in particular are continually advancing, and APA cannot exist without the cooperation of all professionals involved in this field. Educators and practitioners must join those working in medicine, rehabilitation, therapeutic recreation, and sports programs to analyze the quality of existing services.

These proceedings reflect the successful links created between the manifold aspects of APA. It is my hope that the reader will go beyond the traditional understanding of the role of physical education, sports, rehabilitation, motor control, health, and physical fitness to embrace a broader, more comprehensive concept of APA. I am convinced that these proceedings will provide scientists and other APA professionals with a theoretical and practical stimulus that will benefit the implementation of APA research around the world.

J.C. de Potter
IFAPA President

Preface

This volume includes most of the papers presented at the 9th International Symposium on Adapted Physical Activity (9th ISAPA), held in Yokohama, Japan, August 4–7, 1993. The main theme of the symposium was "Stepping Forward Beyond Barriers Through Physical Activity." It was most encouraging that 531 registered participants from 22 countries attended and 244 papers (Poster, 108; Oral, 81; Film, 55) were presented.

This symposium, which was held for the first time in Asia, had two purposes. The first objective was to advance research and education related to the health and physical fitness of people with disabilities, including the elderly. The second aim was to cultivate a deeper understanding of disabled people on the part of those who are not disabled, and of society in general, through physical activity and sports.

Our basic position was the following: "We all have individual differences in ability." On the basis of this principle, we emphasized the idea of "individuality." We also intended to provide an opportunity to improve the quality of life of persons with disabilities through physical activity and sports. This important concept is still relatively new, especially in Asian countries.

In Japan, for example, both the 1964 Olympic Games in Tokyo and the 1972 Olympic Winter Games in Sapporo succeeded in promoting sports activities among Japanese citizens. These two Olympics also stimulated scientific contributions to physical activities and sports. After the Olympics, "sport sciences" developed rapidly in Japan. We hope this ISAPA in Asia will further promote the science and practice of adapted physical activity in Asian countries as well as the rest of the world.

Due to the restriction of pages this volume contains only 39 of the excellent lectures and papers selected by the Program Committee of the 9th ISAPA.

Kyonosuke Yabe
Chairperson of the 9th ISAPA

Contents

Part II Medical Aspects and Rehabilitation

List of Contributors

His Imperial Highness Prince Tomohito of Mikasa

Aihara, Masahiko
Odawara Cardiovascular Hospital, 296-1 Yahagi, Odawara, Kanagawa, 250 Japan

Akataki, Kumi
Institute for Developmental Research, Aichi Prefectural Colony, 713-8 Komiya, Kasugai, Aichi, 480-03 Japan

Akiho, Kenji
Department of Occupational Therapy, Kanagawa Rehabilitation Hospital, The Kanagawa Rehabilitation Center, 516 Nanasawa, Atsugi, Kanagawa, 243-01 Japan

Albat, Bernard
Service de Transplantation Cardiothoracique, Hôpital Arnaud de Villeneuve, 34295 Montpellier, Cedex, France

Arai, Tamon
Kyoto Welfare Center for Aged Citizens, 30 Mibu-Sennen, Nakagyo-ku, Kyoto, 604 Japan

Araya, Haruna
Yokohama Comprehensive Care Continuum, 1735 Toriyama, Kouhoku-ku, Yokohama, Kanagawa, 222 Japan

Asai, Hitoshi
College of Liberal Arts, Kanazawa University, Kakuma, Kanazawa, Ishikawa, 920-11 Japan

Baba, Mikoto
Department of Rehabilitation Medicine, Fujita Health University, Nanakuri Sanatorium, 424-1 Ohtori, Mukaihiro, Hisai, Mie, 514-12 Japan

Barthe, Valérie
Laboratoire Sport Santé Développement, U.F.R.S.T.A.P.S., 700 Avenue du Pic Saint Loup, 34090 Montpellier, France

Bethge, Annett
Department of Cardiology and Cardiac Rehabilitation, Erasmus Teaching Hospital, Free University of Brussels, Route de Lennik 80, 1070 Brussels, Belgium

Bonnet, Michel
Laboratory of Cognitive Neurosciences, National Center for Scientific Research, Chemin Joseph Aiguier, 13402 Marseille, Cedex 9, France

Bressan, Elizabeth S.
Department of Human Movement Studies, University of Stellenbosch, 7600 Stellenbosch, Republic of South Africa

Chang, Kwangchol
Hakuoh Hospital, 270-1 Ushijima, Kaisei, Ashigarakami-gun, Kanagawa, 258 Japan

de Potter, Jean-Claude
Université Libre de Bruxelles, Avenue P. Héger 28, 1050 Brussels, Belgium

Delisle, Marc-André
Faculty of Social Sciences, Laval University, 150 Boul. René Levesque E, Québec, Canada G1R 4Y1

do Carmo, Apolônio A.
Department of Physical Education, Federal University of Uberlândia, Rua Benjamin Constant 1286, Uberlândia 38406-102, Brazil

Dohi, Nobuyuki
Department of Rehabilitation Medicine, Fujita Health University, Nanakuri Sanatorium, 424-1 Ohtori, Mukaihiro, Hisai, Mie, 514-12 Japan

Doll-Tepper, Gudrun
Institut für Sportwissenschaft, Freie Universität Berlin, Schwendenerstraße 8, 14195 Berlin, Germany

Drouin, Denis
Physical Education Department, Faculty of Education, Laval University, 1088 Raymond Casgrain, Québec, Canada G1K 7P4

Ebine, Kunio
Department of Cardiovascular Surgery, Toho University School of Medicine, Ohashi Hospital, 2-17-6 Ohashi, Meguro-ku, Tokyo, 153 Japan

Emes, Claudia
Faculty of Physical Education, University of Calgary, 2500 University Dr. NW, Calgary, Alberta, Canada T2N 1N4

Enzaki, Yuko
University of Tsukuba School for the Physically Handicapped, 2-1-12 Komone, Itabashi-ku, Tokyo, 173 Japan

Filadoro, R.
Department of Preventive and Rehabilitation Sports Medicine, Technical University of Munich, Connollystr. 32, 80809 Munich, Germany

Foster, Bernadette
Department of Human Movement Science, R.M.I.T., Plenty Road, Bundoora, Victoria 3085, Australia

Fujiie, Kaoru
Department of Medical Engineering, Spinal Injuries Center, 550-4 Ikisu Michisaka, Iizuka, Fukuoka, 820 Japan

Fujiwara, Katsuo
College of Liberal Arts, Kanazawa University, Kakuma, Kanazawa, Ishikawa, 920-11 Japan

Goto, Yukihiro
Hyogo University of Teacher Education, 942-1 Shimokume, Yashiro, Kato-gun, Hyogo, 673-14 Japan

Haber, P.
Department of Sports Medicine/Internal Medicine IV, Technical University of Munich, Connollystr. 32, 80809 Munich, Germany

Haishi, Kouichi
Graduate School of Education, Tohoku University, Kawauchi, Aoba-Ku, Sendai, Miyagi, 980 Japan

Hartard, M.
Departments of Sports Medicine/Internal Medicine IV and Preventive and Rehabilitation Sports Medicine, Technical University of Munich, Connollystr. 32, 80809 Munich, Germany

Hase, Hiroki
Third Department of Internal Medicine, Toho University School of Medicine, Ohashi Hospital, 2-17-6 Ohashi, Meguro-ku, Tokyo, 153 Japan

Hentona, Tatsuko
Itoman Municipal Shiohira Elementary School, 634-2 Shiohira, Itoman, Okinawa, 901-03 Japan

Hong, Yang-Ja
Department of Health Education, Ehwa Woman's University, 11-1 Daehyun-Dong, Seodaemun-Ku, Seoul, Korea

Hoshi, Masahiro
Department of Physical Therapy, Kanagawa Rehabilitation Hospital, The Kanagawa Rehabilitation Center, 516 Nanasawa, Atsugi, Kanagawa, 243-01 Japan

Huber, J.
Department of Gynecology, Technical University of Munich, Connollystr. 32, 80809 Munich, Germany

Iida, Masaru
Saitama Prefectural Rehabilitation Center, 148-1 Nishikaizuka, Ageo, Saitama, 362 Japan

Ikeda, Yukiharu
Department of Occupational Therapy, Kanagawa Rehabilitation Hospital, The Kanagawa Rehabilitation Center, 516 Nanasawa, Atsugi, Kanagawa, 243-01 Japan

Ilieva, D.
Department of Sports Medicine/Internal Medicine IV, Technical University of Munich, Connollystr. 32, 80809 Munich, Germany

Imaizumi, Kazuhiko
Department of Living and Health Sciences, Joetsu University of Education, 1 Yamayashiki, Joetsu, Niigata, 943 Japan

Ishii, Kojiro
Department of Health Science, Faculty of Integrated Arts and Sciences, Hiroshima University, 1-7-1 Kagamiyama, Higashi Hiroshima, Hiroshima, 724 Japan

Itoh, Kunihiko
Institute for Developmental Research, Aichi Prefectural Colony, 713-8 Komiya, Kasugai, Aichi, 480-03 Japan

Jeon, Hyae Ja
Department of Physical Education, Soon Cheon Hyong University, Seuol Kang Dong-Ku, Sang Il Dong 124, Joo Kong APT 601-501, Korea

Jeschke D.
Department of Preventive and Rehabilitation Sports Medicine, Technical University of Munich, Connollystr. 32, 80809 Munich, Germany

Kai, Kenji
Department of Rehabilitation, Chugoku Rosai Hospital, 1-5-1 Tagaya, Kure, Hiroshima, 737-01 Japan

Kajiwara, Toshio
Department of Rehabilitation Medicine, Fujita Health University, Nanakuri Sanatorium, 424-1 Ohtori, Mukaihiro, Hisai, Mie, 514-12 Japan

Kazai, Nobuyuki
Bukkyo University, 96 Kitahananobou, Murasakino, Kita-ku, Kyoto, 603 Japan

Kikuchi, Kunio
Department of Health Science, Faculty of Integrated Arts and Sciences, Hiroshima University, 1-7-1 Kagamiyama, Higashi Hiroshima, Hiroshima, 724 Japan

Kim, Jong Seok
Organization for Korean, Atomic Energy Awareness, Korea

Kim, Kwang-Ho
Department of Physical Education, Seoul National University, San 56-1, Shil Rim-Dong, Kwan Ak-Gu, Seoul, 151-742 Korea

Kim, Ui-Soo
Department of Physical Education, Seoul National University, San 56-1, Shil Rim-Dong, Kwan Ak-Gu, Seoul, 151-742 Korea

Kimura, Misaka
Kyoto Prefectural University of Medicine, College of Medical Technology, 410 Nakagoryo, Seiwainguchi Teramachi, Kamigyo-ku, Kyoto, 602 Japan

Kimura, Yasuo
Odawara Cardiovascular Hospital, 296-1 Yahagi, Odawara, Kanagawa, 250 Japan

Kizawa, Tomoko
Saitama Prefectural Rehabilitation Center, 148-1 Nishikaizuka, Ageo, Saitama, 362 Japan

Kokubun, Mitsuru
Faculty of Education, Kanazawa University, Kakuma, Kanazawa, Ishikawa, 920-11 Japan

Komura, Takashi
Department of Health Science, Faculty of Integrated Arts and Sciences, Hiroshima University, 1-7-1 Kagamiyama, Higashi Hiroshima, Hiroshima, 724 Japan

Kotake, Tomomitsu
Department of Rehabilitation Medicine, Fujita Health University, Nanakuri Sanatorium, 424-1 Ohtori, Mukaihiro, Hisai, Mie, 514-12 Japan

Koyama, Yoshiki
Koyama Orthopedics Hospital, 767 Ishinden, Tsu, Mie, 514-01 Japan

Kunimi, Yumiko
Institute of Research, The Kanagawa Rehabilitation Center, 516 Nanasawa, Atsugi, Kanagawa, 243-01 Japan

Kunita, Kenji
College of Liberal Arts, Kanazawa University, Kakuma, Kanazawa, Ishikawa, 920-11 Japan

Kusano, Katsuhiko
Department of Education, Miyazaki University, 1-1 Gakuen Kibanadai Nishi, Miyazaki, 889-32 Japan

Kuster, Markus
Department of Orthopedic Surgery, Kantonsspital St. Gallen, 9000, Switzerland

Larouche, René
Physical Education Department, Faculty of Education, Laval University, 1088 Raymond Casgrain, Québec, G1K 7P4 Canada

Lim, Wan-Ki
Department of Social Physical Education, Hoseo University, San 29-1, Sechul-Ri, Baebang-Myun, Asan-Kun, Chungchungnam-Do, Korea

Livingston, Lori
Department of Physical Education, Wilfrid Laurier University, Waterloo, Ontario, Canada N8L 3C3

Maeda, Kazuya
Department of Health Science and Physical Education, Osaka City University, 3-3-138 Sugimoto, Sumiyoshi-ku, Osaka, 558 Japan

Maruyama, Hirotake
Seibo Junior Women's College, 1 Tayamachi, Fukakusa, Fushimi-ku, Kyoto, 612 Japan

Tsunemi, Kyoko
Saitama Prefectural Rehabilitation Center, 148-1 Nishikaizuka, Ageo, Saitama, 362 Japan

Matsumoto, Takuma
Department of Occupational Therapy, Kanagawa Rehabilitation Hospital, The Kanagawa Rehabilitation Center, 516 Nanasawa, Atsugi, Kanagawa, 243-01 Japan

Matsuzaki, Yasuhiro
Okinawa Prefectural Education Center, 584 Yogi, Okinawa, Okinawa, 904-21 Japan

Mercier, Jacques
Laboratoire de Physiologie des Interactions, 371 av. Doyen Giraud, 34295 Montpellier, Cedex 5, France

Mita, Katsumi
Institute for Developmental Research, Aichi Prefectural Colony, 713-8 Komiya, Kasugai, Aichi, 480-03 Japan

Miyaguchi, Akiyoshi
Kanazawa College of Economics, 10 Gosho, Kanazawa, Ishikawa, 920 Japan

Mizuguchi, Masato
Department of Internal, Kanagawa Rehabilitation Hospital, The Kanagawa Rehabilitation Center, 516 Nanasawa, Atsugi, Kanagawa, 243-01 Japan

Muraki, Satoshi
Department of Health Science, Faculty of Integrated Arts and Sciences, Hiroshima University, 1-7-1 Kagamiyama, Higashi Hiroshima, Hiroshima, 724 Japan

Nakata, Hideo
Institute of Special Education, University of Tsukuba, 1-1-1 Tennohdai, Tsukuba, 305 Japan

Nakaya, Takashi
Nobeoka School for Disabled Children, 1 Matsuyama, Nobeoka, Miyazaki, 882 Japan

Ninomiya, Kenji
Odawara Cardiovascular Hospital, 296-1 Yahagi, Odawara, Kanagawa, 250 Japan

Normand, Roselyne
CLSC Arthur-Caux, rue de la Station Laurier-Station, Québec, Canada GOS 1NO

Odajima, Natu
Saitama Prefectural Rehabilitation Center, 148-1 Nishikaizuka, Ageo, Saitama, 362 Japan

Ogata, Tamae
Odawara Cardiovascular Hospital, 296-1 Yahagi, Odawara, Kanagawa, 250 Japan

Ogawa, Ryokei
Kansai Medical University, 18-89 Uyama Higashi, Hirakata, Osaka, 573 Japan

Ohdoko, Keisuke
Department of Rehabilitation, Koseisogo Hospital, 1427-1 Minamimachi, Mihara, Hiroshima, 723 Japan

Okamoto, Emi
PL Gakuen Women's Junior College, 2680 Kishi, Tondabayashi, Osaka, 584 Japan

Okamoto, Kayoko
Kansai Medical University, 18-89 Uyama Higashi, Hirakata, Osaka, 573 Japan

Okamoto, Tsutomu
Kansai Medical University, 18-89 Uyama Higashi, Hirakata, Osaka, 573 Japan

Okayama, Yasuko
Kyoto Prefectural University of Medicine, College of Medical Technology, 410 Nakagoryo, Seiwainguchi Teramachi, Kamigyo-ku, Kyoto, 602 Japan

Okuzumi, Hideyuki
Graduate School of Education, Tohoku University, Kawauchi, Aoba-ku, Sendai, Miyagi, 980 Japan

Ookubo, Harumi
Saitama Prefectural Rehabilitation Center, 148-1 Nishikaizuka, Ageo, Saitama, 362 Japan

Palsio, Niina
Department of Physical Education, University of Jyväskylä, P.O. Box 35, 40351 Jyväskylä, Finland

Préfaut, Christian
Laboratoire de Physiologie des Interactions, 371 av. Doyen Giraud, 34295 Montpellier, Cedex 5, France

Preisinger, E.
Department of Physical Medicine and Rehabilitation, Technical University of Munich, Connollystr. 32, 80809 Munich, Germany

Quittan, M.
Department of Physical Medicine and Rehabilitation, Technical University of Munich, Connollystr. 32, 80809 Munich, Germany

Rintala, Pauli
Department of Physical Education, University of Jyväskylä, P.O. Box 35, 40351 Jyväskylä, Finland

Saishoji, Hisakazu
Department of Rehabilitation Gymnastics, Kanagawa Rehabilitation Hospital, The Kanagawa Rehabilitation Center, 516 Nanasawa, Atsugi, Kanagawa, 243-01 Japan

Sakurai, Shinji
Research Center of Health, Physical Fitness and Sports, Nagoya University, Nagoya, 464-01 Japan

Sasaki, Hisato
Department of Rehabilitation, Hiroshima Railway Hospital, 3-1-36 Futabanosato, Hiroshima, 732 Japan

Schantz, Otto J.
University of Franche-Comté, 31 rue de l'Epitaphe, Besançon, France

Seidl, G.
Department of Radiology, Technical University of Munich, Connollystr. 32, 80809 Munich, Germany

Setoguchi, Yoshimasa
Koyama Orthopedics Hospital, 767 Ishinden, Tsu, Mie, 514-01 Japan

Sherrill, Claudine
Department of Kinesiology, Texas Woman's University at Denton, Box 23717, TWU Station, Denton, TX 76204, USA

Shinoda, Tatsuaki
Aichi Prefectural Colony, Welfare Center for Persons with Developmental Disabilities, 713-8 Kamiya, Kasugai, Aichi, 480-03 Japan

Simard, Clermont
Physical Education Department, Faculty of Education Laval University, 1088 Raymond Casgrain, Québec, Canada G1K 7P4

Suzuki, Nobuharu
Izu Rehabilitation Welfare Center for Disabled, 202 Jike, Nirayama, Tagata-gun, Sizuoka, 410-21 Japan

Tachiyashiki, Kaoru
Department of Living and Health Sciences, Joetsu University of Education, 1 Yamayashiki, Joetsu, Niigata, 943 Japan

Takagi, Hiroshi
Saitama Prefectural Rehabilitation Center, 148-1 Nishikaizuka, Ageo, Saitama, 362 Japan

Thévenet, André
Service de Transplantation Cardiothoracique, Hopital Arnaud de Villeneuve, 34295 Montpellier, Cedex, France

Tokuhara, Yasuhiko
Osaka International University for Women, 6-21-57 Fujita, Moriguchi, Osaka, 570 Japan

Toyama, Hiroshi
College of Liberal Arts, Kanazawa University, Kakuma, Kanazawa, Ishikawa, 920-11 Japan

Tsukagoshi, Kazumi
Saitama Prefectural Rehabilitation Center, 148-1 Nishikaizuka, Ageo, Saitama, 362 Japan

Tsutsumi, Hiromi
Kansai Medical University, 18-89 Uyama-Higashi, Hirakata, Osaka, 573 Japan

Tsuyuki, Kazuo
Odawara Cardiovascular Hospital, 296-1 Yahagi, Odawara, Kanagawa, 250 Japan

Usui, Sotoyuki
Hokuriku Institution of Wellness and Sports Science, 13-1 Yahata, Komatsu, Ishikawa, 923 Japan

Varray, Alain
Laboratoire Sport Santé Développement, U.F.R.S.T.A.P.S., 700 Avenue du Pic Saint Loup, 34090 Montpellier, France

Vickers, Joan
Faculty of Physical Education, University of Calgary, 2500 University Dr. NW, Calgary, Alberta, Canada T2N 1N4

Vute, Rajko
Faculty of Education, University of Ljubljana, Kard, Pl. 16, Ljubljana, Slovenia

Walkley, Jeff
Department of Human Movement Science, R.M.I.T., Plenty Road, Bundoora, Victoria 3085, Australia

Watakabe, Makoto
Asahikawa Medical College, Nishikagura 4-5, 3-11 Asahikawa, Hokkaido, 078-11 Japan

Winnick, Joseph P.
Department of Physical Education and Sport, State University of New York, College at Brockport, 350 New Campus Drive, Brockport, NY 14420-2994, USA

Wintrebert, Pierre
Service de Transplantation Cardiothoracique, Hôpital Arnaud de Villeneuve, 34295 Montpellier, Cedex, France

Wood, Graeme A.
University of Western Australia, Perth, WA 6009, Australia

Woollacott, Marjorie H.
Department of Exercise and Movement Science, University of Oregon, Esslinger Hall, 1525 University Street, Eugene, OR 97403, USA

Yabe, Kyonosuke
Research Center of Health, Physical Fitness and Sports, Nagoya University, Furo-cho, Chikusa-ku, Nagoya, 464-01 Japan

Yamasaki, Masahiro
Department of Health Science, Faculty of Integrated Arts and Sciences, Hiroshima University, 1-7-1 Kagamiyama, Higashi Hiroshima, Hiroshima, 724 Japan

Yamashina, Tadahiko
Kanazawa Medical College, 1-1 Daigaku Uchinada, Ishikawa, 920-02 Japan

Yamashita, Hideaki
Kansai Medical University, 18-89 Uyama Higashi, Hirakata, Osaka, 573 Japan

Sports for the Disabled

—Special Lecture—

Sports for People with Handicaps

His Imperial Highness Prince Tomohito of Mikasa

The first question I would like to raise is whether there is anyone in the world who is a hundred percent handicapped.

I paraphrase the following illustration which most precisely expresses my thoughts on this point.

"Mr. A is bedridden and needs full care but is a man of great ideas and attractive personality. Mr. B is an all-round sportsman but he has few friends and is a chronic complainer. Compare these two and one notes that Mr. A is handicapped and Mr. B is well where physical activities are concerned. In mental and spiritual matters, Mr. B is the one with the handicap whereas Mr. A is well. No one can be totally handicapped and none of us are perfect."

Doctors invariably begin a physical examination by observation, by touch and by asking questions the first time they see a patient. Only after this is the full medical examination conducted. For those of us engaged in the care of the handicapped, it is extremely important that we look at them, touch them and ask them questions. In other words, when we meet a person who is bedridden or in a wheelchair, or with a white stick or a seeing-eye dog, we must say things like "Tell me all about it," or "Let's see what we can do about this."

We seem to think that people should be judged functionally and categorized as such. For some time, at least for a number of decades, it has been the common practice in Japan to see people as either healthy or handicapped. Those who receive a "Certificate for Physically Disabled Persons" or, in the case of mentally retarded children, a "Certificate of Love" issued by the Ministry of Health and Welfare are defined as handicapped. As I mentioned earlier, no one is totally handicapped—nor totally healthy, for that matter. It is unreasonable, therefore, to classify people with such certificates as handicapped and those without as healthy.

From a medical point of view, these certificates have a valuable function in informing doctors and hospitals if, for example, a child has cerebral or spinal palsy. Apart from this, the simple dichotomy is not desirable for those of us who are involved in the daily care and welfare of the handicapped. Let each of us review what we do in the normal course of a day. How does each of us fare in sports and intellectual pursuits, and what do we score for the state of our health, or for our ability to cook and do the housework? What if those of us who admit we scored 49% were told to carry a certificate and begin rehabilitation? This is what is meant by seeing people "functionally". There are three important points which I beg you to understand well.

We have with us at this conference professional dancers in wheelchairs from Germany, and we may later have the opportunity to enjoy watching them perform. About 20 years or so ago, we first began training programs in the belief that everyone can dance no matter what his or her handicap. One may think that it is too limiting to dance in a wheelchair, but the chair is made to move vertically as well as horizontally. It can even make pivotal turns.

Just as basketball players in wheelchairs are able to perform with acrobatic skills, dancers in wheelchairs can now enter every event. A woman who uses crutches can enjoy a slow dance if I give her a little support. In this way she only needs one stick to support her, and she can enjoy dancing so much more easily then if she were left to dance on her own.

When a visually-impaired person dances, it is usually better to have a partner with good sight so as to avoid collisions. Then he or she can enjoy dancing to the full, even if totally or partially blind.

People with hearing difficulties can usually can feel soundwaves with their bodies. Perhaps the closest we come to this is when the sound of exploding fireworks causes vibrations in our stomachs. By simply adjusting our conventional wisdom, we now have people all over Japan who can enjoy dancing in spite of every kind of handicap. Both those with handicaps and those without have learned that a little imagination can go a long way.

Let me now talk of fashion shows we have organized. We coined a new term, paramode, combining the words "paralysis" and "mode". Friends of ours thought: why not put on a fashion show for people in wheelchairs or with crutches or those who are bedridden? The idea sprang from the need to develop a raincoat for someone in a wheelchair who needs both hands free to turn the wheels. A person with a spinal injury and paralysis of the lower limbs can often easily propel his wheelchair because he has strong upper limbs. However, on a rainy day it is difficult for him to hold an umbrella and turn the wheels at the same time. He needs a raincoat—but not even our biggest department stores carried such an item.

A tailor who is one of our supporting members decided to take up the challenge of designing a raincoat which would cover the whole wheelchair while leaving openings for the rider's arms. There should also be good protection against splashes on a rainy street, and the whole thing should look attractive.

To put on her skirt, a girl or woman normally stands on one leg and puts the other leg inside the skirt, and then repeats the process for the second leg, but if she uses crutches she finds that skirts are difficult to manage. She may have to lie down or twist herself into awkward positions when dressing. Paramode experts had an idea. The edge of a table would be fitted with hooks, while skirts would have unobtrusive rings attached. A skirt can then be hung from the table like a curtain, and the wearer can make a half or full turn with one stick and wrap the skirt around her.

Then there was a young man whose torso was malformed, making it very difficult for him to put on an ordinary jacket. What we did was to devise a jacket with a zipper at the back. He could then put his arms in easily in front, while someone zipped up the jacket behind. When he is seated one cannot tell the difference. It is most important for people with handicaps to be able to enjoy fashionable clothes just the same as anyone else. They do not want their clothes to be designed only for convenience and functionality, for they tend to be unfashionable. They want to look as nice as everybody else.

You may know of the Canadian youth Rick Hansen who travelled around the world in a wheelchair. He suffered a spinal injury when the car in which he was hitchhiking was involved in a crash and he became paralyzed from the waist down. Since the accident, he has entered every sporting championship he can, winning the wheelchair marathon at Beppu in Japan with a world record time. I believe it was 1 h 52 min. He later beat his own record, which now stands at something like 1 h 20 min. After winning many wheelchair sports championships, he decided to go around the world in what was dubbed "The Rick Hansen Man in Motion World Tour". He set out to cover 25 000 miles, which is equivalent to the circumference of the earth. In Japan, I was asked to help coordinate his run which took him around Hokkaido and, after crossing the Tsugaru Straight by ferry, all the way from Aomori to Tokyo, and then on to Aichi prefecture since the Toyota Motor Corporation was sponsoring him. His runs in the three regions totaled a thousand miles. It was a fine feat.

Prior to Rick Hansen's record run, the longest recorded run I knew of was three thousand kilometers. Uemura Naomi, my mountain-climbing partner, the famous Japanese mountaineer and world class alpinist who perished on Mt. McKinley, had planned a 3000 km dogsled expedition in Greenland. Wanting to get the feel of the distance, he walked from Wakkanai at the northern tip of Hokkaido to Kagoshima at the southern end of Kyushu. This was Uemura's personal record, which to my knowledge no other man had equalled. Then along comes Rick Hansen who travels 40 000 km in a wheelchair.

In rallying support for Rick, we introduced him not so much as a handicapped man with a spinal injury and paralysis of the lower limbs but as a great young Canadian setting out to rewrite sporting records. At news briefings and press interviews we made a point of asking newspapers, magazines and television stations to cover his progress in their sports column and not in the social sections. This I believe is an important point as we look to the future of social welfare.

There is a man with one leg who lives in Obihiro, Hokkaido, by the name of Nakao Yasunori. He works in the city office. He has an artificial limb to replace the leg he had to have amputated after being involved in a traffic accident as a child. Fourteen years ago, Inter Ski, an international conference of ski instructors held every 4 years, met in Zao in Yamagata prefecture. As captain of the team of skiers with handicaps Nakao led a fine demonstration.

In teaching a skier with a single leg, we instructors also ski on one leg. In Nakao's case, since his left leg is intact, we use our left ski and remove the one on the right. To ski on one leg we also use an auxiliary device called an outrigger. The outrigger incorporates a 30-cm short ski at the end of a Canadian crutch. Two outriggers are used to assist a skier with a single leg so that he is actually on three skis. Polio victims have both legs but usually lack muscular control. In such cases, two outriggers provide four points of contact with the snow.

As I mentioned, we always left off one of our skis and used outriggers or regular ski poles while coaching Nakao, and in an amazingly short time he became an excellent skier with fine form. Eleven years ago, a timed speed competition was held in which I was asked to go first. Just as I was about to start downhill on my two legs, Nakao called out, "You're a cheat, prince! You have taught us on one leg and today are you going to ski on two. We want you to ski on one leg like the rest of us."

It had taken a whole week to prepare the course, and it was now a formidable world cup class slope, with its icy surface shining in the sun. It was forbidding to ski on one leg but my pride as a coach won and I took my right ski off and started down the slope with outriggers. I knew that the Hokkaido television crews from HBC and STV were waiting near the finish, and as patron of the championship, technical director and course setter, I could not allow myself to fall. Somehow I managed it.

Then I heard Nakao's name being called. He started swiftly, but fell at the most difficult corner where a sharp turn was required on the steepest gradient. After making the turn he was unable to get a grip with the edge of his ski and fell, but because the slope was so steep he hit it hard and bounced back onto his good leg and was able to continue downhill. Usually, a fall like this would slow a skier by three or four seconds. I was sure I had won. However, when I heard Nakao's official time I was shocked. He was faster than me by seven seconds. Any way you looked at it, that was a decisive win. From that day I no longer taught one-legged skiers. "Nakao has mastered the skill and surpassed his coach," I declared. "I will not lose to him on two legs, but on one he is Japan's champion."

Then there are Kudo Takeshi and Fujii Mitsuyoshi. Both men are partially blind and I taught them cross-country skiing. Norway, as you know, is the kingdom of cross-country skiing and for the last 30 years has been organizing world championships for blind skiers. Fourteen years ago, we decided to send skiers to participate in their championships. Whereas we were alpine skiing instructors we decided to learn cross country skiing from Norwegian experts. We therefore invited instructors and competitors from Norway to run a training session in Hokkaido.

Kudo took part and put on skis for the first time in his life. The long, narrow skis were hard to manage. He struggled for a meter and fell, picked himself up, struggled another meter and fell again.

Then he repeated the painful procedure. Three years later he had became a fantastic racer and could ski faster than his coaches. What was inspiring about him was that he did not stop at being the best among the handicapped skiers. He took our coaching seriously and trained with the aim of participating in the All Japan Championships. He now does so and counts among the best of the non-handicapped skiers. Today he has his sights set on improving his own record to catch up with the All-Japan women's record—if not the men's.

For his part, Fujii won three titles in the Senior Skiers' World Championships held in Norway—in the biathlon and the 5 km and 22 km races. After I learned of his great accomplishment I had an opportunity to ski after him in the Hokkaido Championships. He skied so fast that after 1 km I returned to my own pace. After 4 km I saw him slowing down, and smiled to myself. There was no way he could keep up that speed, and with another circuit, I thought, I would easily overtake him. As expected, Mr. Kudo won the championship with Mr. Fujii coming in second.

As his coach, I thus advised Fujii who was wearing his silver medal round his neck: "I skied behind you for one circuit. At that pace you could not possibly complete a long 30- or 40-km race. You should think of distributing your effort." "You are right, Your Highness," Fujii replied, "it was a miserable race today. It was a relatively easy course but I found it a bit taxing. The day before yesterday," he continued apologetically, "I competed in the 86-km Okhotsk marathon. I had not quite recovered from it and miscalculated my pace."

This was unthinkable for normal racers and ski instructors. After completing an 86 km race, even all-Japan class athletes would usually have at least a week or 10 days of rest. Marathon (42.195 km) runners, I believe, usually schedule three races a year. These were the normally accepted limits of the human body. Mr. Fujii, however, raced 86-km, rested for 1 day and competed in our championships. No wonder he did not pace himself as well as he should and felt a little tired. He was a monster of a man. He was then 57 years old and has probably topped 60 today.

To summarize my thoughts, the first rule in teaching skiing to beginner handicapped skiers is to organize programs designed primarily to help them to enjoy the sport and the snow. After three or four days of training, we encourage those who have more or less mastered the basic skills to participate at their level in alpine and cross country competition. Intermediate skiers are urged to participate in small championships organized throughout the country in prefectures with heavy snowfall. I am of course talking now of championships organized especially for handicapped skiers. There is an annual all-Hokkaido championship which is a high-level event. Then there are the all-Japan championships. Beyond these, skiers can aim for the world championships held in Norway or the Winter Olympic games.

After graduating from a series of competitions for the handicapped, skiers are then challenged to compete in no-handicap competitions—again, first at the local level. It is rather like an education that starts a child off in kindergarten, then advances through primary, secondary, and high school, and then finally university. We start, as I have described, with training sessions for handicapped skiers, who are then encouraged to participate in races at different levels. After graduating at the university level—in this case the world championships and Winter Olympic Games for handicapped skiers, we ask them to become full-fledged members of the skiing fraternity by competing among skiers without handicaps. We believe that this is what is meant by the motto "full participation and equality" coined for the International Year of the Handicapped. It is not a high enough aim just to become a champion among other people with handicaps.

You may recall that during the Los Angeles Summer Olympic Games, a female athlete in a wheelchair followed in the wake of the New Zealand delegation as it marched into the stadium. I saw her on television and had enquiries made to find out more about her. She was an archer and did not do too well that year in Los Angeles. The following year, however, she won a well-earned victory in the Commonwealth Games. It does not matter in archery whether an athlete is in a wheelchair or not. She was by any standard an Olympic athlete. For those of us training handicapped people in sports, it is an encouragement and an inspiration that this New Zealand archer has made it to the top in spite of her disadvantage. Rick Hansen is also a champion since no one with or without a handicap has equalled his feat of completing 40 000 kilometers around the world. Likewise, in baseball, there is Jim Abbot who has with great courage and faith in himself overcome daunting odds to become a hero in the American major league.

Finally, 12 years ago, the United Nations in establishing the International Year of the Handicapped announced that there were 450 million people with handicaps worldwide. At that time, the world population was 4.5 billion, so it meant that one person in ten was handicapped. Included were starving children, those wounded in war, those seen by psychiatrists, and alcoholics and habitual users of drugs, hence the large number identified as handicapped. The ratio in Japan is declared to be 60 to 1, since the Ministry of Health and Welfare does not count alcoholics or habitual users of drugs and only includes those with handicaps caused congenitally, by disease or by injury. No matter what criteria one uses, it is obvious that there are far more people without handicaps than with.

Therefore, in a society where the majority are healthy, the challenge is to develop a mechanism which motivates people with handicaps to train, rehabilitate their lost functions, and join the mainstream. For this to be possible, healthy people and those with handicaps should both try hard to support each other through mutually rewarding volunteer activities so that the handicapped can fully participate in the contemporary society which has been shaped by the healthy majority. At the same time, everyone should be educated from childhood not to divide others into two categories, the healthy and the handicapped. Every child must be taught that no one in the world is totally handicapped or, for that matter, a hundred percent healthy. These are the perspectives which must be communicated to as many as possible through this symposium.

Yesterday I was in Tendo city in Yamagata prefecture attending an All Japan Junior High School Shogi Chess Championship. I was there to present my trophy to the champion who would emerge from among the youngsters from the 47 prefectures who had passed the elimination matches. Saitama prefecture was represented by a young man named Nakamura who has osteohypoplasia (a disease, as you may know, which slows the development of the bones). I asked Mr. Yonenaga, the new Shogi champion who was there as the chief judge, to evaluate for me the mastery of the youth in the wheelchair. He spent some time watching the youth, and then said, "The boy should be among the best of the sixty-nine top contestants. There is skill and strength in his moves."

This junior shogi championship is not specifically for young people with handicaps. It is a national championship to nurture future national shogi masters. Master Nakamura, in spite of his physical disadvantage, had passed the elimination and was competing among the nation's best. This made me really happy, because this boy was a living model of what we have been saying for the last 20 years to encourage those with handicaps "to catch up and surpass the others". It was such a wonderful thing that I wanted to share it with you.

Thank you for your attention.

—Part I—

Teaching Methods for Sports, Physical Education, and Recreation

—Keynote Speech—

Adapted Physical Activity Pedagogy: Principles, Practices, and Creativity

CLAUDINE SHERRILL

Abstract. Adapted physical activity pedagogy is dynamic, exciting, and challenging. Beliefs, attitudes, and actions toward people with special needs have changed enormously, demanding new ways of thinking and doing. This paper summarizes current thought about (a) philosophy, theory, and practices; (b) negative attitudes and perceived lack of competence of teachers as the greatest barriers to service; (c) principles to guide public school consultant services; (d) a new definition of adapted physical activity; and (e) emerging pedagogical theory that emphasizes integration of knowledge about individual differences, adaptation, and creativity. Adapted physical education specialists should be employed in every community to work directly with students who are disabled and to act as consultants and administrators to help regular educators change attitudes and practices. Assessment, the foundation of pedagogy, should address both individual differences and environmental barriers. Behavior change should be promoted through application of adaptation and creativity theory. Adaptation theory, first posited by Ernst Kiphard of Germany, stresses working with both the individual and the environment in a continuous, dynamic, and bidirectional manner to achieve educational goals. Creativity theory, advanced by Sherrill, stresses fluency, flexibility, originality, and elaboration as key elements of adapted physical activity pedagogy.

Introduction

Adapted physical activity pedagogy is dynamic, exciting, and challenging. Our beliefs, attitudes, and actions toward people with special needs have changed enormously, demanding new ways of thinking and doing. Even our definitions have changed.

Let's consider briefly the history of adapted physical activity in order to place these changes in proper perspective. This history is difficult to trace because adapted physical activity has been given so many names: medical, therapeutic, rehabilitative, healing, remedial, corrective, curative, special, and developmental [1]. The earliest textbooks in the English language refer to medical gymnastics [2] and special kinesiology [3]. Clearly the origins of adapted physical activity date back into the 1800s. Only recently has a consensus been reached that adapted physical activity is the best name for our profession [4, 5].

Philosophy, Theory, and Practices

Terminology reflects philosophy, theory, and practice. Our philosophy is founded on the belief that all persons can learn and benefit from physical activity if teachers and coaches know how to adapt and are creative in thought and action. Several theories provide guides to service delivery but motor adaptation theory, first posited by Ernst Kiphard [6] of Germany, forms the basis for pedagogy. Adaptation theory stresses assessment of both the individual and the environment and strategically modifying both in a continuous, dynamic, and bidirectional manner to achieve goals. Out of adaptation theory come educational practices like ecological task analysis [7] and various self-concept and attitude change interventions [5, 8].

Physicians, educators, and therapists share ownership of the adapted physical activity knowledge base, because many professions teach, counsel, and mentor in regard to exercise and physical activity as modalities for improving physical, mental, and emotional health [9]. Shared ownership is a strength when school, hospital, and community agencies work together in lifespan physical activity programming that is adapted to the individual needs of each citizen.

The history of adapted physical activity (regardless of the various terminologies used) parallels the evolution of the human rights movement and the subsequent advocacy for acceptance, treatment, and education of people who are ill or disabled. The philosophy of a nation, city, or community in regard to where and how such people should be educated determines adapted physical activity pedagogy.

Research indicates that the greatest barriers to physical education instruction for children and youth with disabilities continue to be negative attitudes and perceived lack of competence [10, 11]. Adapted physical activity pedagogy must therefore address attitudes of everyone concerned (teachers, parents, students) and seek to make all feel competent in adaptation strategies and practices.

Attitudes: The Greatest Barriers

Adapted physical activity pedagogy must be conceptualized first and foremost as attitude change [5, 12]. We must begin to see access to physical education and sport as a basic human right of every individual, worthy of the attention of our governments and of the United Nations. It is noteworthy that an International Charter of Physical Education and Sport, specifying physical education and sport as a fundamental right of all, was enacted by the United Nations in 1978. More recently, on June 25, 1993, the first United Nations World Conference on Human Rights in over 25 years, declared:

The World Conference reaffirms the obligation of states to ensure that persons belonging to minorities may exercise fully and effectively all human rights and fundamental freedoms without any discrimination.

Persons with disabilities represent a viable minority group, many of whom do not have the resources (i.e., money, power, education) to fight for their rights.

If, indeed, our profession believes that vigorous physical activity is a primary factor in physical, mental, and emotional health, we must systematically and persistently work to change society's attitudes about inclusion of people with students. This requires traveling from school to school and meeting regularly with principals, teachers, parents, students, and self-help or advocacy groups.

3. Make this administrator and/or consultant responsible for screening *all* students in the school district in order to identify those with health, fitness, or disability conditions who may benefit from adapted physical activity services.

4. Establish a policy that all students, regardless of the severity of their condition, will receive instruction in sport, dance, aquatics, and fitness exercise that will carry over into their use of leisure time and contribute to an active, healthy lifestyle. This is often called the *zero reject principle*. It is based on the belief that all students can learn if teachers know how to teach.

5. Create a continuum of physical education placements in a variety of environments with different kinds of support services. This is generally called the *least restrictive environment (LRE) placement principle*. The regular classroom is considered least restrictive for most students because it is the norm or average setting and thus considered a basic right in a democratic society. However, the term "least restrictive" denotes the setting in which a student can learn best (i.e., he/she is least restricted by barriers like large class size, architectural inaccessibility, undertrained teachers, negative attitudes, and inappropriate content).

6. Be creative in prescribing least restrictive learning environments and services. Use combinations of separate and integrated settings (e.g., 3 days a week in a small group with basic skills instruction, and 2 days in a regular class size in an integrated setting). A combined placement might also be 6 weeks with support services, in regular education fitness or swimming, followed by 6 weeks of intensive wheelchair sport training.

7. Expect the adapted physical education administrator and/or consultant to use community resources and systematically help students to make the transition from school to community-based programs.

These principles are based on the philosophy that attitudes of the community and of regular educators can be changed only by consistent, persistent advocacy by one or more specially trained, designated professionals within the school system. This philosophy is well supported by staff development and in-service training research [16]. It is not enough to employ adapted physical educators to teach in self-contained or segregated settings. We must set higher standards than this. People with special needs can benefit from adapted physical education services in many settings, and regular educators must be taught the theory and practice of adaptation.

Contemporary Definition of Adapted Physical Activity

The definition of adapted physical activity has clearly changed from pedagogy for students who cannot safely or successfully participate in regular physical education to pedagogy directed toward the entire ecosystem (i.e., people with special needs, their classmates, teachers, families, and significant others). We no longer automatically remove the student from the regular setting. Instead, we consider how the environment can be altered, how attitudes can be changed, and how support services can be provided.

Adapted physical education, once defined as a program, is now conceptualized as a service delivery system with many components: (a) planning for the total school district, the school, and the class; (b) assessment; (c) prescription or placement; (d) teaching, counseling, and coaching; (e) evaluation; (f) coordination of resources; and (g) advocacy. I call this service delivery model PAP-TE-CA, an acronym and memory device in which each letter represents a service delivery component [5].

Adapted physical activity, as a profession and scholarly discipline, requires a broad definition to guide university study and research as well as service delivery. In this definition, we need to consider (a) attritudes and beliefs, (b) the knowledge base, and (c) service delivery. Because definitions are linked with theories, scholars need to synthesize facts in each of these areas into theories to systematize a knowledge base for adapted physical activity.

We do not yet have a short, workable definition of our profession and discipline. I propose, for your consideration: *Adapted physical activity is the crossdisciplinary philosophy, attitudes, knowledge, and skills central to service in the psychomotor aomain for people of all ages whose differences from the norm in function and/or structure require adaptations*. This definition avoids references to problems, disabilities, handicaps, and other terms that some people find offensive. Underlying this definition is an assumption that our basic concern is identification and solution of psychomotor problems, both within the individual and the environment, that constitute barriers to a healthy, active lifestyle and equal access to sport, dance, and aquatics.

Individual Differences, Adaptation, and Creativity

Our focus, as a profession and discipline, should be on individual differences rather than on populations categorized as disabled or special. Many persons in the so-called "normal" population have psychomotor problems that constitute barriers to goal achievement. Attitude theory tells us we should not categorize people as disabled and nondisabled (or by any other global terms) but rather focus on the specific psychomotor variable or cluster of variables (human and/or environmental) that is causing difficulty.

We should not be concerned with characteristics of special populations, as was the practice in the past, because all human beings are different. Adaptation is based on individual assessment, which should not be biased by memorized lists of characteristics.

Now is the time to evolve, expand, and refine theories of individual differences, adaptation, and creativity to guide service delivery practices. This triadic blend (individual differences, adaptation, and creativity theory) forms the acronym, I ACT, reaffirming that adapted physical activity is an action-oriented profession that aims to change attitudes about individual differences, resolve psychomotor problems, and empower people to become the best they can be.

To understand and build on the I ACT triad, several sources are especially recommended [5–8, 12]. The ability to adapt is dependent upon personal creativity and a knowledge of the principles of motor development, biomechanics, exercise physiology, and motor learning/control. Principles of creativity that facilitate effective adaptation include:

1. Fluent thinking. Think of many, many ways to achieve a task.
2. Flexible thinking. Shift categories of problem solving frequently; use diverse philosophies, approaches, principles, and practices to see all sides of an issue or problem.
3. Original thinking. Strive toward novel, unique, and unusual responses. Think of ways no one else has tried.
4. Elaborative thinking. Consider how little details can be changed, stretched, expanded. Use your imagination to make things more meaningful and more fun.

References

1. Sherrill C (ed) (1988) Leadership training in adapted physical education. Champaign, IL: Human Kinetics
2. Wide A (1988) Handbook of medical gymnastics. London, Sampson, Low and Marston
3. Posse N (1901) The special kinesiology of educational gymnastics. Lea and Febiger, Boston
4. Porretta DL, Nesbitt J, Labanowich S (1993) Terminology usage: A case of clarity. Adapt Phys Activity Quart 10(2):87–96
5. Sherrill C (1993) Adapted physical activity, recreation, and sport: Crossdisciplinary and lifespan, 4th edn. Dubuque, Brown and Benchmark
6. Kiphard E (1983) Adapted physical education in Germany. In: Eason R, Smith T, Caron F (eds) Adapted physical activity: From theory to application. Human Kinetics, Champaign, pp 25–32
7. Davis WE, Burton AW (1991) Ecological task analysis: Translating movement theory into practice. Adapt Phys Activity Quart 8(2):154–177
8. Tripp A, Sherrill C (1991) Attitude theories of relevance to adapted physical education. Adapt Phys Activity Quart 8(1):12–27
9. Jochheim KA (1990) Adapted physical activity—An interdisciplinary approach. Premises, methods, and procedures. In: Doll-Tepper G, Dahms C, Doll B, Selzam HV (eds) Adapted physical activity: An interdisciplinary approach. Springer, Berlin Heidelberg New York, pp 15–22
10. Heikinaro-Johansson P, Sherrill C (1994) Integrating children with special needs in physical education: A school district assessment model from Finland. Adapt Phys Activity Quart 11(1):44–56
11. Rizzo TL, Vispoel WP (1991) Physical educators' attributes and attitudes toward teaching students with handicaps. Adapt Phys Activity Quart 8(1):4–11

12. Morisbak I (1990) Adapted physical education: The role of the teacher and pedagogical practices. In: Doll-Tepper G, Dahms C, Doll B, Selzam HV (eds) Adapted physical activity: An interdisciplinary approach. Springer, Berlin Heidelberg New York, pp 235–243
13. Block ME, Krebs PL (1992) An alternative to least restrictive environments: A continuum of support to regulate physical education. Adapt Phys Activity Quart 9(2):97–113
14. Thousand JS, Villa RA (1990) Strategies for educating learners with severe disabilities within their local home schools and communities. Focus on Exceptional Children 23(3):1–24
15. Watkinson EJ (1987) The development and evaluation of integrated programs. Can Assoc Health Phys Ed Rec J 53:13–20
16. Tymeson G (1988) In-service teacher education: A review of general practices and suggested guidelines for adapted physical education teacher trainers. In: Sherrill C (ed) Leadership training in adapted physical education (pp. 401–409). Champaign, IL: Human Kinetics

—Keynote Speech—

Adapted Physical Education Programs for Mentally Retarded Children

GUDRUN DOLL-TEPPER

Abstract. One of the key issues in current research and in practical work in adapted physical activity/education for children with mental retardation focuses on the value of integrative settings. Most recent projects in this area discuss aspects of social integration, motivation, self-determination, and indepdendent living. The so-called normalization principle has addressed the situation and needs of persons with an intellectual disability and has stressed the importance of participation in the mainstream of society. Sports and recreational activities play an important role in the lives of many people. Persons with mental retardation should be given opportunities to participate in games and sports on all levels of performance. Different sports organizations such as Special Olympics International and INAS-FMH present opportunities to participate in international sports events. National organizations are increasingly involved in the development of various sports programs. In addition to leisure activities, different forms of rehabilitative therapeutic activities are being offered aiming at an improvement of the overall situation of the individual. Professionals in physical education and sports as well as in other related fields are facing changes and challenges concerning the inclusion of persons with mental retardation into all areas of life. This study presents current developments and trends in physical activity and sport for these individuals.

Introduction

Immediately after the closing of the 1992 Paralympics in Barcelona—the Games for athletes with physical disabilities or visual impairments/blindness—another world event in sports took place in Spain: the Paralympiada, the Paralympic Games for persons with a mental handicap, were inaugurated in Madrid. For the first time in history, athletes with an intellectual disability participated in a top-level multisport event. In addition, increasing opportunities for physical activities and sports on all levels of excellence are being offered to these people. This is especially true of the sports-for-all movement. These developments demonstrate a change in attitudes towards persons with mental retardation that is taking place in different cultures and societies all over the world.

It is important to mention that worldwide problems of terminology and definition have not yet been solved and categorization criteria differ vastly [1]. This issue has strongly influenced discussions in the area of physical education and sports science. Serious concerns about labelling processes still need to be expressed; however, societal awareness of the needs and interests of persons with mental retardation is growing. Past, present, and future developments have to be examined in this context.

Historical Developments

Many individuals with mental retardation were excluded from sporting activities, from physical education, and even from education in schools for a long period of time. In the 1960s philosophical approaches in many countries, especially in the United States of America, Scandinavian countries and in The Netherlands, stressed the importance of participation of these persons in the mainstream of society. The so-called normalization principle [2, 3], which described the necessity for each individual, despite having a disability, to have access to all areas of life including physical education and sports, played a key role in this process. Wolfensberger [4] and Vermeer [5] pointed out that stigmatization can be reduced on two levels: through heightened competence and through an improvement of social image which can especially be achieved through physical activity and sports.

Despite these serious attempts to contribute to increased social acceptance, the process of inclusion can only be described as very slow. Countries such as the former German Democratic Republic and the former USSR did not include children with mental retardation in their educational system. This led to a total exclusion of these individuals from learning opportunities in school and leisure time settings. In other countries, such as the United States of America, organizations were established, such as the Special Olympics, to offer specific programs of sports and leisure time activities for persons with mental retardation.

Current Situation in Physical Education and Sports for Individuals with Mental Retardation

In the overall development of individuals, the acquisition of independence [6] and self-determination [3] are of crucial importance. These experiences are strongly linked to self-perceived well-being and are important factors contributing to an improved quality of life. Persons with mental retardation can be characterized as individuals who are experiencing more dependence and less autonomy than most other members of society. In the process of education in general, and in particular in physical education and adapted physical education, it is therefore of great significance to offer a broad spectrum of different opportunities in which individuals with mental retardation can experience and achieve more independence.

Adapted physical activities refer to movement, physical activity, and sports in which special emphasis is placed on the interests and capabilities of individuals with limiting conditions. Through these activities, improved competence and thus greater independence can be achieved. Currently, the following four different areas of physical activity can be distinguished in which specific adaptations are being made to meet the needs of persons with mental retardation.

Physical Activities as Part of a Therapeutic or Rehabilitative Setting

Specific programs based on the psychomotor or mototherapeutic approach have been developed. They offer a variety of experiences in the following domains:

- *Personal competence*: perceiving, experiencing, and becoming acquainted with one's own body and knowing how to handle it in different situations
- *Environmental competence*: being able to adjust to one's surroundings, coping with them and being capable of changing them
- *Social competence*: being able to adjust to others, cooperating with them and being capable of influencing them [7, 8]

Physical Education for Children with Mental Retardation in Schools

Despite great differences as far as physical education in special schools and integrated classes/schools is concerned, international comparisons [1] show an increase of mainstreamed programs. To meet the special needs of children with mental retardation, strategies for modifying activities, games, and sports have been developed [9]. In comparing approaches in different countries, it becomes clear that despite current improvements in teaching physical education to children with mental retardation, there is still a lack of competence in many physical education teachers. The unique needs of each individual must be addressed, but this seems to be a heavy burden to some of the teaching staff. In a recent study focusing on attitudes towards the integration of persons with a disability into physical education and sports [10], self-perceived competence on the part of the teaching staff was identified as a crucial factor in succeeding in these difficult teaching situations. These aspects are of similar importance in recreational programs as well.

Recreation and Leisure Time Activities

One of the key issues is, again, the value of integration and how this global aim can be achieved in various areas of education, recreation, and sports. In agreement with Stein [11], it has to be stated: "When all people in the community want mainstreaming to happen, it can be done. But the attitudinal barrlers must come tumbling down. All facilities must become accessible, and every program must accommodate all who desire to participate. Only after we have accomplished this across our nation can individuals with handicapping conditions be integrated into the mainstream of society" [11].

In recent years, we have witnessed an increase in integrated programs offered either by sports clubs, especially in most European countries, or in community-based recreation programs like in the United States of America. In addition, special programs such as the Special Olympics can be found in many parts of the world. In the beginning, almost all of these programs followed the segregated model. Recently, however, segregated and integrated programs have begun to coexist, the preference for one or the other depending on various factors such as support services, number and qualification of staff, and the skill level of the participants. Even sports clubs for the "able-bodied" have opened their doors to individuals with mental retardation, but these are still the exception rather than the rule.

Many recreational programs not only stress the importance of joint action of non-disabled and disabled individuals, but also emphasize family participation as an important factor [12, 13]. In most of these programs, competitive activities are of less importance; instead, they focus on fitness, fun, and sociability. Controversies have arisen since the 1980s when persons with mental retardation were increasingly introduced into competitive sports.

Competitive Sports for Persons with Mental Retardation

In accordance with the normalization principle, Nirje [14] and other representatives of sports organizations for the disabled promoted a sports movement which offered competitive sports to persons with mental retardation. Endeavors to become an integrated part of the sports organizations for the physically disabled failed. This lead to the formation of INAS-FMH (International Sport Federation for Persons with Mental Handicap) in 1986 in The Hague, Netherlands. Ever since, this organization has stressed the importance of elite sports for athletes with mental retardation. In 1989 it introduced World Championships and in 1992 the Paralympic Games in Madrid to these persons.

It is the express wish of the disabled to be part of the Paralympic family in the Paralympic Games in Atlanta, USA, in 1996. However, many problems need to be solved: eligibility, rules, standards of performances, and classification, to name but a few. The Madrid Paralympics have shown great differences concerning the development and impact of high-performance sports among the participating nations.

It is quite remarkable to see Australia, Iceland, Romania, and Sweden in leading positions as compared to their performance in the Barcelona Paralympics where countries such as the United States of America and Germany were dominant. In Germany, physical activities for persons with mental retardation rather focus on recreational programs. In the US, Special Olympics seem to have strongly influenced the development of sports for individuals with mental retardation, applying their own philosophy to sporting activities.

Future Trends

With regard to the controversy of philosophy between INAS-FMH and Special Olympics it has to be hoped that an agreement will be found for coexistence or even cooperation. These developments on the international level could also have a positive influence on physical education and sports programs at the grass-roots level.

To achieve better opportunities, especially for children with mental retardation, three essential problems need to be addressed:

— The *professional training* of physical education teachers, coaches, etc. needs to be improved.
— *A greater number and variety of programs* of physical activity and sports should be offered in schools, sports clubs, and in the community-based initiatives.
— *Research* in this area is urgently needed focusing *on the benefits of physical activities* for individuals with mental retardation (including factors such as health and fitness, segregated versus integrated programs, motor development, motor learning processes, etc.).

The professionals in physical education and sports and in sports sciences are facing the challenge of overcoming barriers and to make participation available for all, including persons with mental retardation.

References

1. Doll-Tepper G (1990) Controversies and current tendencies in physical education and sport for the mentally retarded: An international comparison. In: Vermeer A (ed) Motor development, adapted physical activity and mental retardation. Karger, Basel, pp 78–84
2. Nirje B (1985) The basis and logio of the normalization principle. Aust NZJ Dev Disab 11:65–68
3. Nirje B (1992) The normalization principle papers, Uppsala University, Uppsala
4. Wolfensberger W (1983) Social role valorization: A new term for the principle of normalization. Ment Retard 21:234–239
5. Vermeer A (1988) Der Einfluß von Sport auf persönliche Kompetenz und soziale Stellung von geistig Behinderten. Motorik 11:17–23
6. Hahn M (1981) Behinderung als soziale Abhängigkeit. Reinhardt, Gammertingen
7. Kiphard EJ (1979) Motopädagogik, modernes lernen, Dortmund
8. Doll-Tepper G (1989) Children with special needs—Motodiagnostic test procedures and Kiphard's mototherapeutic approach. Adapt Phys Activity Quart 6:170–175
9. Eichstaedt C, Lavay B (1992) Physical activity for individuals with mental retardation—Infancy through adulthood. Human Kinetics, Champaign
10. Doll-Tepper G, Schmidt-Gotz E, Lienert C, Döen U, Hecker R (1993) Attitudes of students, teachers and coaches towards the integration of persons with a disability into physical education and sport. Bundesinstitut für Sportwissenschaft, Cologne

11. Stein J (1985) Mainstreaming in recreational settings. J Phys Ed Recr Dance 5:25–52
12. Kapustin P (1991) Familiensport als Lebenshilfe. In: Doll-Tepper G, Lienert C (eds) Sport von Menschen mit geistiger Behinderung—Situation und Trends. Lebenshilfe-Verlag, Marburg, pp 71–77
13. Rheker U (1989) Familien-Freizeitsportgruppe mit behinderten und nicht-behinderten Kindern. In: Bös K, Doll-Tepper G, Trosien G (eds) Geistig Behinderte in Bewegung, Spiel und Sport Lebenshilfe-Verlag, Marburg, pp 123–146
14. Nirje B (1993) The origins and purposes of INAS-FMH. INAS News 1–2:5–7

—Keynote Speech—

Legislative Influences on Adapted Physical Activity and Sports in the USA

Joseph P. Winnick

Abstract. This presentation includes an identification and analysis of legislative influences on adapted physical activity and sport in the United States of America since the 1970s. The constitutional basis for and practices leading to important legislation are examined.

Introduction

Although the therapeutic value of exercise has been recognized for centuries, it is clear that the general provision of physical education or physical activity to meet the unique needs of persons considered disabled is a recent phenomenon. Efforts to serve this population through physical activity and sport have only been given significant attention during the 20th century. In the early years of its existence, there were essentially no public provisions for the education of individuals with disabilities in the United States. In the early 1900s, many states began to include special education mandates, special education certification requirements, and other special education provisions in state laws and these spread throughout the country. By 1972, almost 70% of the states had enacted mandatory legislation requiring the education of all handicapped children [1]. In the United States, the education of individuals with disabilities was significantly enhanced by federal legislation passed during and following the 1970s. This presentation is designed to identify some of the practices preceding this legislation, to identify the constitutional basis of the legislation, and to identify some of the provisions of legislation existing today.

Educational Inadequacies Prior to 1970

Although education in residential and regular schools undoubtedly benefitted multitudes of students with disabilities prior to the 1970s and although much progress was being made through state and federal legislation, there still existed many inadequacies related to the education of students with disabilities which were unacceptable to parents, educators, professional groups, and others.

These inadequacies were discussed and advanced in a variety of forums. Some became apparent in right-to-life education court cases. Major precedent-setting decrees came from the following two cases: The Pennsylvania Association for Retarded Children (PARC) v. Commonwealth of Pennsylvania (1971) [2] and Mills v. D.C. Board of Education (1972) [3].

These cases dramatically recorded a variety of inadequacies and questionable practices related to the education of children with handicapping conditions. For example, in PARC v. Commonwealth of Pennsylvania, 13 individuals between the ages of 6 and 21 designated as mentally retarded were excluded by their school districts from programs of public education and training. Children with mental retardation in Pennsylvania could be denied a public education without a hearing or even a notice to parents of their child's exclusion from public school. In one case, the parents of a retarded child were only made aware of their son's exclusion from school when the school bus which regularly brought him to school failed to show up. The facts in the case demonstrated that with mental retardation children could be considered uneducable and/or untrainable and be denied access to a free public program of education and training if the school authority decided that they could not profit from it. In cases in which with mental retardation children were excluded from schools in the public sector, parents rather than the public were required to assume the financial burden of educating their own children. Youngsters with disabilities that were accepted in public education could and were being denied placement in a regular setting without due process or hearing. In Mills v. Board of Education of the District of Columbia, seven children of school age were excluded, suspended, expelled, reassigned, and/or transferred from regular public school classes without due process of the law, i.e., the ability to question or protest.

Constitutional Rights

Thus, although may students with disabilities were being educated in segregated and/or residential schools and/or in special classes in regular schools, the needs of too many were not being met. Further, many who were receiving an education were not receiving an education appropriate to meet their needs. This was undesirable not only because the basic ingredients of a quality education were being violated, but also because the constitutional rights of students with disabilities were being violated. In essence, special education practices were in violation of what America values in education and in regard to the rights of its citizenry. At this point, it is important to briefly consider basic American constitutional rights and relate them to the education of individuals with disabilities.

The 1st, 5th, and 14th constitutional amendments have and continue to influence the educational rights of individuals with disabilities in the United States. Taken separately or in combination, these amendments have led to two major constitutional principles which influence the educational rights of individuals with disabilities. The first of these is "equal protection under the law".

The 14th amendment of the constitution clearly indicates that no state may deny any person within its jurisdiction equal protection of the laws. In brief, equal protection under the law requires that states treat equally situated individuals equally unless it can show a justifiable reason for discrimination. This constitutional principle was influential in the 1954 U.S. Supreme Court case, Brown v. Board of Education [4], which concluded that racial segregation in public schools was unconstitutional and that separate education is inherently unequal. When a state treats students with disabilities differently by denying them an opportunity to attend school or inappropriately assigns them to special education programs, equal protection is violated.

The second constitutional principle which significantly affects the educational rights of children with disabilities is related to due process. The 5th and 14th amendments indicate that no state may deprive any person life, liberty, or property without due process of law. In this context, it is important to emphasize that education is considered by the courts to be property. In regard to individuals with disabilities, this amendment means that no child with a disability can be deprived of an education without the opportunity of exercising the right to protest, i.e., procedural due process. It also means that states may not use more restrictive means than are necessary to accomplish their purpose, i.e., substantive due process. This means that the government must use the least intrusive means to accomplish its goals and the education of children with disabilities should be conducted in the least restrictive, most normal environment possible and appropriate.

These and other federal constitutional amendments; state constitutions; local charters; local, state, and federal laws; and local, state, and federal regulations have guaranteed the educational requirements provided below:

1. The requirement of full educational opportunity for students with disabilities
2. The requirement of an individualized education program for each child that benefits each student
3. Due process if appropriateness of education is in doubt
4. Parental involvement in the education of their children
5. Appropriately prepared teachers
6. A barrier-free appropriate education
7. A free appropriate education
8. Requirement of prior notice regarding educational services
9. Requirement of student evaluation
10. Periodic reevaluation
11. Requirement of child-find
12. Protection from governmental intrusion
13. Requirement of least restrictive alternative when restricting fundamental liberty

Major Legislation from 1970 to the Present

Individuals with Disabilities Act

A major milestone in the education of students with disabilities was the passage of PL 94-142, The Education for All Handicapped Children Act of 1975 [5]. This act is the precursor to the Individuals with Disabilities Act (IDEA). It was designed to assure that children with handicapping conditions, ages 5–21, would have available a free appropriate public education which emphasizes special education and related services designed to meet their unique needs. PL 94-142 clearly specifies that special education, including physical education, must be made available and specially designed, if necessary, to meet unique needs.

The term "free appropriate public education" means special education and related services that are provided at public expense in conformity with an individualized education program (IEP). An IEP is a written statement prepared for each child with a handicapping condition.

The law also provides the right to nondiscriminatory testing, education, and placement procedures. According to the law, tests and other evaluation procedures must be provided and administered in the child's native language or other appropriate mode of communication; tests accordingly reflect and focus on aptitude or achievement rather than the child's disability (unless the test is designed to measure the extent of disability); no single procedure is used as the sole criterion for determining an appropriate educational program for a student; and evaluations are made by a multidisciplinary team.

PL 94-142 also requires that instruction be conducted in the least restrictive environment. Thus, each student with a disability must have the opportunity to participate in the regular educational program available to nonhandicapped children, unless the student is enrolled full-time in separate facilities or needs specially designed education as prescribed in the IEP. Basic to education in the most appropriate setting is a continuum of alternative placements which extends from a setting in which students with disabilities are integrated into a regular class (integrated or mainstreamed setting) to a very restrictive setting (out-of-school segregated placement).

The rules and regulations associated with PL 94-142 also indicate that children with handicapping conditions must be provided equal opportunity for participation in nonacademic extracurricular services and activities, including athletics, intramural, and recreational services.

A second major milestone occurred in 1986 when Congress passed PL 99-457 to amend the Education for All Handicapped Children Education Act of 1975 [6]. In this legislation, two new programs were added. The first required service and intervention programs for infants and toddlers with handicapping conditions and their families. The second program, identified as the preschool program, extended the provisions of PL 94-142 to all children with handicapping conditions, ages 3 to 5.

PL 101-476, The Individuals with Disabilities Education Act of 1990 [7] was another important legislative milestone which added to the provisions of PL 94-142. This act, known as IDEA, replaced the term "handicap" with "disability" and expanded the list of disabilities covered by the legislation by adding autism and traumatic brain injury. PL 102-119 [8] passed on October 7, 1991 was the latest addition to this legislation.

Section 504 of the Rehabilitation Act of 1973

The right of equal oportunity also emerges from another legislative milestone which had an impact on adapted physical education and sport. This legislation is best known as Section 504 of the Rehabilitation Act of 1973 [9]. Section 504 provides that:

> . . . No otherwise qualified handicapped individual . . . solely, by reason of his handicap, be excluded from participation in, be denied the benefits of, or be subject to discrimination under any program or activity receiving federal financial assistance (Department of Health, Education, and Welfare, 1977).

An important intention of Section 504 was to ensure that individuals with handicapping conditions receive intended benefits of all education programs and extracurricular activities.

It is clear that compliance with Section 504 requires program accessibility. The rules and regulations of Section 504 also prohibit exclusion of individuals with handicapping conditions from federally assisted educational programs because of architectural or other environmental barriers. Examples of common barriers to accessibility include facilities, finances, and transportation.

The Amateur Sports Act

In 1978, PL 95–606, the Amateur Sports Act [10], was passed to coordinate American efforts concerning amateur athletic activity, including competition for individuals with disabilities. This legislation led to the establishment of the U.S. Committee on Sports for the Disabled (COSD). As a standing committee of the U.S. Olympic Committee, COSD consists of representatives from special sport organizations serving athletes with disabilities. In addition to its work coordinating and stimulating the sports environment for athletes with disabilities, the COSD has been active in obtaining facilities and other services for these athletes.

Americans with Disabilities Act of 1990

On July 26, 1990, PL 101–336 [11], the Americans With Disabilities Act of 1990, was passed. Whereas Section 504 focused on educational rights, this legislation extended civil rights protection for individuals with disabilities to all areas of American life. The act's provisions include, but are not limited to, employment, public accommodations and services, public transportation, and telecommunications. Related to adapted physical activity, this legislation has

Sources of Enjoyment and Sources of Stress Among Sports Participants with Visual Disabilities

Elizabeth S. Bressan

Abstract. The purpose of this study was to determine sources of enjoyment and sources of stress found in competitive sports as experienced by blind senior men (B1 or B2) participating at the interprovincial level in the team sport of goalball. The major sources of enjoyment could be categorized under the general headings of the physical aspects of participation, the socialization opportunities afforded by goalball, and the process of competition itself. The major sources of stress could be categorized under the general headings of opponents' behavior and self-imposed pressures.

Introduction

The perception of enjoyment has been documented to be an important motivational factor in sports participation for both able-bodied children and adults [1–3]. Research on participants in sports for the disabled has also substantiated claims that enjoyment is an important factor to cultivate in the sports experience. Sherrill [4] discovered that "fun and enjoyment" was one of the most powerful motivational factors for disabled athletes. The identification of the sources of enjoyment becomes important because it will help determine what aspects of the sports experience should be cultivated to encourage a high level of motivation among disabled participants.

Negative Stress

The perception of "negative" stress can lower athletes' motivation to participate as well as their standard of performance [5]. Negative stress may be a particularly important variable to study for disabled athletes. Mastro et al. [6] compared sighted to unsighted beep baseball players and found that the unsighted players scored significantly higher on the tension and the depression dimensions of the Profile of Mood States. This suggests that the unsighted players may be more susceptible to negative stressors. The identification of the sources of stress becomes crucial, then, if these athletes are to learn how to cope effectively with negative stress.

Interview Procedures

The research procedures used in this study follow the format for the long interview described by McCracken [7]. An individual interview of 30–60 min was conducted with 12 interprovincial level senior male goalball players. Each interview was guided by a series of questions. The first cluster of open-ended questions centered upon getting the players to discuss what they enjoy about goalball. The second cluster of open-ended questions asked the players to discuss the source of negative stress that they experience in goalball.

Each interview was recorded on an audio tape and a complete transcript was made of each player's remarks. The content of each transcript was then analyzed to identify similarities in the sources for enjoyment and sources for stress. These patterns of similarity were considered "categories" of sources. The following table presents a summary of the sources of enjoyment and the sources of stress identified in this study. The major headings under which the sources are grouped are the "categories" generated by the researcher.

Sources of Enjoyment

Based on the analysis of the interviews, the physical aspects (11 players/92% of the subjects) and the socialization aspects (11 players/92%) were the most commonly identified general sources of enjoyment among the players. In terms of the physical aspects, 50% of the players mentioned that becoming fit and healthy through goalball was enjoyable for them. "Making you feel better" and "getting tired" were both mentioned by two players each (17%), and one player mentioned that he "liked to sweat".

The socialization aspects mentioned as sources of enjoyment were spread among three comments. The opportunity that goalball provides for the visually impaired participant to "get to know others" was mentioned by 42% of the players; 33% mentioned that goalball gave them the opportunity to communicate with their friends, and 17% simply enjoyed the feeling of "coming together" with others. The positive response of these players to both the health and fitness aspects of participation and the social experience of interacting with opponents and teammates/friends has been supported in other sports motivation research [1, 2, 4, 8].

The act of competition itself was another primary source of enjoyment (83%). The feelings of "competing against others" (8 players/67%) were mentioned most often, while the feelings of "competing physically" and being involved in "strong competition between evenly matched teams" were mentioned by two players/17% each. Feelings found in the process of participation were also identified as sources of enjoyment. Players' remarks in this category were distributed among the feelings of "giving my best", "reaching my peak", "working for everything I get", "improving my skills", and "improving my knowledge of goalball". All of these comments have also been identified as sources of enjoyment among able-bodied sports participants [5].

TABLE 1. Sources of enjoyment and stress identified by goalball players ($n = 12$).

Source of enjoyment	Fr. (*n*)	%	Source of stress	Fr. (*n*)	%
Competition	10	(83%)	Opponents' behav.	8	(67%)
Compete vs. others	8	(67%)	Appeal decisions	2	(17%)
Compete physically	2	(17%)	Mistakes in rules	2	(17%)
Competition with even teams	2	(17%)	Bad attitude	2	(17%)
			Break your concn.	2	(17%)
Participation proc.	7	(58%)	Self-im. pressure	8	(67%)
Give my best	2	(17%)	Avoid mistakes	2	(17%)
Reach my peak	1	(8%)	Not fit enough	2	(17%)
Work for everything	2	(17%)	Play injured	1	(8%)
Improve skill	1	(8%)	Afraid to lose concentration	1	(8%)
Improve knowledge	1	(8%)	Afraid to lose	1	(8%)
			Own mistakes	1	(8%)
Physical aspects	11	(92%)	Rel. w/teammates	5	(42%)
Feel better	2	(17%)	Letting teammates down	3	(25%)
I like to sweat	1	(8%)	Teammates don't show for prac.	2	(17%)
Get tired	2	(17%)			
Become fit/healthy	6	(50%)			
Socialization	11	(92%)	Officials	3	(25%)
Coming together	2	(17%)	Bad judgements	3	(25%)
Commun. w/friends	4	(33%)			
Get to know others	5	(42%)			

Fr., frequency; proc., process; concn; concentration; commun., communication; behav., behavior; im., imposed; prac., practice; rel., relationship.

Sources of Stress

The two categories most frequently mentioned by goalball players as sources of stress were their opponents' behavior (8 players/67%) and self-imposed pressure (8 players/67%). In terms of opponents' behavior, the identification of specific sources of stress were evenly spread among the following (2 players/17% each): "opponents who make appeals following decisions made by officials", "opponents who make mistakes in the rules", "opponents with a bad attitude", and "opponents who do things to try to break your concentration".

The identification of stressors in relation to self-imposed pressure was also distributed over a variety of specific sources. Two players each (17%) mentioned the following self-imposed sources: the "pressure you put on yourself to avoid making mistakes" and "when you are not really fit enough" to play well. One player each (8%) mentioned the following self-imposed sources: "playing when I'm injured", "when I get afraid I will lose my concentration", "when I am afraid I am going to lose", and "when I start making mistakes".

Relationships with teammates were also a possible source of stress (5 players/42%). Three players (25%) specifically mentioned feelings of "letting my teammates down" as a source of stress, while two players (17%) mentioned "when teammates don't show up for practice" as a stressor. The final category of sources of stress was that of the officials, where three players mentioned specifically that "bad judgement" and "bad calls" on the part of the officials caused them stress.

Past research on the sources of stress among able-bodies elite athletes supports the identification self-imposed pressures and interpersonal conflicts as sources of stress [5]. However, opponents' behavior and the behavior of officials are not commonly identified as sources of stress. This may suggest that able-bodied elite athletes have developed the necessary coping strategies to "shut off" these potential stressors. In any case, coping with these two stressors is a psychological skill from which the goalball players in this study would benefit.

Conclusion

The motivational properties of enjoyment have been shown to be powerful. Efforts to get visually impaired athletes involved in sport can become more effective if the sources of enjoyment for them in sports participation can be identified and then emphasized in their sport opportunities. The importance of the identification of the sources of stress they experience is related to the quality of their participation as well. Players must learn specific coping strategies to deal with stress and coaches and administrators must find ways to reduce those stressors that detract from the quality of the competition itself.

There is also a relationship between enjoyment and stress that must be further investigated. Scanlon and Passer [9] found that the most important factor determining the level of post-game stress for girls, was the amount of enjoyment they experienced during the game. If maximizing enjoyment can help moderate stress, it becomes that much more important to find ways to emphasize and enhance the enjoyment aspect of sports competitions.

References

1. Wankel I, Kreisel P (1985) Methodological considerations in youth sport motivation research: A comparison of open-ended and paired comparison approaches. J Sport Psychol 7:65–74
2. May J (1987) Two critical psychological components of ski racing: Fun and feelings. J Sports Sci 5:337–343
3. Scanlon T, Stein G, Ravizza K (1989) An in-depth study of former elite figure skaters: II. Sources of enjoyment. J Sport Exerc Psychol 11:65–83
4. Sherrill C (1986) Social and psychological dimensions of sport for disabled athletes. In: Sherrill C (ed) Sport and Disabled Athletes. Human Kinetics, Champaign, pp 21–33
5. Scanlon T, Stein G, Ravizza K (1991) An in-depth study of former elite figure skaters: III. Sources of stress. J Exerc Sport Psychol 13:103–120

6. Mastro J, Canbal M, French R (1988) Psychological mood profiles of sighted and unsighted beep baseball players. Res Q Exerc Sport 59(3):262–264
7. McCraken G (1988) The long interview. Sage Publications, Newbury Park
8. Cooper M, Sherrill C, Marshall D (1986) Attitudes toward physical activity of elite cerebral palsied athletes. Adapted Phys Activity Q 3:14–21
9. Scanlon T, Passer M (1979) Sources of competitive stress in young female athletes. J Sport Psychol 1:151–159

Effects of Physical Education Programs on Children with Learning Disabilities

PAULI RINTALA and NIINA PALSIO

Abstract. In this study, the term "learning disablity" refers to specific developmental language disorders. Children with language disorders do not perform as well on motor coordination tests compared to children with normal speech. The purpose of this study was to investigate the motor skill level of children with developmental language disorders and to test the effect of three different training programs on these skills. The subjects were 22 elementary special school children with developmental language disorders who were divided into three groups and tested using the nonrandomized control group pretest-posttest design. Training programs were conducted twice weekly for 10 weeks. One group received psychomotor training, the second, body image training, and the control group followed the regular physical education program. The subjects were tested before and after participation in the training programs using a revised version of the Test of Motor Impairment (TOMI). Results indicated that 82% of these children clearly had a motor problem, consisting to a large extent in static balance difficulties. Overall improvement was 54% in the psychomotor training group; 26% for the body image training group; and 41% in the regular physical education group. It is concluded that the motor skills of children with specific developmental language disorders can be improved to a certain degree by intensified training programs.

Introduction

The term "learning disability" is probably the most controversial term among different handicapping conditions. According to Sherrill and Pyfer [1], disagreement over this condition is reflected in the number of terms associated with it:perceptually handicapped, brain injured, minimal brain dysfunctionate, dyslexic, developmentally aphasic, etc. In this study, specifically, learning disability means specific developmental language disorder. However, research on the classification of these "specific developmental disorders" is still in its infancy [2].

Children with language disorders do not perform as well on motor coordination tests compared to children with normal speech [3, 4]. The purpose of this study was to investigate the motor skill level of children with developmental language disorders and the effect of three different programs on their motor skills.

Subjects and Methods

In this field study, 22 students of a special school served as the subjects. All the students had a specific developmental language disorder diagnosed by a doctor. These difficulties hindered them from going to ordinary school.

The students were divided into three study groups and tested using the nonrandomized control group pretest-posttest design. Group I (n = 8; 8–9 years old) followed the psychomotor program which was based on the moto-pedagogic approach [5]; group II (n = 7; 8–10 years old) followed the body awareness/image program, and the control group (n = 7; 7–8 years old) followed the regular physical education (PE) program. The subjects were tested before and after the programs which were conducted twice a week for 45 min, for a total of 20 sessions.

The children were tested using the Henderson revision of the Stott et al. [6] test called the Test of Motor Impairment (TOMI). The aim of the test is to identify and measure impairment of motor function in children 5–12 years of age. It consists of four sets of skill tests, each appropriate for different age levels: 5–6 years of age, 7–8 years, 9–10 years, and 11 years and older. Eight categories of motor functioning are assessed: (1) manual dexterity 1 (speed and sureness of movement of each hand), (2) manual dexterity 2 (coordination of both hands for performance of a single operation), (3) manual dexterity 3 (eye-hand coordination using the preferred hand), (4) static balance (control and balance of the body while immobile), (5) ball skills 1 (catching), (6) ball skills 2 (throwing), (7) dynamic balance 1 (control of the body in rapid movement), and (8) dynamic balance 2 (control and balance in slow movement). Lower scores indicate higher motor skills.

Results

When the total TOMI score was used, 18 of 22 children received a score of 6 or more. This indicates a clear motor problem because the borderline between passing and failing is the score of 6. The remaining 4 children had moderate motor problems, i.e., their score was between 4 and 6.

Table 1 shows the percentage of children who were able to pass the test by various categories of motor functioning: dynamic balance (66%) was the easiest and static balance (15%) the most difficult category to pass.

The Wilcoxon t-test for small samples was performed to assess the effects of different programs within groups. In group I, significant improvement was found in manual dexterity 3 (eye-hand coordination) and ball skills 1 (catching)

TABLE 1. Test of Motor Impairment (TOMI) test results ($n = 22$).

	Pass	Fail
Manual dexterity	41%	59%
Static balance	15%	85%
Ball skills	25%	75%
Dynamic balance	66%	34%

TABLE 2. Percent improvement in total TOMI scores in different groups.

	Pretest	Posttest	Percent improvement
Psychomotor ($n = 8$)	7.6	3.5	54%
Body awareness ($n = 7$)	7.7	5.6	26%
Regular physical education ($n = 7$)	9.2	5.4	41%

($P < 0.05$). In group II, significant improvement was found in manual dexterity 2 (coordination of both hands). Also in the control group, there was significant improvement in ball skills 1 and static balance.

When examined individually, all children in the control group improved their score from pre- to posttest. In the experimental groups, all except one of the children improved in the measured items. The Wilcoxon *t*-test, revealed a significant difference between two experimental groups in manual dexterity 3. Overall improvement based on total TOMI scores are presented in Table 2. The greatest improvement was seen in group I which followed the psychomotor program.

Discussion

Earlier results [7] have indicated that only 5% of children in the general population receive a total TOMI score of 6 or more. The percentage in this study was 82% among children with specific language disability. This finding supports Cermak's statement [3] that children with speech/language disorders do not perform as well on motor coordination tests as children with normal speech. However, the percentage of children whose total score was 6 or more had diminished to 32% at the posttest. That is an indication of the effectiveness of the intensive physical education programs.

The specific effect of different programs is seen between the psychomotor program and the body awareness program: children in the psychomotor program improved by 54% compared with 26% in the body awareness program. The control group, which followed the official PE curriculum, improved by 41%. This implies that the psychomotor and standard PE programs may have contained similar skill training items, but also that children's natural development is a part of all these improvements.

Conclusion

Children with specific developmental language disorders often have major problems with their motor skills. These skills can be improved to a certain degree by intensified physical education programs within the existing special schools. These types of programs illustrate the need for structured physical education programs for students with motor and language delays.

References

1. Sherrill C, Pyfer J (1985) Learning disabled students in physical education. Adapt Phys Activity 2:283–291
2. Bishop D, Rosenbloom L (1987) Childhood language disorders: Classification and overview. In: Yule W, Rutter M (eds) Language development and disorders. Mac Keith, London, pp 16–41
3. Cermak S, Ward E, Ward L (1986) The relationship between articulation disorders and motor coordination in children. Am J Occup Ther 40:546–550
4. Merriman WJ, Barnett BE, Kofka JB (1993) The standing long jump performances of preschool children with speech impairments and children with normal speech. Adapt Phys Activity 10:157–163
5. Kiphard EJ (1990) Motopädagogik (Motopedagogy). Modernes lernen, Dortmund
6. Stott DH, Moyes FA, Henderson SE (1984) Manual: Test of motor impairment. Brook Educational, Guelph
7. Maeland AF (1992) Identification of children with motor coordination problems. Adapt Phys Activity 9:330–342

Sports for the Disabled in Slovenia—New Directions: Institutionalized Physically Disabled Youth in Slovenia and Their Preferences in Active and Passive Sports Participation

RAJKO VUTE

Abstract. It can be said of young people in general that they are very good "consumers" of sports. This also applies to physically disabled youth. The aim of this study was to investigate the attractiveness of various sports disciplines for 85 individuals aged 12 to 21 living in an institution for the physically disabled. The data were collected in September, 1992. Using contingency tables, we present the most popular sports that were actively participated in; the sports the youths would most wish to play if they had a chance; and the sports they most frequently watched on television.

Introduction

Many studies have been undertaken to examine the effects of various sports programs on the performance of individuals with disabilities. Sports disciplines chosen by the physically disabled present useful and interesting information which enables us to plan work in this specific area better and offers us the possibility of considering the personality of the participants and their demands. The benefits of participation in physical activity—physical education, sports, and therapy—were found to include improved fitness, flexibility, strength, social interaction, and self-concept [1]. Self-esteem is probably the most frequently used indicator of mental well-being, and sports and exercise may be important vehicles for its promotion [2]. A successful sports program should include all youth, and we should respect their wishes regarding their choice of sports whenever possible. Truthful cooperation and understanding can help the youth better cope with success and failure, develop habits of good living, cooperation, mutual trust, teamwork, and tolerance, and encourage them to form good relationships [3].

When choosing their favorite sports, the disabled face both objective and subjective barriers. In spite of all that, they participate in various activities including extreme ones. If skiing is like chugging a shot glass of adrenalin after every trip up the lift, rock climbing is like sipping it from a beer stein all day long [4].

The youth are very impressionable and can be influenced by various spheres of social life. One potentially influential area is sports. Some important reasons for becoming involved in sports are to take advantage of the possibilities which are offered, the emulation of sports idols, and the youth's own interest in sports. To physically disabled youth, active participation in sports imparts a feeling of power and importance which contributes to greater independence, and it is also an important means of using one's free time.

Children aged 8 to 14 prefer games which they organize themselves over those dominated by adults in [5]. In 1985, the most popular sports in Slovenia in which physically disabled male youth actively participated were: table tennis, wheelchair hockey, football (soccer), air rifle shooting, basketball, swimming, and skiing [6].

From the above, it is apparent that we should take into consideration the extremely sensitive period of adolescence in the long-term planning of sports for the disabled. The starting point for sports participation, and also when choosing sports disciplines, in many cases depends on the decisions made during this particular period in life.

Methods

The purpose of this study is to find out how the physically disabled youth living in an institution choose sports activities according to their active and passive participation. The study group is comprised of the institutionalized physically disabled youth at ZUIM (institution for physically disabled youth) Kamnik. The part we are presenting here includes 85 youths, aged 12 to 21, consisting of 66 boys and 19 girls. In autumn 1992, we started a study which is still on-going and is part of a wider research project called "Sport activities and quality of life of the physically disabled in Slovenia" which we hope will eventually include about 500 physically disabled people with different levels of mobility and different disabilities, of both sexes and different ages.

Because the work has not been finished yet, we are trying to predict the current trends in preferences of popular sports events based on a relatively small sample. Using the questionnaire STP-1, [7], the subjects were asked to name and rank (from 1 to 3) their most liked sports according to their own active participation, the sports they would wish to participate in if they got a chance, and the most frequently watched sports on television. Contingency tables were used for presenting the results.

Results and Discussion

Sports Participation: Active Participation

The first, second, and third most liked sports in which the physically disabled boys we studied take an active part are ranked as follows: First choice: (1)

table tennis (15/22.7%), (2) basketball (10/15.2%), and (3) wheelchair hockey (9/13.6%). Of these, table tennis is the only game which is played individually or in pairs and, as such, is placed at the top of the list. The attractiveness of this game is due to the wide variety of disabilities that can be accommodated, and to different levels of participation. It is based on relatively simple equipment and is popular also according to the tradition and facilities of the institution in which the participants live. Basketball in all its variations has a good influence on the development of participants' physical abilities; it provides an opportunity for an intensive cognitive and emotional experience of a game. It is also a very dynamic and attractive game which demands cooperation from the players. These elements are important for the disabled; besides, basketball is one of the most popular sports in Slovenia. The popularity of wheelchair hockey confirms that this event is very attractive with many exciting situations. Those taking part in this sport have an opportunity to feel the spirit of the game in a very short time and it is suitable for a very wide range of disabilities. Thus, with respect to the first choice, we notice the following cohesive elements: accessibility, attractiveness, and tradition.

The following sports were listed as the second choice: (1) basketball (13/19.7%), (2) football (11/16.7%), and (3) table tennis (9/13.6%). These choices confirm the popularity of basketball and table tennis and the more recent addition of football. Football is a rather simple game and certainly still the most popular sport in our country. It is also best covered by the media which has an important influence on the disabled who choose this popular sport. Football with its basic idea to get the ball into the opponent's goal also gives a variety of different disabilities a chance to play and fulfill this idea.

The third choice was given as follows: (1) football (8/12.1%), (2) basketball (7/10.6%), and (3) volleyball (5/7.6%). The first two, common and well-liked sports, are joined by a fourth sport—volleyball. Numerically poorly represented, it is nevertheless well-known as a universal game suitable for men and women, young and old, and it plays an important role in physical education, sports recreation, and as a competitive sport. It is also useful in the process of rehabilitation. The result of the efforts to make the game accessible to a majority of the disabled is sitting volleyball. Those with leg problems, amputees, and some light cases of cerebral palsy can easily play this game. Volleyball completes the choices of liked and popular team sport events where the role of an individual in the team is important but not ultimately decisive. In a team, the response of the group to an individual is also important. These are sports where, depending on the number of players in the game, a distribution of the roles is possible and thus the compensation of different disabilities.

The relatively small number of girls questioned enables us only to generalize regarding the sports in which they like to participate. The list of the chosen sports includes: boccia, table tennis, volleyball, field hockey, basketball, and nature trips. The choices are similar to those of the boys, but there is a noticeable emphasis on activities which given them more opportunities for relaxation and enjoyment rather than on competition.

Sports Participation: Wish to Participate

Wishes for sports participation among the disabled boys living in the institution were expressed as follows: First choice: (1) swimming (14/21.2%) and (2) horseback riding and motor racing (10/15.2%); second choice: (1) swimming (7/10.6%), (2) horseback riding (6/9.1%), and (3) motor racing (5/7.6%); and third choice: (1) swimming (8/12.1%), (2) horseback riding (6/9.1%), and (3) skiing (5/7.6%).

At the top of the list of sports wishes, rather unexpectedly, is swimming. According to many experts this is one of the most suitable sports for the disabled. Water offers an opportunity for independent movements, which is of extreme importance. We would therefore also expect swimming to be on top of the list of sports actively participated in. It seems there is a gap between the youths' recognition of the importance and benefits of swimming and the opportunities to go swimming at a pool or at the beach. For someone in a wheelchair to be able to swim requires that they have access to the pool, transportation, and related support services. If the institution organizes a swimming camp during the summer, the chances of accomplishing this goal are better. We should be aware of the fact that living in an institution also means being limited by the available facilities, programs, teachers, finances, etc.

Horseback riding activates the whole body of the rider. It is important for the development of balance and coordination, which is a weak point of many disabled. This is why the chance to develop these skills is highly appreciated. Horseback riding is consistent among all three choices. In the institution, horseback riding plays an important role in leisure time activity programs. The youths have experienced staff, their own horses, and this makes their wishes relalistic and feasible. It seems that more and more young people want to take part in this exciting activity. Those who have positive experiences obviously spread the popularity of this sport to their schoolmates. A successful horseback riding program generates new participants. As a relatively new sport and therapeutic option, horseback riding has quickly become one of the most sought-after activities in the institution.

Wishes to take part in motor racing are also high on the list. This sport seems to be interesting not only because of its dynamics and attractiveness but also as a symbol of independent movement. In motor sports such as Formula One, there are also prominent people in wheelchairs involved who play a significant role (F. Williams, C. Regazzoni), which has some influence as well. The chances of fulfilling this sort of wish for active participation in the institution are almost nil. However, a chance to learn to drive as a first step could be of major importance with respect to independent movement. When this step has been accomplished, further steps are always possible. Rally driving is known and also practiced among the disabled. To get a driver's license should become the first goal. To try to reach this goal and fulfill some expectations about driving should not be an obstacle for physically disabled youth in the institution.

Skiing seems to be very difficult for those using orthopedic aids, but we should be aware that skiing is possible today even for those in wheelchairs. So-called monoski have been constructed which are maneuverable by a sophisticated mechanism allowing all styles of ski-like descent. In winter, an increasing number of the disabled can be seen using adapted skiing equipment for various forms of skiing. There are no reasons not to encourage participation in this sport in the institution because skiing has been available for quite some time, the skiing tradition is strong, and last but not least, skiing is our national sport.

The girls questioned indicated choices similar to those of the boys. Their chosen sports are swimming and horseback riding; the additional ones are nature trips and table tennis.

Sport Preference: Most Watched on Television

The sports most watched on television by physically disabled youth are: First choice: (1) basketball (13/19.7%), (2) football (12/18%), and (3) motor racing and skiing (both 8/12.1%); second choice: (1) basketball and football (both 11/16.7%) and (2) ice hockey (10/15.2%); and third choice: (1) basketball (10/15.2%), (2) football (8/12.1%), and (3) gymnastics (5/7.6%). Among girls, the sports most watched on television are basketball, skiing, swimming, and tennis.

The selection of best-liked sports watched on television by the youth in the institution is similar to the results of the survery done by Slovene National Television. According to M. Lah/Dnevnik (March, 1993) the most-watched sports on TV Slovenia are: skiing, basketball, tennis, motor racing, athletics, football, figure skating, and ice hockey. Last year, national television covered 46 different sports. Choices of physically disabled youth fit into the general frame of the most popular sports watched on television in Slovenia.

At the top of the list of the chosen sports are team sports with their attractiveness and unpredictable situations. Watching television presents easy access to sports entertainment. For television viewers, all relevant information is "ready to use" as prepared by the commentators. For the youth, sports presented on television could have a significant influence on their future active role in sport participation. The reverse is also true: active participants in sports are stimulated to watch more sports programs on television. This could explain why basketball and football rank so high on the list of active participation among the physically disabled youth.

Conclusion

We should take into consideration that these results are part of the beginning phase of broader research. Nevertheless, they give us a closer view of a real situation and enable us to predict contemporary trends. On all three levels of engagement, active participation, wishes to participate, and sports most watched on television, we noticed a strong influence of the surroundings where the persons questioned live and of traditional Slovene sports. Accessibility and practical-financial possibilities for participation also play an important role when choosing a suitable sport. The preferences are directed towards dynamic team sports which especially attract the youth. We should strive to enrich sports possibilities and provide conditions that make sports a lifelong activity.

References

1. De Pauw KP (1992) Current international trends in research in adapted physical activity. In: Williams T, Almond L, Sparkes A (eds) Sports and physical activity—moving towards excellence. Spon, London, pp 221–228
2. Fox KR (1992) The complexities of self-esteem promotion in physical education and sport. In: Williams T, Almond L, Sparkes A (eds) Sports and physical activity—moving towards excellence. Spon, London, pp 383–389
3. Burton C, Kent G (1993) Inspiration for physical education. Scholastic Publications, Leamington Spa
4. Ross M (1991) Pass the adrenalin please, Palaestra, vol 8, no 1, pp 44–46
5. Johns DP, Eldridge G (1992) Fair play and the organization of sport. In: Williams T, Almond L, Sparkes A (eds) Sports and physical activity—moving towards excellence. Spon, London, pp 499–503
6. Vute R (1985) Physical education and physically disabled. Telesna Kultura 85(4): 10–12
7. Vute R (1992) Students of the faculties of education in Slovenia and their attitudes toward sports for the disabled. Pedagoška obzorja 22(VII):53–58

Physical Disability: The Brazilian Society Creates, "Rehabilitates", and Stigmatizes

APOLÔNIO A. DO CARMO

Abstract. In general, disabled people, and especially the physically disabled in Brazilian society, have been discriminated against, particularly with respect to work, educational, and recreational opportunities. This study provides a critical review of the proposals that have been made and realized within the framework of Brazilian social policies concerning the physically disabled from 1981 to 1987. Also discussed herein is the integration of the disabled into the educational system, affirming the need to guarantee access to knowledge to all persons with handicaps, no matter what their social condition or physical limitation. Finally, this study examines the psychological mechanisms that have led to the creation, stigmatization, and rehabilitation of the "handicapped".

Introduction

My concern about the physically disabled began in 1982 when I taught physical education at the University of Uberlândia. I was teaching swimming to children 5–10 years old when three handicapped children were enlisted in the group. From then on, I started to develop new methods of teaching swimming to assist those children. Although I did not have enough knowledge at the time, I never thought it was impossible or that the children were unable to do it.

This event in my life made me think more deeply about the situation of the disabled, above all because the needs of those children differed from everything I had learned at college. At the time, most graduate schools in Brazil had never dealt with the problems of people with handicaps.

Today it is clear to me that this phenomenon is due to society's dominant conception of "physical fitness", i.e., an image of body, health, beauty, and performance that has always prioritized the normal, the beautiful, the perfect, and the best.

What most people forget is that each of us has a specific part and a general part.

It is important to consider both the specific and the general parts in movement, of dynamic form, where there is neither primacy of the specific over the general nor of the general over the specific. For example, the general part of the human being, i.e., the aspect that is common to everyone, is the species-being who cries, loves, suffers, thinks, feels, etc.; the specific aspect consists of the differences in terms of skills, intelligence, performance, development, etc.

Generally speaking, people tend to separate the general from the specific abilities and, in the case of handicapped persons, we only see their disabilities because these are more easily noticed, and the person's general aspects are not considered.

This study aims to identify the mechanisms generated by Brazilian society which have contributed to create, rehabilitate, and stigmatize the "handicapped".

Study Design

Three randomly selected regions of Brazil were studied: the Northeast, Southeast, and South. In each region, using the same process, one handicap association was selected, in which about 10 persons were interviewed. The study comprises a total of 30 persons of different levels of education, age, professions, and socioeconomic standard, both male and female. All interviews were tape recorded. The interviews tried to identify the subject's viewpoint on education, work, leisure, and governmental rehabilitation policy for disabled persons, aiming to confront the governmental policy with the reality lived by the handicapped.

Results and Discussion

Concerning education, we can state that two kinds of thinking are prevalent. One advocates education for the handicapped in special schools, while the other is for education in regular schools. Despite this, the great majority of handicapped people have no access to *either* kind of school. Statistically speaking, according to the United Nations Organization, approximately ten million people have various kinds of disabilities.

These findings have led us to struggle for a school for the handicapped, either integrated or segregated, because what really counts is to give the handicapped a chance to prove they can make a difference, and because knowledge is an important weapon against domination, stigmatization, etc.

Something that also deserves to be stressed is the fact that Brazil's constitution guarantees free school education to all children below 14 years of age; however, the great majority of public schools do not have adequate facilities to accommodate the handicapped. The teachers have no specialized training, and there are no teaching materials, especially for deaf, blind, and mentally retarded persons.

To reverse this situation, our department is developing training programs for teachers who work at elementary schools. We are also struggling to get the government to provide the badly needed school facilities.

Regarding work, we began our study by trying to understand the capitalistic system in Brazil philosophically, especially because working relationships in this country have mostly been unfair and inhumane, since in the capital-labor relationship, workers are treated as objects. Besides, most Brazilian workers receive unfair wages: 60% of Brazilian working people make less than the minimum wage, which is below $100 per month. Another shocking example is that a PhD university professor with a 20-year career and published books makes less than $2000 per month. One the other hand, a good-quality book costs around $40 and a new car around $25 000.

This economic situation still persists in Brazil and has contributed to discrimination against the handicapped. The great majority of the handicapped survive on donations and underpaid jobs. Therefore, handicapped persons, due to the lack of an education or any technical training, find it very difficult to get a job. In spite of all this, the disabled have organized themselves to minimize these obstacles. Physical education and sport have aided in these organizations, promoting championships, political debates, and aiming to inform the handicapped of their rights.

The few handicapped that manage to get a job in Brazil seldom stay at the job long, which is due above all to the numerous obstacles they are confronted with, such as architectural barriers, lack of appropriate transportation, lower wages, and condescension on the part of their boss, even though the handicapped are sometimes more productive than normal workers.

The capitalistic system in Brazil is such that it is able to use the disabled for its own interests. At present, for example, the bosses have given preference to deaf persons for work in extremely noisy environments because they do not need to pay extra fees for high-risk jobs. However, by virtue of receiving normal pay rather than high-risk pay, the deaf are effectively being underpaid because of their disabilities. This has a doubly damaging effect, because the disability which in this case should be considered an asset is once more being used as a discriminating factor.

Until 1950, the Brazilian state took no measures to assist or "rehabilitate" disabled people, and it was not until 1970 that a consistent policy toward equal opportunities for the disabled was established. In regard to what the government says and what it really does in terms of helping the handicapped, however, we detected in our study that it has not done enough. For example, there are only three public rehabilitation centers in the entire country. This deficit is an open violation of the constitutional rights of the handicapped.

It was with this sad picture in mind that we started our work at the University of Uberlândia in 1982, trying, above all, to reverse the situation regarding the practice of physical activities. You might ask: How has that been possible?

Our first step was to define the philosophical framework of the rehabilitation program. Next, we set reasonable goals for what we thought we could accomplish. We started out only with the physically disabled, and now we are already working with various other types of disabilities.

The program consists of document research, technological advancement, and special teaching methods. This program presently assists around 150 disabled persons a day. In addition, it has already trained about 150 teachers from several Brazilian universities at the postgraduate level.

In practical terms, this program, by the use of physical education, has already accomplished some significant gains for the handicapped, including two lift-adapted buses and restricted parking spaces at various spots in the city. Furthermore, housing department engineers have designed special adaptations for new schools, and we have designed and manufactured, along with the University Engineering Department, lighter and cheaper wheelchairs. Regarding sport, we have contributed to the teaching of swimming, basketball, and other athletic modalities.

Finally, we are able to say that physical activity has greatly contributed to the recovery of equal citizenship status for disabled persons. It is encouraging that the very movement that has generated much of the discriminating mechanisms can also contribute to their elimination.

—Part II—

Medical Aspects and Rehabilitation

—Tutorial Lecture—

The Handicapped as Depicted in the Art of Japan

TATSUAKI SHINODA

Abstract. Disorders that are mentioned in ancient Japanese literature include congenital hypotonia, Down syndrome, and speech disturbances. With the birth of Japanese culture in the ninth century, the sick are depicted increasingly in scenes where they are being visited and nursed. In a collection of scrolls from a later period, dwarfism, obesity, and spastic gait can be seen. Pictures from the sixteenth century show disorders including polydactyly, apoplexy, cerebral palsy, and ataxia. To this day, votive pictures of the handicapped can be seen in Buddhist temples all over Japan.

Introduction

Looking back on the history of Japan, it may be said that the mentally and physically handicapped were subjected to miserable conditions. In the ancient period, people with any handicaps were thought to be useless, and they often became outcasts or were even killed by their family or society.

Kojiki and Nihon-Shoki

In the ancient literatures of "Kojiki" and "Nihon-Shoki", there was a story of "Hiruko". Hiruko was the first child of Izanagi and Izanami, the rulers of the mythological age. Because of congenital hypotonia, Hiruko could not creep or roll over without help. When he was three years old, his parents abandoned him in the river by placing him on a boat made of reeds (Fig. 1). We now believe Hiruko was a child with cerebral palsy or congenital myopathies.

The second child of Izanagi and Izanami was also handicapped, and the description of him suggests he may have had mental retardation as a result of Down syndrome.

One of the chapters of "Kojiki", describes a handicapped person named "Kuebiko" who was unable to stand or walk without support. "Kuebiko" means "scarecrow" in old Japanese. He would sit by the fireplace all day long, consulting about various things with village people. It is interesting that a

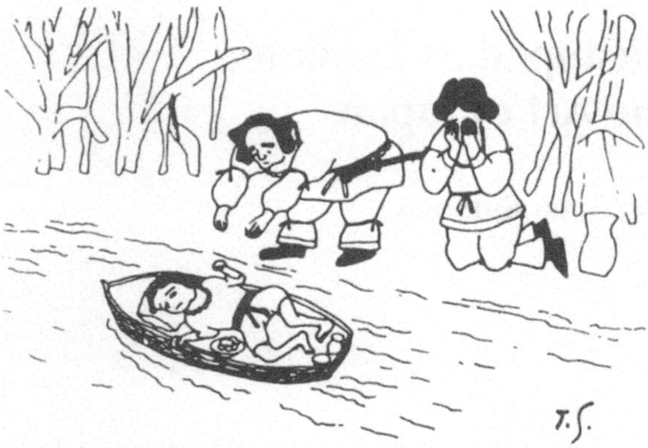

FIG. 1. An ancient Japanese legend tells the story of a handicapped child abandoned by his parents. It is now believed the child was suffering from cerebral palsy or congenital myopathies

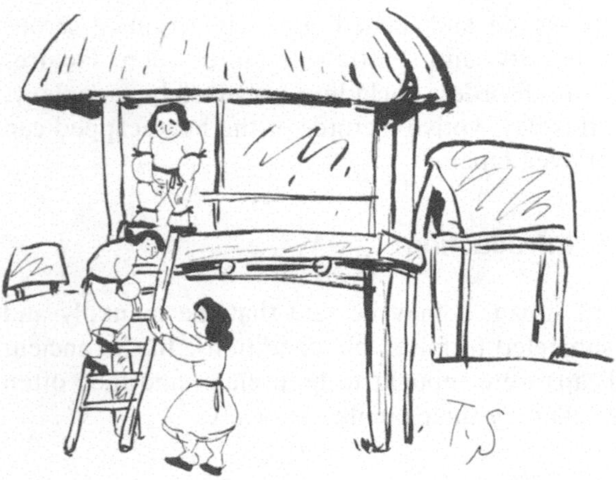

FIG. 2. Another Japanese legend describes the use of play therapy to cure mental deficiencies. The retarded son of a ruler was taught to climb up and down the ladder to his cottage

handicapped person could act as a kind of case worker in a village of old Japan.

A case of speech disturbance was also described in "Kojiki". "Homuchiwake-no-mikoto", the son of Suinin-Tennoh, was unable to speak since birth. When he became an adult, he cried "B-i-irrd" looking at a big swan flying in the sky.

"Izumo-Hudoki", another character in the literature of ancient Japan, described the play therapy of a retarded child. "Ajiskitakahiko", the son of the ruler, had been taught to climb up and down the ladder on the high cottage to cure a mental deficiency (Fig. 2).

Historical Perspective

Buddhism arrived in Japan from China at the end of the sixth century. In China, there already existed a systematic science of medicine. Many political systems and laws were brought to Japan by the immigrants and missionaries from China.

The enaction of the "Taiho-Ritzuryo" in the eighth century was the first law which provided for the handicapped. According to that law, handicaps were classified into three groups according to the type of disorder, and, if the disorder was severe, they were freed from paying tax ("So", "Yo", and "Choh") by the governor.

This excellent law was based on T'ang law, although it is uncertain to what extent it was actually followed. However, it is surprising that such advanced systems were set up in such an early century.

The ninth century saw the transfer of the capital of Japan from Nara to Kyoto and the birth and flourishing of Japanese culture. During this era, scenes of visiting of the sick and of nursing could be seen in a pictorial version of "The Tale of Genji" by Lady Murasaki.

From the end of the Heian period to the beginning of the Kamakura period, the "Pictures of Disease" ("Yamai-no-soshi") were drawn by unknown Japanese artists. These picture scrolls, which remain a national treasure, depict epileptic attacks, dwarfism due to vertebral caries, an obese woman, the spastic gait of a man, and so on.

In the history of Japan, the sixteenth century is called the "Years of Battle". The great shogun Hideyoshi was born in that century and he had congenital polydactyly of the right hand.

In the Edo era, there were some handicapped persons in the Tokugawa family of shoguns. I'emitsu—3rd Shogun and Yoshimune—8th Shogun showed "Mann-Wernicke's posture" due to apoplexy. I'eshige, the son of Yoshimune, and I'esada—13th Shogun had cerebral palsy. I'eshige had a speech disturbance, so nobody around him could understand his commands except one samurai named Ohoka Tadamits. The ataxic posture of I'eshige can be seen in his portrait drawn in the Edo era.

It was believed that Buddha could heal unknown chronic diseases and some kinds of handicaps. This belief persisted until the end of the Edo era. The handicapped and their families sought to cure their disorders by offering votive pictures named "ema" after praying to the Buddha of Healing. These votive pictures almost came to be fixtures in temples devoted to Buddha. Even today, "ema" of the handicapped may be seen in temples all over Japan.

Study of the Longitudinal Evaluation of Physical Activity and Sports in Cardiac Transplant Recipients

ANNETT BETHGE

Abstract. The goal of this study was to give an account of a persons' abilities to practice one or more physical activities or sports after an invasive surgical procedure such as cardiac transplantation.

Introduction

The principal goals of the present work are to set forth the longitudinal evolution of the physiological and physical capacity of a cardiac transplant recipient after the operation and to present the multiple reasons why in practice the cardiac transplant recipient sets out to assume or resume the physical activity of a sport or a completely different physical activity demanding good physical condition and stamina.

Study Design

The study is based on a population of 47 people and brings together two directions of research, different in nature but necessary to meet the principal goals formulated above. One orientation is purely physiological. It is a longitudinal study over a post operative period of at least 5 years and, depending on the case, extending to a period of 10 post operative years. Here, we seek to define the changes in the physiological variables registered during the postperative period, from the 1st month to 10 years, as well as the evolution of the recovery of the physical condition of the cardiac transplant recipient.

The physiological variables are ascertained in two ways:

1. In tests of maximal exertion on the ergometric cycle
2. By means of meticulous consultation of the medical files of each person

The reflections as well as the conclusions deduced from this first branch of the study will be analyzed in the light of the statistical test P.C.S.M. (the Conversation Program of Statistics for Sciences and Marketing), and more particularly Wilcoxon's nonparametric test.

Se : leaving school
T : work
SM : military service
M : weding
D : moving
E : birth of a child
Div. : divorce
PT : first cardiac disorders
Hosp: hospitalization
TC. : transplantation

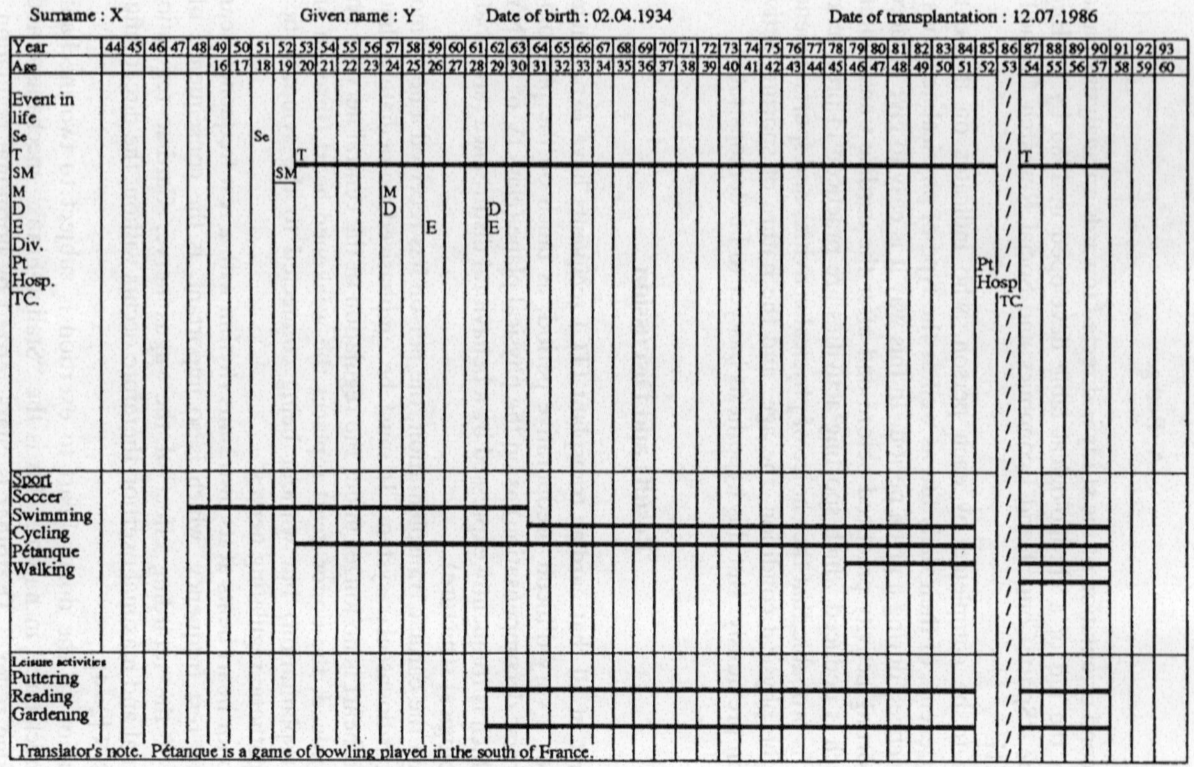

FIG. 1. Chronological table

The second orientation of the study is directed towards an analysis of a social type with the aid of a chronological table developed in 1986 by an English group, the "Sport Council and Economics and Social Research Council" of London [1].

This is to be completed by each person, who indicates on it the most important events of their daily life as well as the type of physical activities and sports practiced during a given period. In this way it is easy to give an account of the sporting activity practiced before and after the cardiac transplantation, from which is deduced which sporting activities are practiced in preference to others. It is probable that the choice of physical activities and sports depends at once on the physical condition, the age, and the nature of sporting activities engaged in previously. But this hypothesis has yet to be demonstrated.

Results and Discussion

Recall first of all that cardiac transplant (TC) recipients have experienced in most cases a very difficult preoperative period, as much on the physiological level (cardiac decompensation) as on the physical plane (class IV of the NYHA scale), which is frequently expressed by a behavioral disturbance (an imbalance in psychological structure).

Through the cardiac transplantation, the person has received a new "motor" for the cardiovascular system. It must be emphasized immediately that the implanted heart is no longer under the regulation of the central nervous system (CNS). Indeed, the donor heart replaces the weakened heart (through orthotopic transplantation) but without being connected to the sympathetic and parasympathetic regulating nerves.

The donor heart beats at its own sinus rhythm with a rest frequency near 100 bpm. This rest frequency, which is so important, is the consequence of the absence of the retarding effect of the vagus nerve. Cardiac regulation at submaximal and maximal exertion therefore occurs without the direct influence of the CNS [2–4].

Adaptation of the donor heart to exertion is subject to two mechanisms. One is mechanical in nature. This is the "Staling-Frank" mechanism and the "Bainbridge reflex." The other is characterized by hormonal regulation. The concentration and the nature of circulating catecholamines (epinephrine and norepinephrine) secreted by the medullae of the adrenal glands regulate cardiac work at exertion [5].

The absence of the CNS in the direct regulation of the heart generates modifications in cardiovascular adaptation to exertion. For example, acceleration of the heart rate (HR) during exertion is slower, since it depends principally on the two mechanisms described above and no longer on the direct link with the CNS [6].

Through a longitudinal physiological study of 5 years dealing with a population of 47 TC recipients, we obtained the following results noted in the table

TABLE 1. Physiological variables measured during exertion tests.

Variables	Submaximal exertion	Maximal exertion
HR (bpm)	113 ± 11.51	154 ± 12.74
$\dot{V}O_2$ (ml/min)	890 ± 100	1.86 ± 0.39
ERO_2	31.73 ± 3.54	40.4 ± 5.17
QR	0.91 ± 0.07	1.19 ± 0.11
SBP (mmHg)	170 ± 16.69	204 ± 16.35
DBP (mmHg)	99 ± 14.01	105 ± 11.34
Effort (watt)		155 ± 25

HR, heart rate; $\dot{V}O_2$, oxygen uptake; ERO_2, respiratory equivalent in oxygen; QR, respiratory quotient; SBP, systolic blood pressure; DBP, diastolic blood pressure.

below. Table 1 reflects the cardiovascular adaptation typical of a cardiac transplant recipient.

We have observed a very significant evolution (statistically speaking) over the first 12 postoperative months. Beyond this 1st year (APO1), we did not observe very striking changes [5, 7, 8].

It is very important to emphasize the fact that this study concerned sedentary people. The results we obtained therefore reflect the "natural" physiological evolution which has not been encouraged by a specific training program but by the one proposed and initiated during the reeducational phase.

What does the expression "specific training" call to mind? Specific training emphasizes the need to consider the physiological and physical abilities and limitations of a population to be able to create a training plan specifically adapted to it.

We observe that what has been formulated is the principal objective of the teaching of adapted physical activity (APA). Its goal is to provide access, by an individualized approach, to a sports activity for a specific population characterized by a reduced physical capacity.

The cardiac transplant recipient undergoes a physiological deficiency which engenders, according to the case, a physical deficiency. The important points that must be taken into consideration when proposing a physical activity or sport to a cardiac transplant recipient are the physiological predispositions, the intensity of physical work, and the frequency of sessions [9].

As a function of the information obtained from the longitudinal study of the physiological variables, we ascertained that the cardiac transplant does not have the physiological predispositions to practice basically anaerobic physical activities. It is therefore very highly recommended to propose activities relying essentially on endurance (aerobic activities), such as cycling, walking, downhill skiing, etc.

When a training program is being set up, it is fundamental to take account of certain aspects. The first bears on the essential role of the warmup phase, for it is during this phase that the cardiovascular system progressively adapts to exertion. Physical work of growing intensity not exceeding 50% of maximal aerobic capacity (PMA) is required.

The second aspect bears on the intensity of physical work during training properly so called. There exists a space that delimits the intensity of the physical work. Its limits are calculated in the following manner:

$$\text{lower limit} = \text{rest HR} + 60\% \ (\text{max. HR} - \text{rest HR})$$
$$\text{upper limit} = \text{rest HR} + 90\% \ (\text{max. HR} - \text{rest HR}),$$

where HR refers to heart rate.

The third and final aspect concerns the frequency of sessions of training per week. Three sessions of 20–60 min are recommended.

Above all, we must never forget that a transplant recipient's physical capacity is and will always remain reduced compared with that of a "healthy" person. Their maximal HR will not exceed 80% of their theoretical cardiac frequency and will thus affect the maximal cardiac debt. Therefore, training programs should have moderate goals to avoid undue demand upon the cardiovascular system [4].

A sports training program must essentially have these two objectives:

1. Improvement in physical condition which accommodates the physiological limits of the transplant recipient
2. This person's opening up to a sporting activity

Evidence for this has been supplied by this study dealing with our population of 47 people, in the course of which we discovered with the aid of the chronological table that 55.32% of the people have resumed a physical activity or sport after transplantation.

The favorite activities are walking, cycling, swimming, and tennis. The principal expectations expressed in relation to physical activity and sport, of which I totally approve, are summarized by these six key words: preservation, prevention, conviviality, pleasure, sport, and recognition.

Acknowledgements. The author would like to express her gratitude to all members of the Department of Cardiology of the Erasmus Teaching Hospital, particularly to Dr. Degré (cardiologist) and Dr. Niset (physiotherapist); to Dr. DePotter (lecturer in adapted physical activities at the University of Brussels); to all patients with the hearts of "champions", who have taught her invaluable lessons; and to her parents.

References

1. Hedges B (1986) Personal leisure histories. Social and Community Planning Research, The Sport Council and Economic and Social Research Council, London
2. Kavanagh T (1991) Exercise training heart transplanted patients. Herz 16(4):243–250

3. Kavanagh T, Yacoub MH, Campbell B, et al. (1988) Cardiorespiratory responses to exercise training after orthotopic cardiac transplantation. Circulation 77:162–171
4. Niset G (1991) Rééducation fonctionnelle de l'opéré cardiaque adulte. Frison-Roche, Paris
5. Squires RW (1991) Exercise training after cardiac transplantation. Med Sci Sports and Exercise 23(6):686–694
6. Shephard RJ (1991) Responses to acute exercise and training after cardiac transplantation: a review. Can J Sport Sci 16(1):9–22
7. Degré S, Niset G, Desmet JM, et al. (1988) Cardiorespiratory response to early exercise testing after orthotopic cardiac transplantation. Am J Cardiol 60:926–928
8. Niset G, Hermans L, Depelchin P (1991) Exercise and hourt transplantation: a review. Sports Med 12(6):359–379
9. Broustet JP (1978) Cardiologie sportive. Masson, Paris

Development of Pressure Sores in Active and Inactive Persons with Spinal Cord Injury

Masahiro Yamasaki, Takashi Komura, Kaoru Fujiie,
Hisato Sasaki, Kenji Kai, and Keisuke Ohdoko

Abstract. To investigate the benefits of sports participation on the prevention of pressure sores, a questionnaire was mailed to 668 men and women with spinal cord injury. The questionnaire was designed to clarify the effects of physical activity and lifestyle on the development of pressure sores. Usable questionnaires were received from 466 persons, representing a response rate of 70%. Thirty-eight percent were quadriplegic and 62% paraplegic, with incomplete injuries accounting for 26% of the combined group. About half of the 466 subjects reported the development of pressure sores during their wheelchair life. There was a clear tendency for the subjects with severe and frequent spasms of their legs to have no pressure sores. Forty percent of the subjects (active subjects) participated in sports regularly, including basketball, tennis, table tennis, swimming, and road racing. When the development of pressure sores for the 5 years before sports participation was compared with the 5-year period after commencement of sports participation, no significant difference was noted. Thus, whether sports participation has a positive benefit in the prevention of pressure sores in paraplegics and quadriplegics could not be determined from the present study.

Introduction

Persons with spinal cord injury (SCI) are at increased risk for the development of pressure sores, which can cause serious complications and increase disability [1]. Thus, pressure sores often prevent paraplegics and quadriplegics from taking advantage of opportunities to increase their independence and to widen their participation in work, community, and sports activities.

It has been suggested that regular physical activity such as sports participation is of benefit in the prevention of pressure sores in persons with SCI, because exercise of the upper limbs can increase skin blood flow of the lower limbs during arm exercise [2]. However, our unpublished data showed little increase in skin blood flow of the paralyzed lower limbs during arm cranking exercise at work loads of 10, 30 and 50 watts.

Curtis et al. [3] reported that 29.85% of subjects whose average sports involvement was 5.38 h/week had decubitus ulcers, and subjects with 8.59 h/week of sports participation had no pressure ulceration. From this result, it cannot be concluded that sports participation is useful for the prevention of pressure sores, since persons without pressure sores may be able to spend a longer time in sports participation.

Therefore, the purpose of this study was to investigate the benefits of sports participation on the prevention of pressure sores. For this purpose, a questionnaire was mailed to men and women with SCI. The questionnaire was designed to clarify the effects of physical activity and lifestyle on the development of pressure sores.

Methods

Subjects

This retrospective sampling frame consisted of paraplegics and quadriplegics living in the western part of Japan, including the districts of Chugoku, Shikoku, and Kyushu. Names and addresses were obtained from two distinct populations. The first population consisted of members of the Japanese Association of Spinal Cord Injury. The second population comprised participants in wheelchair athletics.

Between November, 1991 and January, 1992, a questionnaire was sent to 668 men and women with SCI. Usable questionnaires were received from 466 persons, representing a response rate of 70%. Thirty-seven percent were quadriplegic and 63% paraplegic, with incomplete injuries accounting for 23% of the total. Table 1 shows the general characteristics of the subjects. In

TABLE 1. General characteristics of subjects.

	Number of subjects		Age (years)		Time since injury (years)	
	n	%	Mean	SD	Mean	SD
Neurologic status						
Quadriplegic	173	37.1	45.2	14.7	11.0	6.9
Complete	94	20.2	42.3	13.6	11.7	6.9
Incomplete	61	13.1	48.6	14.9	10.0	6.3
Unknown	18	3.8	49.6	15.9	10.8	8.2
Paraplegic	293	62.9	47.3	14.3	15.3	9.0
Complete	220	47.2	47.3	14.3	15.9	8.9
Incomplete	47	10.1	47.2	14.1	14.4	8.8
Unknown	26	5.6	47.3	15.2	11.6	10.0
Sex						
Male	431	92.5	47.2	14.3	14.1	8.7
Female	35	7.5	39.2	14.6	10.2	6.2

comparing these groups, age and time since injury were found to be similar. Only 7.5% of paraplegics and quadriplegics were female.

Questionnaire

All subjects completed a four-page questionnaire which was specifically designed to clarify the effects of physical activity and lifestyle on the formation of pressure sores.

The questionnaire was divided into five sections which related to general characteristics of subjects, experience of pressure sores, wheelchair sports participation, spasms, and life style. In this study, the following items were utilized for analysis: (1) physical characteristics of subjects including age, neurologic status, and time since injury, (2) experience of pressure sores, (3) effect of sports participation, and (4) effect of spasms.

Statistical Analysis

The data were analyzed by chi-square test. Differences were considered to be significant if the 5% level of confidence was achieved ($P < 0.05$).

Results

Figure 1 shows the subjects' experience of pressure sores in their wheelchair life: 42.9% of the quadriplegics, 60.2% of paraplegics, and 53.6% of the total subjects reported pressure sores.

Spasms are widely observed in quadriplegics and paraplegics. In fact, 73.1% of subjects reported spasms of various intensities and frequencies. Thus, according to the intensity and frequency of spasms, subjects were divided into three groups: (1) frequent and severe spasms, (2) less frequent and weak spasms, and (3) no spasms. Figure 2 shows the relationship between pressure

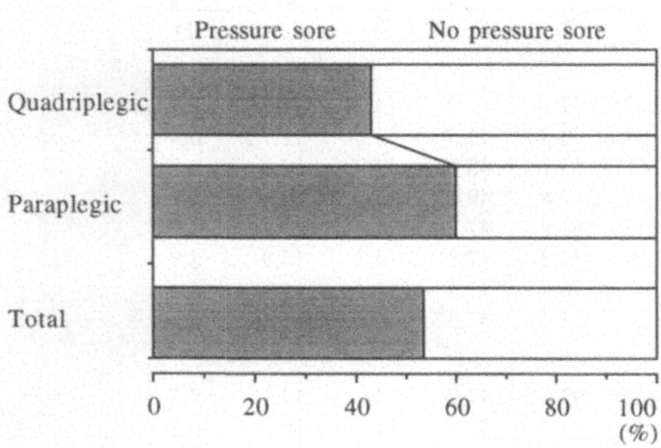

FIG. 1. Experience of pressure sores in wheelchair life

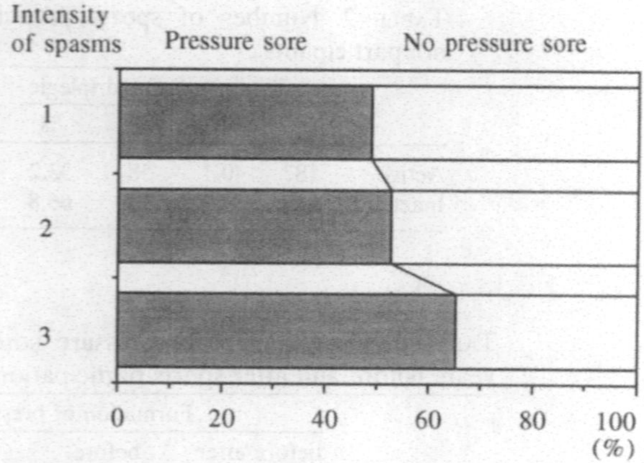

FIG. 2. Relationship between pressure sores in wheelchair life and spasms. 1, Frequent and severe spasms; 2, less frequent and weak spasms; 3, no spasms

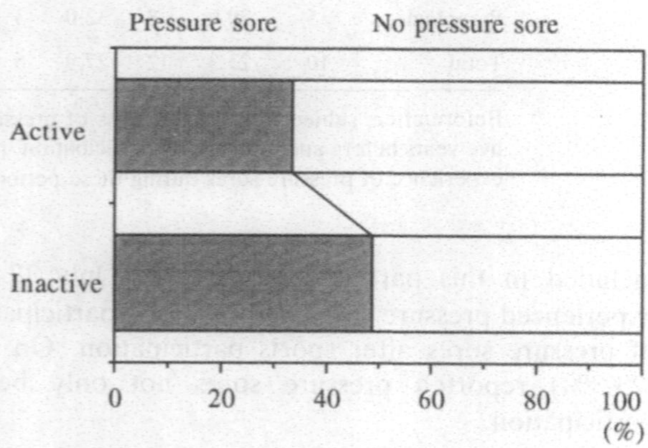

FIG. 3. Pressure sores in active and inactive subjects

sores in wheelchair life and spasms. When the number of subjects without pressure sores was compared between groups 1 and 3, a significant difference was found ($P < 0.05$).

The subjects were also divided into active and inactive groups. The former comprised competitive wheelchair athletes or subjects who regularly participated in recreational sports, including basketball, tennis, table tennis, swimming, and road racing. The latter comprised nonparticipants or irregular participants in sports. Forty percent of all subjects were active (Table 2). Figure 3 compares pressure sores in the active group with those in the inactive group. A significant difference was found in the formation of pressure sores between active and inactive subjects ($P < 0.05$).

To clearly demonstrate the effects of sports participation on the prevention of pressure sores, the development of pressure sores during the 5 years before sports participation was compared with that during the 5-year period after commencement of sports participation (Table 3). Forty-three subjects were

TABLE 2. Number of sports participants and nonparticipants.

	Total		Quadriplegic		Paraplegic	
	n	%	*n*	%	*n*	%
Active	187	40.1	58	33.2	129	44.3
Inactive	279	59.9	117	66.8	162	55.7

TABLE 3. Development of pressure sores during the five years before and after sports participation.

	Formation of pressure sore							
	before/after		before		after		non	
	n	%	*n*	%	*n*	%	*n*	%
Quadriplegic	5	27.8	4	22.2	2	11.1	7	38.9
Paraplegic	5	20.0	8	32.0	3	12.0	9	36.0
Total	10	23.3	12	27.9	5	11.6	16	37.2

Before/after, subjects had experiences of pressure sores during the five years before and after sports participation, respectively; non, no experience of pressure sores during these periods.

included in this part of the analysis. Only 12 subjects (27.5%) who had experienced pressure sores before sports participation showed no development of pressure sores after sports participation. On the other hand, 10 subjects (23.3%) reported pressure sores not only before but also after sports participation.

Discussion

Pressure sores are one of the most frequent medical complications in quadriplegics and paraplegics. The reported frequency of pressure sores ranges from 25% [4] to 85% [5]. In this study, many subjects also reported pressure sores (Fig. 1). Although many persons with SCI suffer from pressure sores, there are only a few investigations on the prevention of pressure sores [6, 7].

One of the causes of pressure sores is considered to be tissue ischemia due to continuous pressure. Therefore, increased blood flow in the affected tissue may prevent pressure sores. In fact, pressure sores were observed less frequently in the subjects with frequent and severe spasms, which can also increase the blood flow to paralyzed muscles, as compared to the subjects without spasms.

Sports activity may be an effective method to prevent pressure sores because it can also increase the blood flow of tissues [2]. In fact, fewer active subjects had pressure sores than inactive subjects (Fig. 3). This is in good agreement with the results of Curtis et al. [3], who reported that subjects with greater sports participation (8.59 h/week) had no pressure sores. These results alone, however, are not conclusive as to whether sports partcipation is effective for prevention of pressure sores, because it is possible that the greater participation in sports activity may have been due to the absence of pressure sores.

If indeed sports involvement does prevent pressure sores, the subjects should report less pressure sores after sports participation. To clarify this point, the development of pressure sores during the 5 years before sports participation was compared with the 5-year period after commencing sports participation (Table 3). There was no evidence of a trend for pressure sores to occur less frequently after sports participation. Therefore, although quadriplegics and paraplegics without pressure sores had a greater tendency to participate in sports activity, there were no clear positive benefits of sports involvement on pressure sores.

It is obvious that more work needs to be done on the impact of sports participation on the prevention of pressure sores. In addition, careful physiological study of blood flow of paralyzed muscle during sport is needed in addition to a random study with long-term follow-up.

References

1. Vaziri ND, Cesario T, Mootoo TK, Zeien L, Gordon S, Byrne C (1982) Bacterial infections in patients with end-stage renal disease associated with spinal cord injury. Arch Intern Med 142:1273–1276
2. Ogata H (1991) Relationship between wheelchair sport and rehabilitation (in Japanese). Rehabilitation Igaku 28:3–10
3. Curtis KA, McClanahan S, Hall KM, Dillon D, Brown KF (1986) Health, vocational, and functional status in spinal cord injured athletes and nonathletes. Arch Phys Med Rehab 67:862–865
4. Munro D (1940) Care of back following spinal cord injuries: consideration of bed sores. N Engl J Med 223:391–398
5. Kuhn WG (1947) Care and rehabilitation of patients with injuries of spinal cord and cauda equina: preliminary report on 113 cases. J Neurosurg 4:40–68
6. Carpendale M (1974) A comparison of four beds in the prevention of tissue ischaemia in paraplegic patients. Paraplegia 12:21–32
7. Souther SG, Stephen DC, Vistnes LM (1974) Wheelchair cushions to reduce pressure under bony prominences. Arch Phys Med Rehab 55:460–464

Effects of Feeding Levels and Body Weight Loading on Muscle Size and Visceral Organ Sizes in Rats

KAORU TACHIYASHIKI and KAZUHIKO IMAIZUMI

Abstract. The effects of feeding levels and body weight loading on the soleus muscle size and visceral organ sizes in rats were studied by using the whole-body suspension technique. Body suspensions in the free-feeding and chow-restraint conditions were maintained for 18 and 11 days, respectively. The rats were divided into three groups: cage control (CON), body suspended (BS), and BS plus continuous weight-bearing of the hind limbs on the floor of the cage (BSW). In the free-feeding conditions, the body weights of the BS and BSW rats decreased during the first 4 days. The initial loss of weight correlated with a reduced chow intake during this period. In the chow-restraint conditions, however, the body weight of BS and BSW rats decreased with prolongation of the suspension period, indicating that factors other than chow intake participated in the weight decrease. In both feeding conditions, the adrenal weights of the BS and BSW rats were 2 times higher than those of CON rats, suggesting that suspension stress may produce adrenal hypertrophy. The rectal temperatures of BS and BSW rats were also significantly higher than those of CON rats, showing that a higher metabolic state may be induced by suspension. In both feeding conditions, the weights and protein concentrations of soleus muscles of BSW rats were significantly higher than those of BS rats, suggesting that the weight bearing by the soleus muscles during suspension may maintain the size and protein levels of muscles.

Introduction

Skeletal muscle atrophy and reduced work capacity are characteristic of the prolonged hypokinesia (i.e., decreased motor activity) and/or hypodynamia (i.e., decreased mechanical loading) resulting from joint immobilization [1, 2], restricted movement [3], prolonged bed rest [4], limited muscular function [5], and space flight [6]. The causes may be disuse, inadequate functional loading, insufficient food intake, and/or lack of exercise [1, 7, 8]. Muscle atrophy, especially of those muscles that counteract Earth's gravity, has been an important problem in the field of rehabilitation, sports medicine, physical fitness, and space biology [9, 10].

Many reports have shown changes in physiological, histological, and biochemical properties of atrophied muscle [1, 8, 11]. However, its mechanism is still uncertain [10]. It is, therefore, essential for the complete elucidation of muscle atrophy to study the intracellular changes of atrophic muscle in an animal model. A variety of animal models can be utilized to simulate such muscle changes, including whole-body suspension [12], tail suspension [13], limb casting [14], denervation [15], and small-cage restraint [16]. Here, we used the whole-body suspension of rats [17, 18]. It is very important to study the mechanism underlying hypokinesia and hypodynamia on skeletal unloading [19–22], because such examination will contribute to health and safety before, during, and after joint immobilization, restricted movement, and limited muscular function, and to a solution of the many physiological problems of prolonged bed rest [19].

However, few reports are available on the effects of feeding levels (chow- and water-intake) and constraint stresses accompanied with suspension on muscle size, organ size and physiological functions, by using the whole-body suspension model of rats [8, 17]. The aim of the present paper is to evaluate the effects of feeding levels and body weight load on muscle size in the rat.

Materials and Methods

Animals

Specific-pathogen-free male Sprague-Dawley rats (7 weeks old: Japan SLC, Hamamatsu Japan) were used (body weight range: 219–222 g). The rats were fed for 3–5 days for adaptation to the new environment. The following morning, the rats were divided into three groups (n = 8 per group): cage-control (CON), whole-body suspended group (BS), and BS plus continuous weight-bearing of the hind limbs on the floor of the cage (BSW) [18].

Experimental Procedures

This experiment was carried out using whole-body suspensions in the free-feeding and in the chow-restraint conditions which were maintained for 18 and 11 days, respectively. The rats were anesthetized with ethyl ether and those in the BS and BSW groups were each placed in a suspension harness made of denim material and fastening tape. The denim harness was cut to fit around the torso, and the legs extended through the openings. The denim suit was fastened with tape on the dorsal surface and held by clips to conform to the dorsal surface of the animal [7, 15]. This unit was attached to a swivel [19]. The suspended rats of BS and BSW groups were able to use their forelimbs to eat food (CE-2 type, CLEA Japan, Tokyo, Japan) and drink once-boiled water. Rats in the CON group were not suspended at all and served as cage-control (nonsuspended group). The suspension apparatus used was a modified version of a type used by Musacchia et al. [12]. Experiments were conducted so as to inflict the least possible pain or discomfort to the animals [23, 24]. Animals were checked daily for signs of leg, nose, and eye lesions, unusual breathing patterns, or undue discomfort. A rat showing any of these signs was removed immediately from the study [25].

The room temperature was maintained at 24 ± 1°C and at a relative humidity of 55 ± 5%. A 12-h light-dark cycle was controlled automatically (lights on from 8:00 to 20:00). All the rats were individually supported or housed, and weighed every day during the experimental period. The present studies were carried out according to "Guiding Principles for the Care and Use of Animals in the Field of Physiological Sciences", in The Physiological Society of Japan [26]. On the morning of the final day in each experiment, the rats were anesthetized with sodium pentobarbital (50 mg/kg), and muscles (soleus and gastrocnemius), some organs (liver, testis, adrenal, spleen, thymus and kidney), and blood were immediately removed [23, 24, 27]. The water content of both muscles was the same, and we measured wet weight instead of dry weight. The serum and muscle protein contents were determined according to the method of Lowry et al. [28].

Statistical Analysis

Results were expressed as the means ± SE. The statistical significance of the differences between values was estimated by Student's *t*-test. P values of less than 0.05 were considered to be statistically significant.

Results

Body Weight

In free-feeding conditions (Fig. 1A), there was an initial decrease of body weight during the first 4 days in the BS and BSW groups and it remained nearly constant between days 5–18 of suspension in the BS group. In the BSW group, however, there was a slight but progressive body weight increase. This correlated with reduced chow intake and water intake during the first 4 days of suspension (Fig. 1C,D). In fact, as shown in Fig. 2, a high positive correlation between daily chow and water intake and daily change in body weight was observed under free-feeding conditions. Conversely, in chow-restraint conditions (Fig. 1B), there was a progressive decrease of body weight in both the BS and BSW groups. The body weights of the CON group were nearly constant between the 1st and 11th days of suspension. These results suggest that factors other than chow and water intakes were involved in the decrease of body weight. The body weight of rats at 18 days of suspension was 13% higher ($P < 0.05$) in the BSW group than in the BS group.

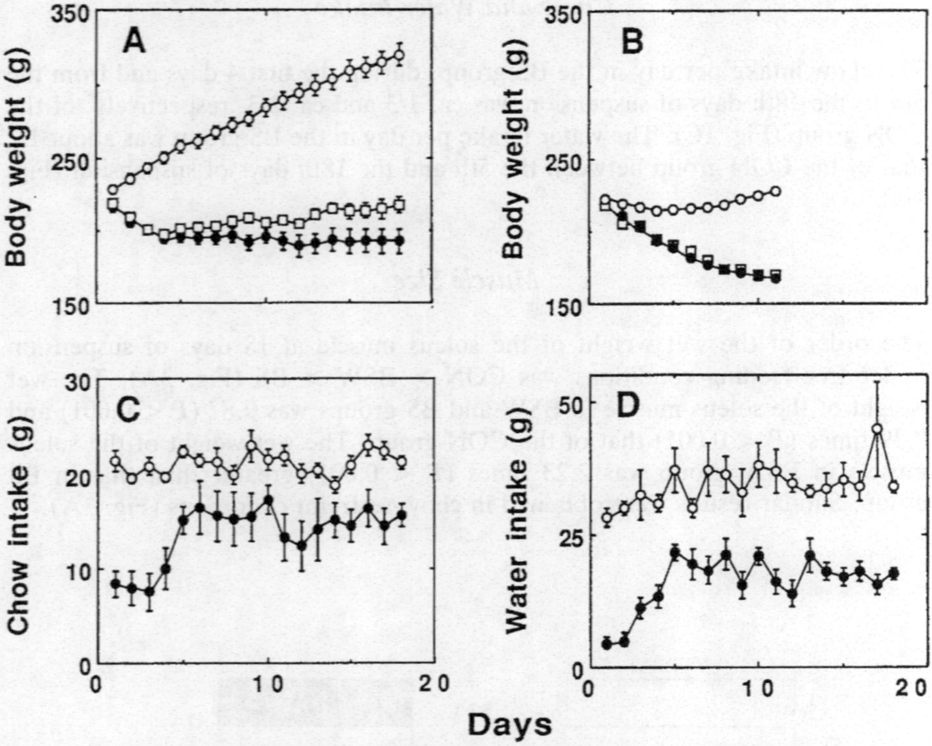

FIG. 1. Changes in the body weight (**A** and **B**), chow intake (**C**), and water intake (**D**) during body suspension. **A**, **C** and **D** Free-feeding conditions. **B** Chow-restraint conditions. Values are Means ± SE. *Open circles*, CON; *closed circles*, BS; *open squares*, BSW

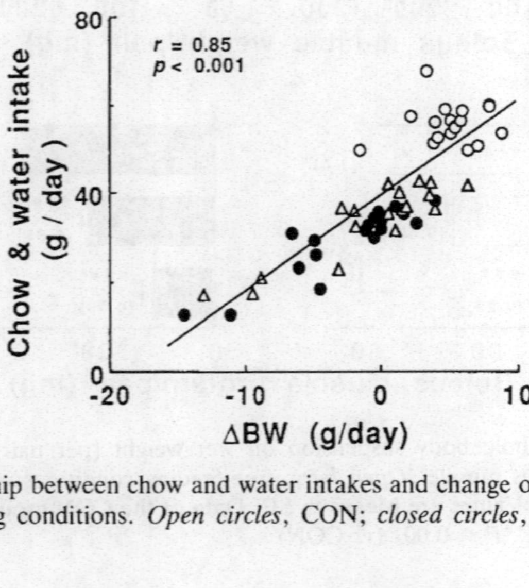

FIG. 2. Relationship between chow and water intakes and change of body weight (*BW*) under free-feeding conditions. *Open circles*, CON; *closed circles*, BS; *open triangles*, BSW

Chow and Water Intake

The chow intake per day in the BS group, during the first 4 days and from the 5th to the 18th days of suspension was ca. 1/3 and ca. 2/3, respectively, of the CON group (Fig. 1C). The water intake per day in the BS group was about 1/2 that of the CON group between the 5th and the 18th days of suspension (Fig. 1D).

Muscle Size

The order of the wet weight of the soleus muscle at 18 days of suspension under free-feeding conditions was CON > BSW > BS (Fig. 3A). The wet weight of the soleus muscle in BSW and BS groups was 0.87 ($P < 0.001$) and 0.39 times ($P < 0.001$) that of the CON group. The wet weight of the soleus muscle in BSW group was 2.23 times ($P < 0.001$) greater than that in BS group. Similar results were obtained in chow-restraint conditions (Fig. 3A).

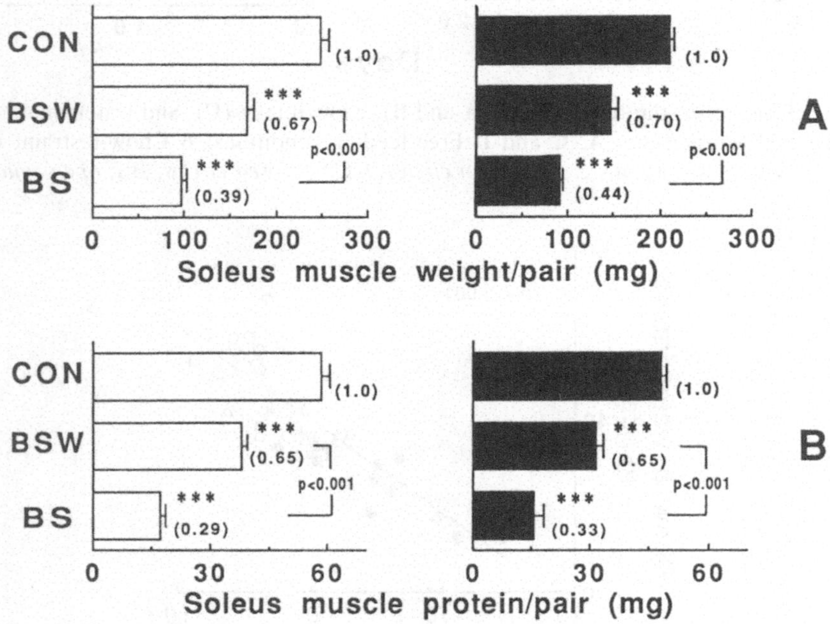

FIG. 3. Effect of whole body suspension on wet weight (per pair) (**A**) and protein content (**B**) of soleus muscle. *Open bars*, free-feeding conditions; *closed bars*, chow-restraint conditions. Values are Means ± SE. Data of the CON group are employed as the standard ratio. ***$P < 0.001$ (*vs* CON)

Muscle Protein Content

The order of soleus muscle protein content (per pair) was CON > BSW > BS (Fig. 3B) in both experimental conditions. Soleus muscle protein in the BSW and BS groups at 18 days of suspension, in free-feeding conditions, was 0.65 ($P < 0.001$) and 0.29 times ($P < 0.001$) of the CON group, respectively. The soleus muscle protein in the BSW group was 2.24 times ($P < 0.001$) greater than that in the BS group, suggesting that the weight bearing by the soleus muscle, during whole-body suspension, may prevent muscle protein loss. Similar results were observed in chow-restraint conditions (Fig. 3B).

Although data are not shown, muscle protein concentration was significantly lower in the BS group than the CON and BSW groups, suggesting that body weight bearing to hind limb muscles can help maintain soleus muscle protein concentration.

Visceral Organ Sizes

As shown in Fig. 4A,B, the ratio of adrenal wet weight (per pair) to body weight was significantly higher in the BSW and BS groups than the CON group. These results suggest that whole-body suspension stress may produce adrenal hypertrophy. Although data are not shown, we observed hypertrophy of the testis, kidney, and heart, and atrophy of the thymus induced by the whole-body suspension method.

Rectal Temperatures

The rectal temperature of rats at 11 days of suspension, in chow-restraint conditions, was significantly higher in the BSW and BS groups than the CON

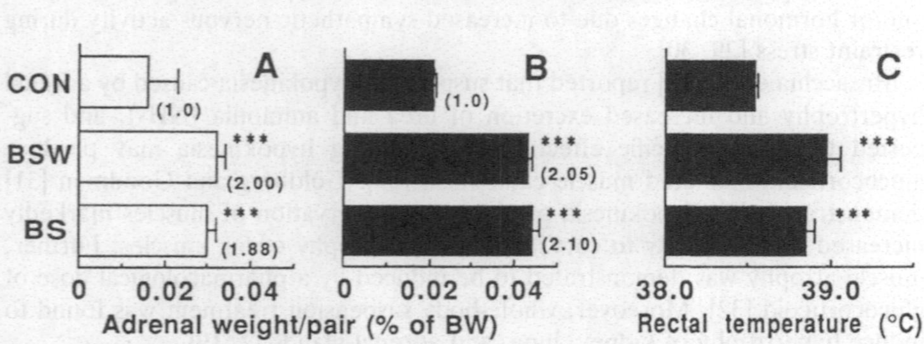

FIG. 4. Effects of whole body suspensions on the ratio of wet weight (per pair) of adrenals to body weight (*BW*) (**A** and **B**) and rectal temperature under chow-restraint feeding (**C**). **A** Free-feeding conditions. **B** and **C** Chow-restraint conditions. Values are Means ± SE. Data of the CON group shown in **A** and **B** are shown as the standard ratio. ***$P < 0.001$ *vs* CON

group (Fig. 4C). These results are consistent with our previous observations [17, 18].

Discussion

The present study showed that whole-body suspension (BS and BSW groups) hypokinesia in rats was associated with skeletal muscle atrophy (Fig. 3). Further, we showed that weight bearing by the soleus muscles during whole-body suspension may help maintain the size and protein levels of muscles (Fig. 3). These results suggest that muscle unloading is involved in suspension-induced atrophy of soleus muscle. The soleus muscle, a major antigravity muscle, was found to be the most susceptible to suspension [12]. This is consistent with the results of previous studies [7, 10, 12, 17, 19, 20]. It is generally accepted that increased urinary [^{7}N]methylhistidine excretion, higher muscle degradation rate, and increased lysosomal protease activity in muscle were induced by suspension [7, 10, 12, 17]. These findings suggest that increased protein breakdown and decreased protein content are involved in the muscle atrophy [12, 28].

In the present study, rectal temperatures of rats at the 18th day of suspension were demonstrated to be significantly higher in BS and BSW rats than in CON rats (Fig. 4C), suggesting that a higher metabolic state may be induced by whole-body suspension. Because there was no significant difference between BS and BSW rats in terms of rectal temperature, the effects of restraint stress to rats may affect body temperature at a deeper level in both suspension groups [7, 17, 18]. On the other hand, a marked decrease in body weight in both BS and BSW rats was observed (Figs. 1 and 2). The decrease in body weight in both suspension groups (BS and BSW) cannot be explained by chow and water intake alone (Fig. 1B and Fig. 2), suggesting that the decrease in body weight during suspension is induced at least in part by higher metabolic and/or hormonal changes due to increased sympathetic nervous activity during restraint stress [29, 30].

Musacchia et al. [12] reported that suspension hypokinesia caused by adrenal hypertrophy and increased excretion of urea and ammonia (NH_3), and suggested that a nonspecific effect of stress during hypokinesia may produce glucocorticoid-mediated muscle catabolism [29]. Goldberg and Goodman [31] demonstrated that hypokinesia produced by denervation of muscles markedly increased the sensitivity to cortisone-induced atrophy of leg muscles. Further, muscle atrophy was demonstrated to be induced by a pharmacological dose of glucocorticoid [32]. Moreover, whole-body suspension treatment was found to induce hypertrophy of kidney, lung, and adrenal glands [7, 19].

In the present study, we showed hypertrophy of testis, kidney, and adrenals, and atrophy of the thymus (data not shown), induced by whole-body suspension. These findings, together with the present ones, suggest the likelihood of involvement of glucocorticoid in the changes of protein metabolism occurring in suspension hypokinesia. Further studies, however, are necessary to investigate these possibilities in greater detail.

Acknowledgements. We thank Dr. Yoshinobu Ohira (National Institute of Fitness and Sports) for his excellent technical advice. Thanks are due to Ms. Mika Shirata and Ms. Akiko Mori for their collaboration. We are also grateful to Ms. Saori Harada, Ms. Tomoko Sano, and Mr. Akira Shiraishi for the preparation of this manuscript. This study was supported in part by the Fund (U-20) for Basic Experiments Oriented to Space Utilization from the Institute of Space and Astronautical Sciences, Japan, and by a Grant-in-Aid from the Special Scientific Research Fund of the Joetsu University of Education.

References

1. Booth FW (1977) Time course of muscular atrophy during immobilization of hindlimbs in rats. J Appl Physiol: Respirat Environ Exercise Physiol 43:656–661
2. Kondo H, Miura M, Nakagaki I, Sasaki S, Itokawa Y (1992) Trace element movement and oxidative stress in skeletal muscle atrophied by immobilization. Am J Physiol 262 (Endocrinol Metab 25):E583–E590
3. MacDougal JD, Ward GR, Sale DG, Sutton JR (1977) Biochemical adaptation of human skeletal muscle to heavy resistance training and immobilization. J Appl Physiol: Respirat Environ Exercise Physiol 43:700–703
4. Conbertino VA, Keil LC, Greenleaf JE (1983) Plasma volume, renin, and vasopressin responses to graded exercise after training. J Appl Physiol: Respirat Environ Exercise Physiol 54:508–514
5. Oganov VS, Patapov AN (1976) On the mechanisms of changes in skeletal muscles in the weightless environment. Life Sci Space Res 19:137–143
6. Ilyina-Kakueva EI, Portugalov VV, Krivenkova NP (1976) Space flight effects on the skeletal muscle of rats. Aviat Space Environ Med 47:700–703
7. Yokogoshi H, Takase S, Goda T, Hoshi T (1990) Effects of suspension hypokinesia/hypodynamia on the body weight and nitrogen balance in rats fed with various protein concentration. Agric Biol Chem 54:779–789
8. Thomason DB, Booth FW (1990) Atrophy of the soleus muscle by hindlimb unweighting. J Appl Physiol 68:1–12
9. Darr KC, Schultz E (1989) Hindlimb suspension suppresses muscle growth and satellite cell proliferation. J Appl Physiol 67:1827–1834
10. Booth FW, Thomason DB (1991) Molecular and cellular adaptation of muscle in response to exercise: Perspectives of various model. J Appl Physiol 71:541–585
11. Cooper RR (1972) Alterations during immobilization and regeneration of skeletal muscle in cats. J Bone Jt Surg Am 54-A:919–953
12. Musacchia XJ, Deavers DR, Meininger GA, Davis TP (1980) A model for hypokinesia: Effects on muscle atrophy in the rat. J Appl Physiol 48:479–486
13. Morey-Holten E, Wronski TJ (1981) Animal models for simulating weightlessness. Physiologist 24[Suppl VI]:S45–S48
14. Witzman FA, Kim DH, Fitt RH (1983) Effect of hindlimb immobilization on the fatigability of skeletal muscle. J Appl Physiol 54:1242–1248
15. Ohira Y (1989) Effects of denervation and deafferentation on mass and enzyme activity in rat skeletal muscles. Jpn J Physiol 39:21–31
16. Baranski S, Kwarecki K, Szmigielski S, Rozynski J (1971) Histochemistry of skeletal muscle fibers in rats undergoing long term experimental hypokinesia. Follia Histochem Cytochem 9:381–386

17. Imaizumi K, Tachiyashiki K, Shirata M (1992) Hindlimb suspension-induced changes of skeletal muscles and physiological functions in rats. Jpn J Physiol 42 [Suppl]:S255
18. Imaizumi K, Tachiyashiki K, Jikihara K (1993) Responses of the sizes of visceral organs and muscles to whole body suspension, and recovery in rats. Jpn J Physiol 43 [Suppl]:S324
19. Hayase K, Yokogoshi H (1991) Effects of suspension hypokinesia/hypodynamia on tissue protein turnover in rats. Jpn J Physiol 41:473–482
20. Ohira Y, Jiang B, Roy RR, Oganov V, Ilyina-Kakueva EI, Marini JF, Edgerton VR (1992) Rat soleus muscle fiber responses to 14 days of spaceflight and hindlimb suspension. J Appl Physiol 73[Suppl]:51S–57S
21. Jiang B, Ohira Y, Roy RR, Nguyen Q, Ilyina-Kakueva EI, Oganov V, Edgerton VR (1992) Adaptation of fibers in fast-twitch muscles of rats to spaceflight and hindlimb suspension. J Appl Physiol 73[Suppl]:58S–65S
22. Thomason DB, Morrison PR, Oganov V, Ilyina-Kakueva EI, Booth FW, Baldwin KM (1992) Altered actin and myosin expression in muscle during exposure to microgravity. J Appl Physiol 73[Suppl]:90S–93S
23. Tachiyashiki K, Imaizumi K (1992) Lowering and delaying actions of bovine bile on plasma ethanol levels in rats. J Nutr Sci Vitaminol 38:69–82
24. Tachiyashiki K, Imaizumi K (1993) Effects of vegetable oils and C_{18}-unsaturated fatty acids on plasma ethanol levels and gastric emptying in ethanol-administered rats. J Nutr Sci Vitaminol 39:163–176
25. Hauschka EO, Roy RR, Edgerton VE (1987) Size and metabolic properties of single muscle fibers in rat soleus after hindlimb suspension. J Appl Physiol 62: 2338–2347
26. The Physiological Society of Japan (1990) Guiding principle for the care and use of animals in the field of physiological sciences. The Physiological Society of Japan, Tokyo
27. Imaizumi K, Tachiyashiki K, Sekiya M (1990) Quantitative analysis of skeletal muscles in dystrophyic mice as a model of non-exercise muscle atrophy. In: Kaneko M (ed) Fitness for the aged, disabled and industrial worker. Human Kinetics, Champaign, pp 169–177
28. Lowry OH, Rosebrough NJ, Farr AL, Randall RL (1953) Protein measurement with the Folin phenol reagent. J Biol Chem 193:265–275
29. Ballard FJ, Tomas FM (1983) 3-Methylhistidine as a measure of skeletal muscle protein breakdown in human subject: The case for its continued use. Clin Sci 65:209–215
30. Tsuchiya K, Matsumoto I, Kosaka M, Aikawa T (1992) Rise in core temperature and changes in plasma catecholamines level during restrained stress in rats. Jpn J Physiol 42[Suppl]:S291
31. Goldberg AL, Goodman HM (1969) Relationship between cortisone and muscle work in determining muscle size. J Physiol (London) 200:667–675
32. Odedra BR, Bates PC, Millward DJ (1983) Time course of the effect of catabolic doses of corticosterone on protein turnover in rat skeletal muscle and liver. Biochem J 214:617–627

Exercise-Induced Temperature Changes in the Tympanic Membrane and Skin of Patients with Spinal Cord Injury

Kojiro Ishii, Masahiro Yamasaki, Satoshi Muraki, Takashi Komura, Kunio Kikuchi, and Kazuya Maeda

Abstract. The kinetics of thermoregulation mechanisms were observed in patients with spinal cord injury (SCI) during exercise. Five patients with paraplegia (T4–T12/L1) due to spinal cord injury underwent arm cranking exercise after 60 min of rest in the sitting position. The exercises were conducted with incremental increases (5 watts/min) in external workload starting at 0 watts (50 rpm). They were performed in a climato-therapeutic chamber at 25°C and a relative humidity between 50%–60%. The patients were worked to exhaustion. Tympanic membrane (Tty) and the skin (Tsk; head, arms, chest, thigh, and shin) temperatures were measured at rest and during exercise. Results of the measurements showed that Tty in the SCI group was lower both at rest (36.15°–36.65°C) and during exercise (36.15°–36.70°C) than in the healthy control group. Tsk were also lower at all measured sites. The differences in the temperatures were especially marked at sites where dermal sensation was impaired such as the thighs and shins. It is concluded that the lower temperatures were due to disturbances in the input of thermal information to the thermoregulatory nucleus as well as the generation and modification of output command signals and responses with regard to the regulation of temperature which were caused by the spinal cord injury.

Introduction

Exercise is important in patients with spinal cord injury (SCI) as a means of physical rehabilitation and as an integral part of the training program for residual motor functions. It also plays an important role in the social rehabilitation and occupational training of patients with SCI. However, patients with SCI often develop various complications due to alterations in the autonomic system. Impaired thermoregulation is one such complication. In patients with SCI, adaptation to environmental changes is difficult because of both the reduction or complete loss of the reflex and sweating functions of the cutaneous blood vessels, and the complete loss of the shivering function in body surface areas where the cutaneous senses have been impaired. For this reason, exercise often leads to difficulties such as excess body temperature elevation and discomfort due to an imbalance between heat generation and heat diffusion. A review of the literature revealed only a few reports dealing with thermoregulation in patients with SCI during exercise [1–3]. The purpose of this study was to clarify the kinetics of thermoregulation in patients with SCI during exercise and to obtain data that will be useful for the prevention of heat exhaustion in such patients.

Subjects and Methods

Subjects

Five patients with paraplegia (T4–T12/L1) due to spinal cord injury were selected as subjects (Table 1). They had been participating in athletic programs for the handicapped using wheelchairs (basketball, marathon, and tennis). Five healthy male college students were chosen as controls and underwent the same arm cranking exercise as the paraplegics.

Experimental Procedure

The subjects had the upper half of their bodies and their legs fully exposed during the tests. The experiments were performed in a climato-therapeutic chamber at 25°C and a relative humidity between 50%–60%. Before the experiments, the subjects rested in the sitting position for over 60 min. Subsequently, they performed arm cranking exercise which consisted of incremental increases (5 watts/min) in external workload starting at 0 watts (50 rpm). The exercise test was performed until exhaustion.

Items and Methods for Measurement

For assessment of core temperature, tympanic membrane temperature (Tty) was measured using the device developed by Masuda and Uchino [4] for measurement of the tympanic membrane temperature during exercise. Tty was serially measured starting 5 min before exercise until cessation of the exercise (R280; Technol Seven, Japan). Since the external auditory meatus was stenotic

TABLE 1. Characteristics of the paraplegics.

Subject	Age (years)	Time since injury (yr)	Spinal cord lesion level
A	45	25	T12/L1
B	46	20	T7/T8
C	27	4	T6
D	24	3	T4
E	51	15	T10

in 1 control subject, the temperature recording device could not be inserted and placed inside it. Therefore, the control group with regard to the measurement of Tty consisted of only 4 subjects. Skin temperature (Tsk) was measured at 5 sites: the head, arm, chest, thighs, and shins. Measurements were started 5 min before exercise and once every minute thereafter until cessation of the exercise using the thermocouple method (Data Collector AM-2000; Anritsu Meter, Japan). Oxygen uptake, respiratory rate, and heart rate were also monitored during exercise. Expired air was collected at rest (5 min before initiation of exercise) and during exercise once every minute using the Douglas bag method. The gases were weighed using a desiccated gas meter; O_2 and CO_2 concentrations were analyzed using a Respina IH 26 analyzer (NEC-San-ei, Tokyo, Japan). Values obtained 5 min before exercise were converted to those 1 min before the initiation of exercise. A thermistor element was fixed in the mask used for gas collection. The respiratory rate was calculated based on changes in the temperature within the mask which occur as a result of ventilation. Heart rate was determined every minute using a heart rate recording device, PE-3000 (Polar Electro, Finland).

Results

Changes in Tty at rest and during exercise are shown in Fig. 1. Tty in the SCI group was lower both at rest (36.15°–36.65°C) and during exercise (36.15°–36.70°C) than in the healthy control group. There were individual differences in Tty in both the SCI and healthy control groups whose subjects exhibited various patterns of changes. When Tty was plotted against oxygen uptake, a similar tendency was observed (Fig. 2).

The changes in Tsk at rest and during exercise are shown in Fig. 3. Measured values at all sites were lower in the SCI group than in healthy controls. Tsk in

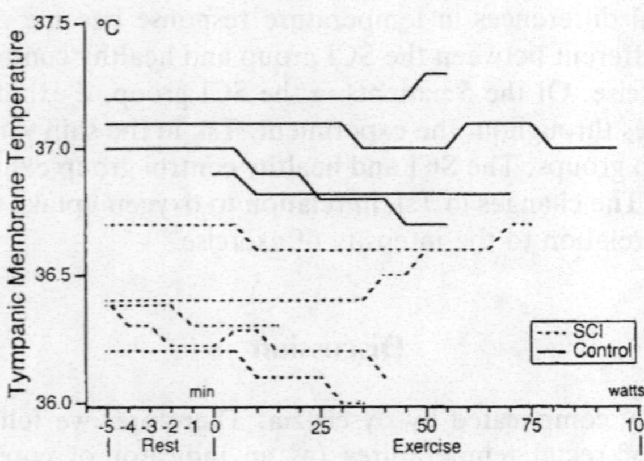

FIG. 1. Tympanic membrane temperature before and during arm cranking exercise

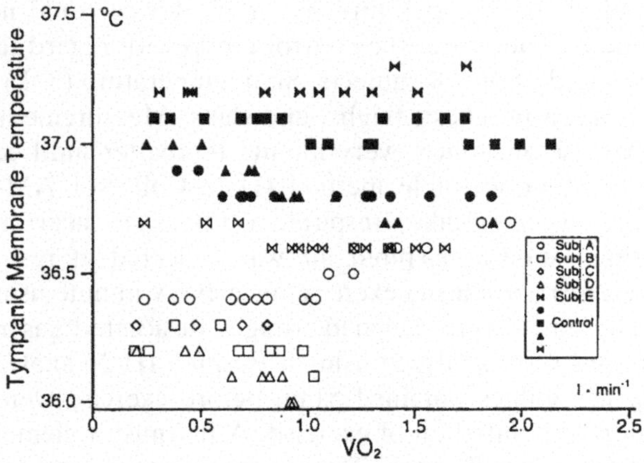

FIG. 2. Relationship between tympanic membrane temperature and oxygen uptake

the head region in healthy controls was flat at the initiation of exercise, but individual differences appeared after increases in the exercise load. In contrast, Tsk in the head region in the SCI group exhibited marked individual differences from the start of the exercise program. Some showed a flat response, others demonstrated a rise in temperature after an initial drop in temperature. Those in the SCI group who were able to continue the exercise at increased external loads exhibited temperature elevations that were similar to those seen in the healthy controls. There was no significant difference in Tsk in the arm between the SCI group and the healthy controls at rest. Tsk in the arm in all healthy controls was in the range of 34°–35°C, 10 min after initiation of exercise. However, in the SCI group, individual differences became greater with the progression of the exercise test. Tsk in the chest was also similar in the SCI and healthy control groups before initiation of exercise. After initiation of exercise, all healthy controls demonstrated temperature elevations whereas in the SCI group individual differences in temperature response became evident. Tsk in the thigh was different between the SCI group and healthy controls both at rest and during exercise. Of the 5 patients in the SCI group, 2 exhibited extremely low temperatures throughout the experiment. Tsk in the shin was also different between the two groups. The SCI and healthy control group exhibited different Tsk in the legs. The changes in Tsk in relation to oxygen uptake were similar to Tsk changes in relation to the intensity of exercise.

Discussion

SCI is frequently complicated by dyschezia. Therefore, we felt that repeated measurements of rectal temperatures (as an indicator of core temperature) were not feasible in our patients from a psychological perspective. This is the

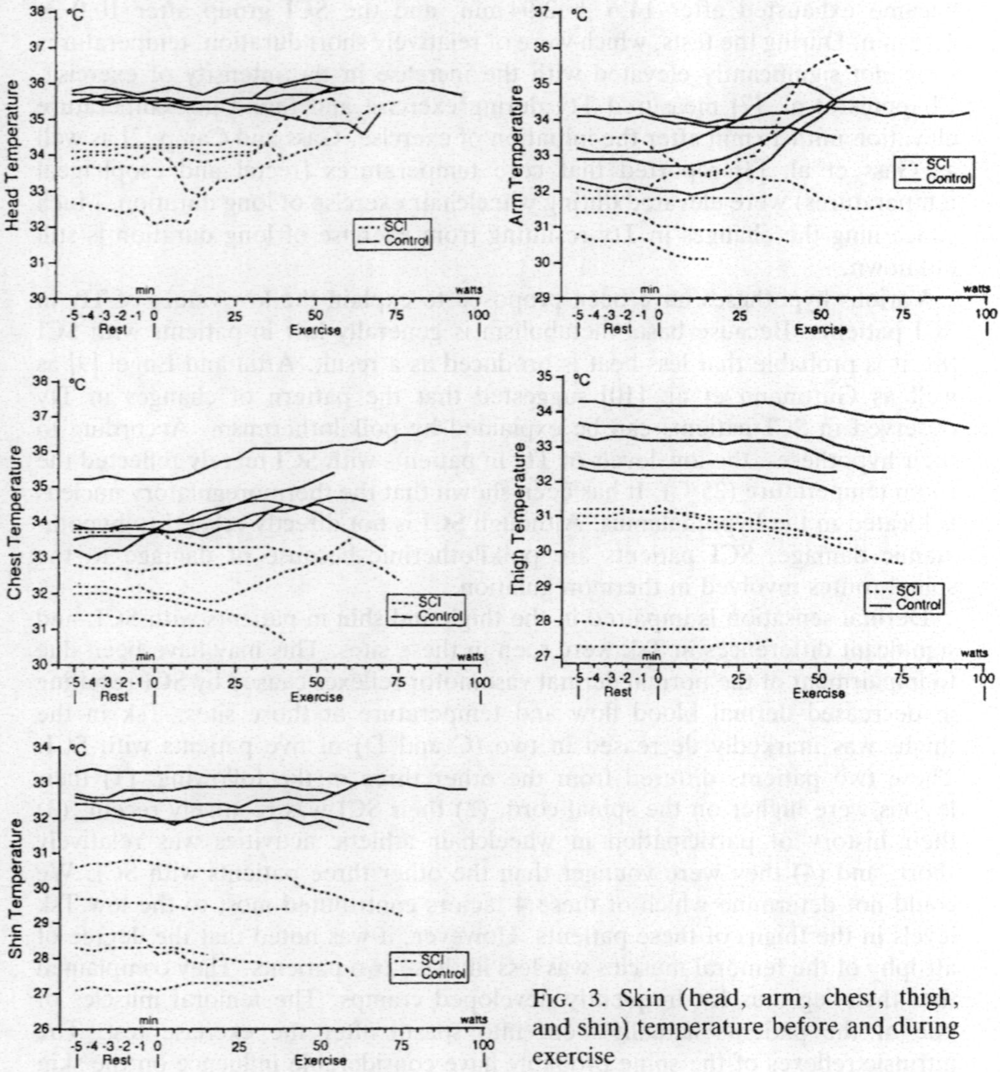

FIG. 3. Skin (head, arm, chest, thigh, and shin) temperature before and during exercise

reason we measure Tty instead of the rectal temperature as an indicator of core temperature. Previous reports describing changes in core temperatures during exercise in patients with SCI used rectal and esophageal temperatures as indicators [2, 3].

Temperature elevation is proportional to oxygen uptake (VO_2) [5]. Exercise involving the arms causes the same degree of temperature elevation as does exercise involving the legs if the VO_2 is similar [6]. The exercise tests in the present study were not of long duration. The external load was increased every minute so that the subjects reached exhaustion quickly. The normal controls became exhausted after 14.6 ± 2.94 min, and the SCI group after 10.0 ± 4.15 min. During the tests, which were of relatively short duration, temperatures were not significantly elevated with the increase in the intensity of exercise. Chappuis et al. [7] measured Tty during exercise and found no temperature elevation until 15 min after the initiation of exercise. Gass and Camp [2] as well as Gass et al. [3] reported that core temperatures (rectal and esophageal temperatures) were elevated during wheelchair exercise of long duration. Much concerning the changes in Tty resulting from exercise of long duration is still unknown.

Various hypotheses have been proposed to explain the low values of Tty in SCI patients. Because basal metabolism is generally low in patients with SCI [8], it is probable that less heat is produced as a result. Attia and Engel [9] as well as Guttmann et al. [10] suggested that the pattern of changes in Tty observed in SCI patients can be explained by poikilothermism. According to their hypotheses, the low levels of Tty in patients with SCI merely reflected the room temperature (25°C). It has been shown that the thermoregulatory nucleus is located in the hypothalamus. Although SCI is not directly related to hypothalamic damage, SCI patients are poikilothermic because of damage to the spinal routes involved in thermoregulation.

Dermal sensation is impaired in the thigh and shin in patients with SCI, and significant differences in Tsk were seen in these sites. This may have been due to impairment of the normal dermal vasomotor reflexes caused by SCI resulting in decreased dermal blood flow and temperature at those sites. Tsk in the thighs was markedly decreased in two (C and D) of five patients with SCI. These two patients differed from the other three in the following: (1) their lesions were higher on the spinal cord, (2) their SCI was relatively recent, (3) their history of participation in wheelchair athletic activities was relatively short, and (4) they were younger than the other three patients with SCI. We could not determine which of these 4 factors contributed most to the low Tsk levels in the thighs of these patients. However, it was noted that the degree of atrophy of the femoral muscles was less in these two patients. They complained that their leg muscles frequently developed cramps. The femoral muscles of one of the patients actually went into spasm after the exercise test. The intrinsic reflexes of the spine probably have considerable influence on the skin temperature of the legs.

Dermal sensation in the head, arm, and chest are not impaired by SCI, but Tsk in these regions is lower than in normal controls because it is influenced by heat convection and conduction from the paralytic areas which are transmitted via the blood flow in the skin and muscles. It is also possible that the autonomic nervous system is impaired even in the non-paralytic areas in patients with SCI. Our findings indicate that disturbances in the input of thermal information to the thermoregulatory nucleus as well as the generation and modification of output command signals and responses with regard to the regulation of body temperature are present in SCI.

The nervous system distal to the level of the spinal injury becomes isolated from the central nervous system (isolated spinal segment) in SCI. The peripheral nervous system can no longer be controlled by the central nervous system. Moreover, information from the peripheral nervous system will not reach the central nervous system. Thus, patients with SCI have difficulty maintaining the homeostatic mechanism. In many situations, existing data cannot be always relied upon in the care of patients with SCI. Pathological responses in patients with SCI merit further investigation.

Acknowledgements. We are indebted to the Y. Nakamura, M.D. Memorial Fund whose sponsorship made this research possible.

References

1. Fitzgerald PI, Sedlock DA, Knowlton RG (1982) Cardiovascular responses of spinal cord injured women to prolonged submaximal wheelchair activity (abstract). Med Sci Sports Exer 14:166
2. Gass GC, Camp EM (1984) Prolonged exercise response in trained male paraplegics. Thermal Physiol 9:429–432
3. Gass GC, Camp EM, Nadel ER, Gwinn TH, Engel P (1988) Rental and rectal vs. esophageal temperatures in paraplegic men during prolonged exercise. J Appl Physiol 64:2265–2271
4. Masuda M, Uchino K (1978) A device for tympanic membrane temperature in man. Jikeikai Med J 25:95–99
5. Nielsen M (1938) Die Regulation der Körpertemperatur bei Muskelarbeit. Scand Arch Physiol 79:193–230
6. Nielsen B (1966) Regulation of body temperature and heat dissipation at different levels of energy and heat production in man. Acta physiol Scand 68:215–227
7. Chappuis P, Pittet P, Jequier E (1976) Heat storage regulation in exercise during thermal transients. J Appl Physiol 40:384–392
8. Ogata H, Asayama K, Morita H, Hashimoto T, Akatsu T (1979) The adaptation to seasonal environmental variatations seen in patients with spinal cord injury. J University of Occupational and Environmental Health 1:351–359
9. Attia M, Engel P (1984) Thermoregulatory set-point in paraplegics. In: Hales JRS (ed) Thermal physiology. Raven, New York, pp 79–82
10. Guttmann L, Silver J, Wyndham CH (1958) Thermoregulation in spinal man. J Physiol (Lond) 142:406–419

Comparative Study on the Response of Cardiopulmonary Function Between the Spinal Cord Injured and the Normal Sedentary During Maximal Exercise and Rest

WAN-KI LIM and YANG-JA HONG

Abstract. The purpose of this study was to analyze the response of cardiopulmonary function between the spinal cord injured and the normal sedentary during maximal exercise and rest. The subjects were 10 spinal cord injured who did not participate in regular exercise and 10 normal sedentary college students. Incremental exercise testing to the point of exhaustion was done on all 20 subjects. The cardiopulmonary variables—$\dot{V}O_{2peak}$, $\dot{V}e_{peak}$, HR_{peak}, and O_2pulse_{peak}—were measured by auto gas analyzer. Independent *t*-tests between the two groups were done to detect mean differences in these variables. The results were as follows: (a) significant differences between the spinal cord injured and the normal sedentary were found in $\dot{V}O_{2peak}$, $\dot{V}e_{peak}$, O_2pulse_{peak} during maximal exercise; (b) no significant differences were found in HR_{peak}, VE_{peak} during maximal exercise; and (c) there were no statistical differences among all the variables in this study during rest.

Introduction

Technological advances, including widespread use of the automobile, the continuing horrors of modern warfare, and sports injuries, have caused many spinal cord injuries. The use of antibiotics and modern techniques of rehabilitation have greatly enhanced the survival prospects of individuals with paraplegia, thus increasing the overall portion of such people in the community [1].

Research on physical rehabilitation of the spinal cord injured has been conducted since World War II, the Korean War, and the Vietnam War to take care of the injured veterans. Today, research is performed to help them maintain a normal life and to lengthen their life expectancy. The spinal cord injured lose motor abilites secondary to the damage to the central nervous system which can lead to problems associated with the muscle system such as paralysis, paresis, and spasticity, thus resulting in muscular atrophy and disuse due to a sedentary lifestyle. The acute fatigue experienced by the spinal cord injured while moving in a wheelchair or on crutches is due to reduced working muscle mass, cardiovascular function, and venous return capacity [2–5].

The cardiopulmonary function in response to activity among the spinal cord injured were studied by several researchers [6–8]. According to these previous studies, regular exercise might maintain or enhance the cardiopulmonary capacity, and thus lengthen life expectancy of human.

However, there are few systematic studies of the physiological responses following exercise among the spinal cord injured. Therefore, in this study, we investigated cardiopulmonary changes and the differences between the spinal cord injured and normal sedentary persons during maximal exercise and during rest.

Patients and Methods

Patients

Ten spinal cord injured (SCI) who were otherwise healthy and who were not engaged in regular exercise comprised the study group. Ten graduate students who were preparing for the civil service exam served as controls. The subjects selected were those who could perform the required exercise, and informed consent was obtained in writing from each subject. The physical characteristics of the subjects are listed in Tables 1 and 2.

Experimental Procedures

The subjects were requested to arrive at the laboratory by 10 o'clock in the morning. After the experiment was explained to them, they were instructed to warm up for a 10-min adaptive period, followed by 10 min of rest. At the same time, the assistant recorded the ambient temperature and air pressure of the laboratory.

TABLE 1. Physical characteristics of the sedentary subjects.

Subjects	Age (yr)	Height (cm)	Weight (kg)	$\dot{V}O_{2peak}$/kg
K.T.W.	24	175	57	37.31
L.D.H.	24	172	93	31.72
K.J.H.	21	178	62	39.12
H.J.H.	24	173	73	25.33
C.B.D.	27	170	65	37.71
C.S.K.	37	169	53	44.42
K.Y.J.	33	168	68	20.39
P.H.C.	32	182	75	27.20
A.S.H.	30	173	76	28.48
J.S.H.	30	181	74	28.41
M	28.2	174.1	69.6	32.01
SD	5.0	4.9	11.4	7.40

$\dot{V}O_{2peak}$, peak oxygen uptake.

TABLE 2. Physical characteristics of the spinal cord injured.

Subjects	Age (yr)	Height (cm)	Weight (kg)	$\dot{V}O_{2peak}$/kg
K.S.W.	23	174	68	19.09
H.C.T.	28	177	58	22.25
H.J.H.	27	175	67	34.63
L.K.O.	26	176	60	29.72
L.J.Y.	29	170	72	18.15
K.K.H.	37	167	36	21.08
L.B.G.	35	180	67	26.43
P.J.C.	31	168	50	31.09
L.Y.K.	31	170	47	23.57
K.S.B.	38	172	59	18.02
M	30.50	172.90	58.40	24.40
SD	4.90	4.20	11.21	5.83

$\dot{V}O_{2peak}$, peak oxygen uptake.

Figure 1 shows the detailed experimental procedures in a block diagram.

Prior to beginning the exercise, each subject had a warm-up period with the speed of 50 rpm at 1 kp for 1 min, and then took a 1-min rest. No resistance was given at the beginning and the work intensity was gradually increased by 0.5 kp/min until exhaustion. When the heart rate exceeded 170 bpm, the subjects' condition was observed continuously, and the subject was encouraged to make his best effort. When the subject signalled that he reached the all-out state, the researcher let him stop the exercise.

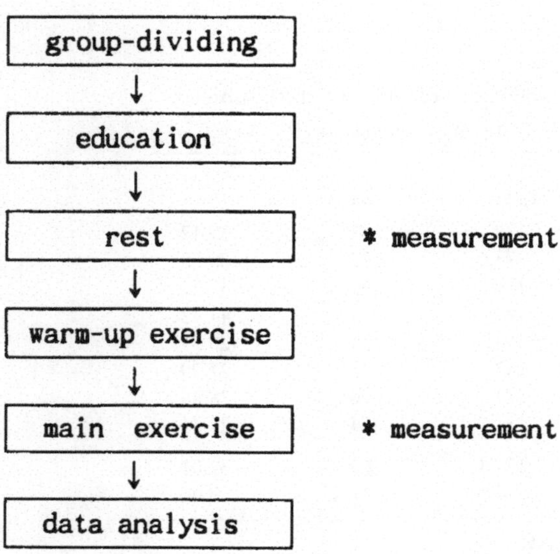

FIG. 1. Experimental procedures

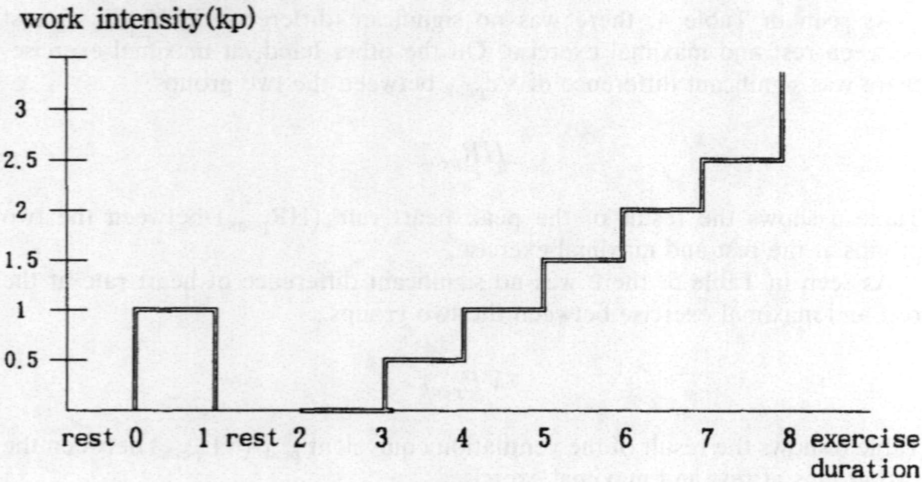

FIG. 2. Exercise test

Results

$\dot{V}O_{2peak}/kg$

Table 3 shows the result of the $\dot{V}O_{2peak}$/kg between the two groups at rest and during maximal exercise.

As seen in Table 3, there was no significant difference of $\dot{V}O_{2peak}$/kg between rest and maximal exercise. On the other hand, at maximal exercise there was significant difference of $\dot{V}O_{2peak}$/kg between the two groups.

$\dot{V}e_{peak}$

Table 4 shows the result of the ventilation $_{peak}$ ($\dot{V}e_{peak}$) between the two groups at rest and at maximal exercise.

TABLE 3. Test results of peak oxygen consumption ($\dot{V}O_{2peak}$/kg).

	Group	n	$\dot{V}O_{2peak}$ (ml/kg·min^{-1})	df	t-value	P
Rest	SCI	10	6.86 ± 1.53	9	2.04	0.33
	Sedentary	10	6.01 ± 2.19			
Maximum exercise	SCI	10	24.40 ± 5.83	9	1.61	0.02*
	Sedentary	10	32.01 ± 7.40			

SCI, spinal cord injured.
* $P < 0.05$ SCI *vs* sedentary.

As seen in Table 4, there was no significant difference in $\dot{V}e_{peak}$ at rest between rest and maximal exercise. On the other hand, at maximal exercise, there was significant difference of $\dot{V}e_{peak}$ between the two groups.

HR_{peak}

Table 5 shows the result of the peak heart rate (HR_{peak}) between the two groups at the rest and maximal exercise.

As seen in Table 5, there was no significant difference of heart rate at the rest and maximal exercise between the two groups.

VE_{peak}

Table 6 shows the result of the ventilation equivalent $_{peak}$ (VE_{peak}) between the two groups at rest and maximal exercise.

TABLE 4. Test results of ventilation peak (Ve_{peak}).

	Group	*n*	Ve_{peak} (l/min)	df	*t*-value	*P*
Rest	SCI	10	14.36 ± 2.67	9	−0.45	0.66
	Sedentary	10	13.84 ± 2.54			
Maximal exercise	SCI	10	53.73 ± 20.10	9	3.33	0.04*
	Sedentary	10	82.82 ± 18.98			

SCI, spinal cord injured.
* $P < 0.05$ SCI *vs* sedentary.

TABLE 5. Test results of peak heart rate (HR_{peak}).

	Group	*n*	HR_{peak} (bpm)	df	*t*-value	*P*
Rest	SCI	10	84.50 ± 12.41	9	−1.86	0.08
	Sedentary	10	74.30 ± 12.16			
Maximal exercise	SCI	10	24.40 ± 5.83	9	−1.93	0.07
	Sedentary	10	32.01 ± 7.40			

SCI, spinal cord injured.

TABLE 6. Test results of ventilation equivalent (VE_{peak}).

	Group	*n*	VE_{peak}	df	*t*-value	*P*
Rest	SCI	10	31.03 ± 6.29	9	−0.20	0.84
	Sedentary	10	30.41 ± 7.22			
Maximal exercise	SCI	10	32.65 ± 6.18	9	−0.07	0.95
	Sedentary	10	32.82 ± 5.30			

SCI, spinal cord injured.

TABLE 7. Test results of the oxygen pulse peak (O_2pulse_{peak}).

	Group	n	O_2pulse_{peak} (ml/beat·min^{-1})	df	t-value	P
Rest	SCI	10	4.1800 ± 0.811	9	2.04	0.39
	Sedentary	10	5.2000 ± 1.378			
Maximal exercise	SCI	10	8.6100 ± 2.673	9	3.49	0.003*
	Sedentary	10	12.5800 ± 2.410			

SCI, spinal cord injured.
* $P < 0.05$ SCI *vs* sedentary.

As seen in Table 6, there was no significant difference in VE_{peak} at rest and during maximal exercise between the two groups.

O_2pulse_{peak}

Table 7 shows the oxygen pulse peak (O_2pulse_{peak}) between the two groups.

As seen in Table 7, there was no significant difference in O_2pulse_{peak} at rest between rest and maximal exercise. On the other hand, at maximal exercise, there was significant difference in O_2pulse_{peak} between the two groups.

Discussion

In this study, the $\dot{V}O_{2peak}$/kg of the control group were greater than those of the SCI group, whose result is in agreement with previous studies. The reason for this result is that SCI have less opportunity and desire for exercise than the healthy control subjects, resulting in limited physical activities [2, 9].

The cardiac functions of individuals with spinal cord injury is influenced by the lesion level; those with spinal cord lesions at a higher level carry disturbances of sympathetic vaso-motor tone. Hence, decreased stroke volume and venous return cause limited cardiac output.

In this study, $\dot{V}e_{peak}$ was significantly higher in the control group than in the SCI group. Generally speaking, $\dot{V}e$ depends on the pulmonary contracting force and the airway diameter, and it is generally accepted that the pulmonary contracting force and the airway diameter are greater among normal sedentary patients than in the SCI, thus resulting in greater $\dot{V}e$.

Generally, SCI patients consume less energy than the normal sedentary, because the change of center of gravity is much smaller during the wheelchair ambulation than during walking in the general population. However, because the SCI use small muscle groups of the upper body, the heart rate of the SCI is greater than that of the sedentary [10]. This result agrees with previous studies.

VE is used to estimate the ventilation efficiency. It is usually greater in the upper extremity exercises than in the lower extremity exercises. The greater the $\dot{V}e$. the greater the VE due to increased metabolic acidosis [11]. In this study, VE among SCI patients is similar to that of normal sedentary patients. This result agrees with previous studies [12]; however, it is produced because of significantly higher $\dot{V}e$ as well as $\dot{V}O_{2peak}$ of the sedentary compared to the SCI patients.

Even if the VE_{peak} value between the two groups were the same, this does not necessarily mean that the ventilation efficiency between the two groups is the same.

O_2pulse_{peak} was significantly higher in the sedentary than in the SCI patients. The low O_2pulse_{peak} observed in the SCI patients is due to low cardiac output, insufficient blood flow to the working muscles, and low a-vO_2 difference resulting from weakness of the sympathetic nerve impulse [13].

However, Van Loan et al. [14] reported that there is no significant difference in a-vO_2 difference during maximal exercise between the SCI and sedentary patients.

Coutts et al. [12] reported that the greater the O_2 pulse, the greater the stroke volume and venous return. Sympathetic nerve impairment can be a major factor limiting cardiopulmonary functions in SCI patients. Generally, the SCI has reduced vasoconstriction below the lesion level and reduced venous return which directly limits stroke volume.

References

1. Shephard RJ (1990) Fitness in special populations. Human Kinetics Books, Champaign
2. Zwiren L, Bar-Or O (1975) Responses to exercise of paraplegics who differ in conditioning level. Med Sci Sports Exer 7:94–98
3. Glaser RM, Foley DM, Laubach LL, et al. (1978–79) An exercise test to evaluate Fitness for wheelchair activity. Paraplegia 16:341–349
4. Engel P, Hildebrant G (1973) Long term spiro-ergonometric studies of paraplegic during the clinical period of rehabilitation. Paraplegia 11:105–110
5. Glaser RM, Sawka MN, et al. (1981) Energy cost and cardiopulmonary responses for wheelchair locomotion and walking on tile and on carpet. Paraplegia 19:220–226
6. Coutts KD (1990) Peak oxygen uptake of elite wheelchair athletes. APA Quart 7:62–66
7. Glaser RM, Davis GM (1989) The wheelchair dependent individual. Exercise in Modern Medicine, pp 237–267
8. Wells CL (1990) The spinal injured athlete. APA Quart 7:265–285
9. Pollock ML, Miller HS, Linnerud AC, Laughridge E, Coleman E, Alexander E (1974) Arm pedalling as an endurance training regimen for the disabled. Arch Phys Med Rehab 55:418–424
10. Hildebrandt G, Voight E, Bahn D, et al. (1970) Energy costs of propelling a wheelchair at various speeds: Cardiac responses and effect on steering accuracy. Arch Phys Med Rehab 51:131–136
11. Pimental, Nancy A, Michael N, Sawka, et al. (1984) Physiological responses to prolonged upper-body exercise. Med Sci Sports Exer 16:360–365
12. Coutts KD, Rhodes EC, McKenzie DC (1983) Maximal exercise responses of tetraplegics and paraplegics. J Appl Physiol 55(2):479–482

13. Hoffman MD (1986) Cardiorespiratory fitness and training in quadriplegics and paraplegics. Sports Med 3:312–330
14. Van Loan M, McCluer S, Loftin JM, et al. (1987) Comparison of physiological responses to maximal arm exercise among able-bodied, paraplegics and quadriplegics. Paraplegia 25:397–405

Circulatory Response During Isokinetic Training on Upper Extremity in Coronary Heart Disease Patients

Kazuo Tsuyuki, Masahiko Aihara, Kenji Ninomiya, Tamae Ogata, Yasuo Kimura, Kwangchol Chang, Hiroki Hase, and Kunio Ebine

Abstract. The purpose of this study was to investigate the circulatory response during muscular training in coronary heart disease patients. Thirty-five male patients with effort angina pectoris and a history of myocardial infarction were studied. All patients performed a cardiopulmonary exercise test (SL-GXT) and isokinetic training at elbow flexion. The pressure rate product (PRP) during training approached the PRP level at the endpoint on SL-GXT as myocardial aerobic impairment increased. Additionally, ST changes appeared when PRP during the training equalled or exceeded the PRP endpoint on SL-GXT. In conclusion, patients showing low exercise tolerance and poor cardiac function must be carefully monitored during isokinetic training.

Introduction

In the past, aerobic training has been used in cardiac rehabilitation due to improved exercise tolerance and reduced coronary risk factors. However, this type of training involved not only aerobic effort but also muscular strength. The increase in myocardial load due to effort requiring muscular strength might cause a cardiac accident. This accident is more easily caused in patients having less muscular strength. Recently, muscular training has been assigned to cardiac patients as a precaution against cardiac accidents [1]. The purpose of this study was to investigate the circulatory response during muscular training in coronary heart disease patients.

Patients and Methods

Patients

Thirty-five male patients with effort angina pectoris and a history of myocardial infarction (MI) were studied. Informed consent was obtained from each patient. Their ages were 58.9 ± 6 years (mean ± SD; range, 48–69 years). All patients were clincally stable and free of heart failure on clinical examination.

Of these 17 patients had been taking antihypertensive drugs. Thirteen had been taking antiarrhythmics, 7 had been taking digoxin, and all had been taking vasodilators, but none were taking β-blockers. These patients had no previous history of musculoskeletal dysfunction or other conditions that would contraindicate isokinetic training.

Cardiopulmonary Exercise Test

Symptom limited graded exercise test (SL-GXT) was performed using the modified Bruce protocol. Oxygen uptake, blood pressure, and heart rate (calculated from ECGs) were measured continuously during the exercise. Test endpoints included the presence of angina, ST segment depression or elevation (±0.1 mV or more), abnormality in blood pressure, or serious arrhythmia. Functional aerobic impairment (FAI) and myocardial aerobic impairment (MAI) were calculated using Bruce's formula [2].

Isokinetic Training Model

The isokinetic exercise at right elbow flexion was performed using the CBX 350 isokinetic exercise machine (Lumex, New York, N.Y.) under recording ECGs and measuring blood pressure. All patients performed three sets of 60% peak torque elbow flexions, and each set was repeated ten times with a 2-min rest period between each set (Fig. 1). The elbow flexed from 0 to 90 degrees (0 degree = fully extended elbow). The angular velocity was set at 30 deg/sec. Elbow joint flexion started at end expiration with a verbal signal, and was performed during air breathing.

Statistical Methods

Statistical significance was established at the 0.05 probability level. The data were presented as mean ± SD and analyzed using an unpaired student's *t*-test and the chi-squared test.

Results

Cardiopulmonary Exercise Test

A total of 35 patients were examined by exercise ECG. Of these, 31 (88.6%) were shown to have ST changes, and 8 (22.9%) were shown to have premature ventricular contraction (PVC). The peak oxygen uptake (peak $\dot{V}O_2$) was 24.7 ± 5.1 ml/kg per min; the FAI was 15.6 ± 18.6%; and the MAI was 27.5 ± 21.3% in SL-GXT.

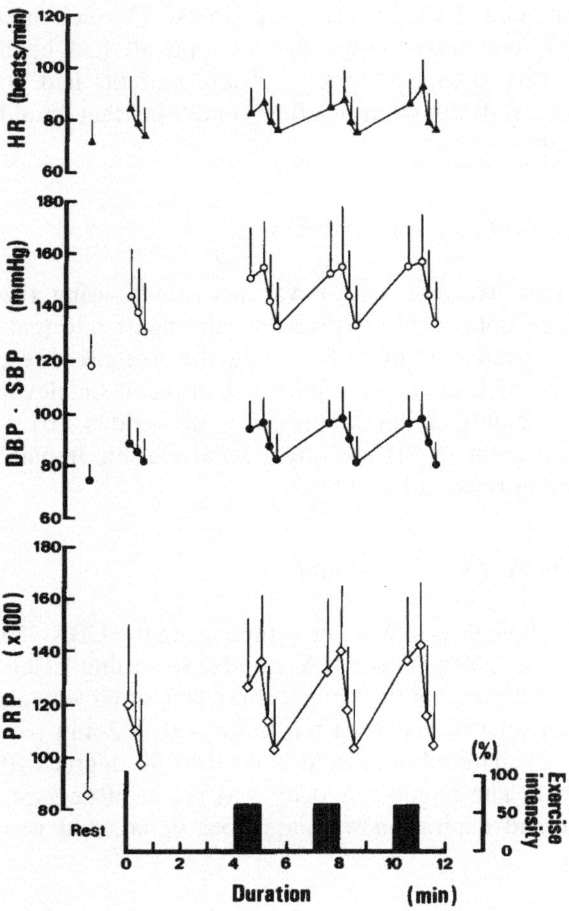

FIG. 1. Circulatory response during isokinetic training. *HR*, heart rate; *SBP*, systolic blood pressure; *DBP*, diastolic blood pressure; *PRP*, pressure rate product

Circulatory Response During Isokinetic Training

The increases in systolic blood pressure (SBP) and in diastolic blood pressure (DBP) were proportionally higher than the increase in heart rate (Table 1). The peak SBP during isokinetic training in the hypertensive group (n = 17) was compared with the normotensive group (n = 18). There was no significant difference between the two groups. The same result was obtained in peak DBP during isokinetic training. There was a significant correlation between SBP at rest and peak SBP during training. The same result was obtained for DBP.

ECG Findings During Isokinetic Training and MAI

Two patients (5.7%) exhibited ST changes during isokinetic training. This appearance rate was significantly lower than GXT, and 8 patients (22.9%) had

TABLE 1. Comparison of rate of change in each parameter.

Parameter	Rest	Peak	Rate of change (%)
HR (beats/min)	72.3 ± 9.6	92.0 ± 10.9	28.1 ± 12.5
SBP (mmHg)	117.4 ± 11.9	164.9 ± 19.4	40.5 ± 12.2
DBP (mmHg)	75.1 ± 6.4	100.5 ± 11.4	34.0 ± 13.7
PRP (×100)	84.8 ± 16.2	151.0 ± 27.9	78.4 ± 24.6

HR, heart rate; SBP, systolic blood pressure; DBP, diastolic blood pressure; PRP, pressure rate product.

PVCs during isokinetic training. This appearance rate was equivalent to GXT. PRP during training approached the PRP level at the endpoint on GXT as MAI increased. Additionally, ST changes appeared when PRP during training equalled or exceeded the PRP endpoint on GXT. However, the appearance of PVC was unrelated to the value of MAI or the level of PRP during training (Fig. 2).

Discussion

Elbow flexion occurs frequently in daily life and was chosen for muscular training. Isokinetic training is ideal muscular training. Ordinarily, maximal

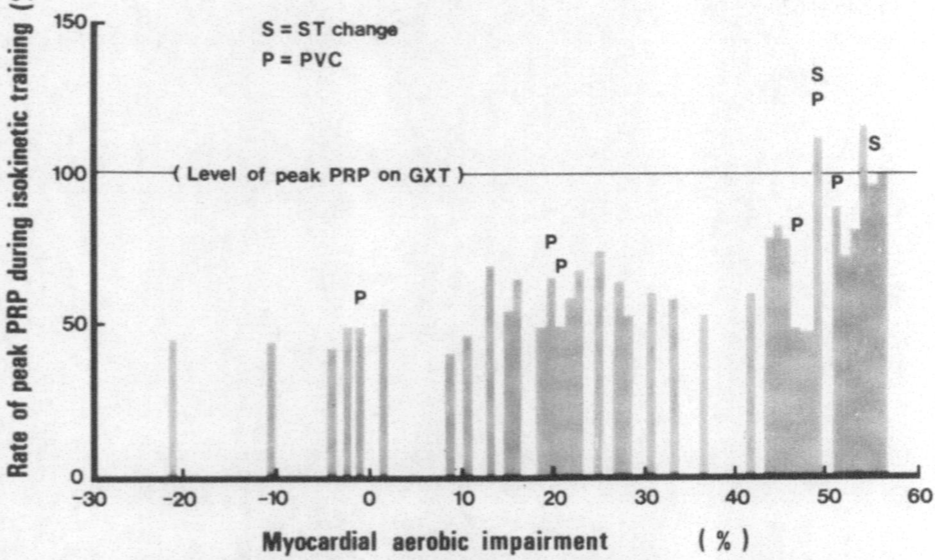

FIG. 2. Relationship between pressure rate product (*PRP*) during isokinetic training, myocardial aerobic impairment, and ECG findings. *PRP*, pressure rate product; *GXT*, graded exercise test

voluntary contraction (MVC) is performed in isokinetic training. However, because of the danger of cardiac accident, a training model with an exercise intensity of 60% MVC was designed.

The results of the training model indicate that the rate at which SBP and DBP increased was greater than the rate of increase of heart rate. These results suggest that the rise in SBP and DBP should be carefully monitored during isokinetic training. There was a significant correlation between SBP at rest and the peak SBP during training, regardless of whether the patient had hypertension. The importance of blood pressure control at rest was confirmed. Two patients had ST changes during isokinetic training. Their ST change appeared in the case that the PRP during the training equalled or exceeded the PRP endpoint level on GXT. The appearance of ST changes appear to result from ischemia due to the rise in myocardial load mainly caused by rise in SBP and DBP. MAI was high in these two patients.

In conclusion, the patients with lower exercise tolerance and poor cardiac function must be carefully monitored during isokinetic training to avoid cardiac accidents.

References

1. Franklin BA, Bonzheim K, Gordon S, Timmis GC (1991) Resistance training in cardiac rehabilitation. J Cardiopulmon Rehab 11:99–107
2. Bruce RA, Kusumi F, Hosmer D (1973) Maximal oxygen intake and normographic assessment of functional aerobic impairment in cardiovascular disease. Am Heart J 85:546–562

Different Forms of Body Activity as Therapeutical Concepts in Osteopenia

M. HARTARD, P. HABER, D. ILIEVA, E. PREISINGER, M. QUITTAN, G. SEIDL, J. HUBER, R. FILADORO, and D. JESCHKE

Abstract. The effects of two different forms of body activity on bone density of the lumbar vertebrae (L2–4) and the left hip (neck) were observed in a group of 39 women (age 50 and over) with osteopenia. For 20 weeks over a six-month period, 16 women engaged in systematic weight training (T), 8 followed a program of therapeutic gymnastics (G), and 15 served as controls (C). Bone density was measured using DEXA before and after the observation period. In groups G and C, the extent of bone density loss was approximately the same. A significant bone density loss did not occur in group T. Therefore, in this study, systematic weight training was the only form of therapy that was able to maintain bone mass density of the lumbar vertebrae and hip in women with osteopenia.

Introduction

Current knowledge about the effects of different forms of training and of body activity on bone density leads us to believe that certain training concepts are able to counteract further bone destruction in cases of bone density loss [1–8]. Research reviews on this subject raise doubts about the methodical principles used in many studies [3, 5, 9]. Up to now, it has been difficult to define therapeutic movement measures in relation to adequate individual dosages, as is the case with all medical therapy concepts. The purpose of this study was to investigate the effects of sytematic muscle training on bone mass density in comparison with a therapeutic gymnastics program. A high value was given to training prescribed according to precise qualitative and quantitative rules.

Patients and Methods

Patients

Thirty-nine women (64.5 ± 6.9 years of age) were included in the study. All of the patients included in this study demonstrated a bone tissue loss of over 30%, shown before the beginning of training by means of X-rays of the hip and of the lumbar vertebral column (a-p, and lateral projection). Abnormalities that affect bone metabolism such as fractures of the femoral neck or of a vertebral body, or pronounced hyperostosis leading to secondary osteoporosis were considered exclusion criteria.

The 39 participants were divided into three groups: 16 (63.6 ± 6.2 years of age) carried out 20 weeks of systematic weight training (T group), 8 women (66.2 ± 7.8 years of age) a therapeutic gymnastics program (G group), and 15 women (67.4 ± 9.7 years of age) served as controls (C group).

Training Organization

The T group carried out a 20-week course of systematic training of muscle strength within a 6-month period, while the G group performed a therapeutic gymnastics program over the same time period. The 20-week training units for the small groups were equally distributed over a period of 1 year. Therefore, seasonal fluctuations of bone density were considered to be negligible.

Training Methods

The T group trained the muscle groups of 11 clearly defined joint movements: extension, flexion, abduction, and adduction by means of a traction apparatus in the area of the shoulder and hip joint; knee and hip extension by means of a leg press, and ante- and retroflection of the vertebral column by means of an adjustable individual training bench (abdomen and back muscles).

Each training unit (2 per week) began with a warm-up program and ended with stretching exercises of the trained muscle groups. Each training unit lasted approximately 45 min. The training load was dosed according to the rules of medical training theory, in an optimal individual relation to the actual functional capacity. This was possible with a quantitative and qualitative exact definition of the training load. The intensity of the training load was fixed at 70% of the actual maximum muscle strength. Before the beginning of training, maximal strength of each muscle group was determined in the form of the One-Maximum-Repetition (OMR: load at which an exercise can just barely be repeated once). The duration of the training load was defined as the sum of repetitions carried out without a pause. An optimal efficacy was reached when 8–12 repetitions led to an extensive fatigue of the tested muscle group. This unit corresponds to a set. If, during training, an exercise with the initial defined load could be repeated more than 14 times, the load was increased. The pause interval between training of two sets of the same muscle group was at least 2 min. The frequency of the training load amounted to 2 units per week. The total weekly training load (TWTL), the total sum of the effective sets per week and per muscle group, was gradually increased from two in the beginning (individually adapted) to a maximum of four. This system is known as Continuously Adapted Strength Training (CAST).

In the G group, the frequency of the training load amounted to three units per week. The therapeutic gymnastics included exercises for the trunk as well as for the extremities. The aim was to balance the muscle forces for the whole body and to avoid overloading the ligaments and joints. Three exercise programs were offered and each program had to be carried out at least once a week: The first program included 12 exercises for muscle tension and stretching for the trunk and the extremities carried out in supine position, sitting upright on the floor, and kneeling on all fours. Every exercise lasted about 1–3 min. The second program included 12 exercises with the big "Pezzi" ball (an air-filled rubber ball, diameter: 50–70 cm). The women trained with the ball in a sitting position (dipping upright on the ball) or in a supine position, the ball being used as training instrument for the upper or lower extremities and for the trunk. Each exercise lasted about 3–5 min. The third program included 6 exercises (mainly for the upper extremities) with an elastic band. The exercises were carried out in a sitting position (on a chair) or standing, with the elastic band fixed under the feet or at the wall. Again, each exercise lasted about 1–3 min.

Bone Density Measurement

Bone density was measured by means of an instrument of the type Norland XR-26, at the beginning and end of training. The measurement was carried out in conformity with the DEXA technique. With the evaluation software (automatic profile finding program) two particularly interesting regions were defined and the densities estimated: in the region of the vertebral column, the lumbar bone density (LBD L2–L4); and in the region of the left hip, the femoral neck bone density (FNBD). The results were indicated as BMD (bone mineral density) in grams Ca/cm^2.

Statistics

Statistical analysis was carried out on a PC (Macintosh plus) with the software Stat View 512 plus: Student's *t*-test for paired and unpaired sample tests. $P < 0.05$ was chosen as the level of significance. The initial and final measurements were taken at an interval of 6 months.

Results

The results (Table 1) are given as mean values (x) with standard deviation (sd) of bone mineral density ($g\,Ca/cm^2$) in the areas of control (L2-4 and left hip). The measurements before (1) and after (2) the observation time showed constant BMD levels in the training group (T) and a comparable BMD loss in the gymnastic (G) and control group (C).

TABLE 1. BMD measurements (g Ca/cm^2).

Section	Group	1		2		2–1
		x	sd	x	sd	
L2-4	T	0.871	0.201	0.874	0.204	+0.003
	G	0.869	0.176	0.829	0.183	−0.040
	C	0.876	0.141	0.822	0.125	−0.054
Left hip	T	0.747	0.129	0.742	0.140	−0.005
	G	0.742	0.103*	0.690	0.113	−0.052
	C	0.732	0.092*	0.670	0.080	−0.062

* $P < 0.05$.

Conclusion

Numerous cross-section and intervention studies support the hypothesis that bone mineral density is able to increase with body activity [6–8, 10–13]. The importance of mechanical stress factors on bone reorganization becomes evident when comparing bone mass density development in the absence of gravity and under high performance sports training [2, 14–17]. The localization of mechanical stress and the intensity of the load stimulus seem to have a key function in the process of new bone formation [10, 12, 13, 15]. Special importance has to be given to the degree of load intensity and less to a very high number of repetitions of a single load [18]. Cross-section studies with corresponding formulations confirm these results [2, 17–22]. Lanyon and Rubin [23, 24] described that bone formation was dependent on the cycles of mechanical stimulus, the observation of which shows a positive correlation between intensity and frequency of stimuli per day, the number of days and the bone formation. Frost [19] and Carter [21] postulated that bone metabolism is dependent on the degree (intensity), the duration (number of load stimuli), and the volume of the load (number of load cycles over time). In this regard, the results of the studies of Margulies et al. [25] and Sinaki et al. [26] are of interest. The existence of a threshold dose is impressively confirmed by the results of the investigation of Sinaki et al. [26]. They tested the influence of a "nonloading" training (home training of the back extending muscles with an intensity of 30% of maximum strength which included one set with 10 repetitions per day, 5 days a week) to prevent a bone density loss. Dual photon absorptiometry (DPA) measurements of L2–L4 were done every 6 months) on 65 postmenopausal women in a 2-year controlled study. Increased muscle strength in the training group was evident, but both groups showed comparable significant bone density loss. The authors concluded that "modest, nonloading exercise" programs do not effectively counteract bone density loss.

In our study, the effects of two different forms of body activity on bone mass density of the lumbar vertebrae and hip in a group of women with osteopenia were observed and compared with controls. The systematic training of muscular strength alone was enough to maintain bone mineral density of lumbar vertebrae and hip in women with osteopenia. The muscle groups of all important joint movements (especially in the region of the hip joint) were included in the systematic training. A significant bone density loss in this area of control did not occur in the T group as it did in the G and C groups. In the G and C groups, a nearly comparable bone density loss could be observed.

Therefore, the methodical conditions described are optimally fulfilled by (maximum muscle strength) training according to the method of the Continuously Adapted Strength Training (CAST). A highly significant increase of muscle power was achieved as a further desirable side effect. While the purpose of increasing bone density is to avoid bone fractures when falling, increased muscle strength in old people helps prevent falling in the first place. The presented muscle training model can be adopted in any well-equipped fitness center without fundamental changes, although specialized qualified supervision is recommended.

References

1. Chirschilles EA, Butler CD, Davis CS, Wallace RB (1991) A model of lifetime osteoporosis impact. Arch Intern Med 151:2026–2032
2. Le Blanc A, Schneider V (1991) Can the adult skeleton recover lost bone? Ext Gerontol 26:189–201
3. Dalsky GP (1989) The role of exercise in the prevention of osteoporosis. Comprehensive Therapy 15(9):30–37
4. Prince RL, Smith M, Dick IM, Price RI, Webb PG, Henderson NK, Harris MM (1991) Prevention of postmenopausal osteoporosis—a comparative study of exercise, calcium supplementation, and hormone replacement therapy. N Engl J Med 325:1189–1195
5. Aloia JF, Vaswania N, Yeh JK, Cohn St. H (1988) Premenopausal bone mass is related to physical activity. Arch Intern Med 148:121–123
6. Beverly MC, Rider TA, Evans MJ, Smith R (1989) Local bone mineral response to brief exercise that stresses the skeleton. BMJ 299:233–235
7. Gleeson PB, Protas EJ, LeBlanc AD, Schneider VS, Evans HJ (1990) The effects of weight lifting on bone mineral density in premenopausal women. J Bone Miner Res 5(2):153–158
8. Dilsen G, Berker C, Oral A, Varan G (1989) The role of physical exercise in prevention and managment of osteoporosis. Clin Rheum 8(2):70–75
9. Block JE, Smith R, Friedlander A, Genant HK (1989) Preventing osteoporosis with exercise: A review with emphasis on methodology. Med Hypotheses 30:9–19
10. Chow R, Harrison JE, Notarius C (1987) Effect of two randomised exercise programmes on bone mass of healthy postmenopausal women. BMJ 295:1441–1444
11. Dalsky GP, Stocke KS, Ehsani AA, Slatopolsky E, Lee WC, Birge St. J (1988) Weight-bearing exercise training and lumbar bone mineral content in postmenopausal women. Ann Intern Med 108(6):824–828
12. Krolner B, Toft B, Nielsen SP, Tondevold E (1983) Physical exercise as prophylaxis against involutional vertebral bone loss: A controlled trial. Clin Sci 64:541–46
13. Simkins A, Ayalon J, Leichter I (1987) Increased trabecular bone density due to bone-loading exercise in postmenopausal osteoporotic women. Calcif Tissue Int 40:56–63

14. Schultheis L (1991) The mechanical control system of bone in weightless spaceflight and in aging. Exp Gerontol 26:203–214
15. Colletti LA, Edwards J, Gordon L, Shary J, Bell NH (1989) The effects of muscle-building exercise on bone mineral density of the radius, spine, and hip in young men. Calcif Tissue Int 45:12–14
16. Schoutens A, Laurent E, Poortmans JR (1989) Effects of inactivity and exercise on bone. Sports Med 7:71–81
17. Suominen H (1988) Physical activity and bone. Ann Chir Gyn 77:184–188
18. Wahlen RT, Cater DR, Steel CR (1987) The relationship between physical activity and bone density. Trans Orthop Res Soc 12:464–467
19. Frost HM (1989) Transient-steady state phenomena in microdamage physiology: A proposed algorithm for lamellar bone. Calcif Tissue Int 44:367–381
20. Viceconti M, Seireg A (1990) A generalized procedure for predicting bone mass regulation by mechanical strain. Calcif Tissue Int 47:396–301
21. Carter CR (1987) Mechanical loading history and skeletal biology. J Biomech 20(11,12):1095–1109
22. Shangold MM (1990) Exercise in menopausal women. Obstet Gynecol 75[Suppl IV]:53–58
23. Lanyon LE, Rubin CT (1984) Static vs dynamic loads as an influence on bone remodelling. J Biomech 12(17):897–905
24. Lanyon LE (1987) Functional strain in bone tissue as an objective, and controlling stimulus for adaptive bone remodeling. J Biomech 20(11/12):1083–1093
25. Margulies JY, Simkin A, Leichter I, Bivas A, Steinberg R, Giladi M, Stein M, Kashtan H, Milgrom C (1986) Effect of intense physical activity on the bone mineral content in the lower limbs of young adults. J Bone Joint Surgi 68A(7): 1090–1093
26. Sinaki M, Wahner HW, Offord KP, Hodgson St. F (1989) Efficacy of nonloading exercise in prevention of vertebral bone loss in postmenopausal women: A controlled trial. Mayo Clin Proc 64:762–769

A Computed Tomography Study of Skeletal Muscle in the Thigh in Hemiplegics

Tomomitsu Kotake, Mikoto Baba, Nobuyuki Dohi,
Toshio Kajiwara, Yoshiki Koyama, and Yoshimasa Setoguchi

Abstract. Transverse CT scans were used to calculate the ratios of each muscle group in the thighs of healthy subjects and patients with hemiplegia due to cerebrovascular diseases. No significant differences were observed between the affected and unaffected sides in the gracilis muscle, but significantly lower ratios were observed among the other muscle groups of the affected side.

Introduction

It is possible, using computed tomography (CT), to perform quantitative transverse analyses of various muscle areas. In this study, scans were taken of the quadriceps femoris, femoral flexor muscle group, femoral adductor muscle group, sartorius, and gracilis at the middle of the thigh in healthy controls as well as in subjects with hemiplegia due to cerebrovascular disease.

Subjects

One sample each was taken from a group of 14 healthy volunteers, which included nine men and five women (group 1). Subjects ranged in age from 22 to 34 years of age, with a mean of 30.4. All subjects were hospital employees, and none of them were unusually active in sports or other kinds of vigorous physical activities.

In group 2, 34 CT scans were taken from 13 men and 4 women subjects in their 50's, 60's, and 70's (mean age was 62.4 years) with hemiplegia due to cerebrovascular disease. One sample each was taken from both the affected and unaffected sides. Subjects for this group were chosen among hemiplegia patients whose cranial CT scans revealed only one supratentorial lesion. Further, no neurological or other irregularities were observed in the unaffected sides. Brunnstrom stages for the lower extremity of each subject were as follows: stage II, ten subjects; stage III, four subjects; and stage IV, three subjects. Five subjects were unable to walk, seven subjects required assistance while walking, and five subjects could walk unassisted.

Methods

In groups 1 and 2, CT was performed in the area encompassing the central thigh region, halfway between the knee joint space to the greater trochanter of the femur.

The CT used was a Hitachi CT-W 1000GR (Hitachi Medical Corporation, Tokyo, Japan). Images were taken at 5-mm width with a 200 mA, 120 kVp X-ray; scanning times were 2.9 s. A tracer was employed for outlining the target muscle group during scanning. The image was then measured by computer and

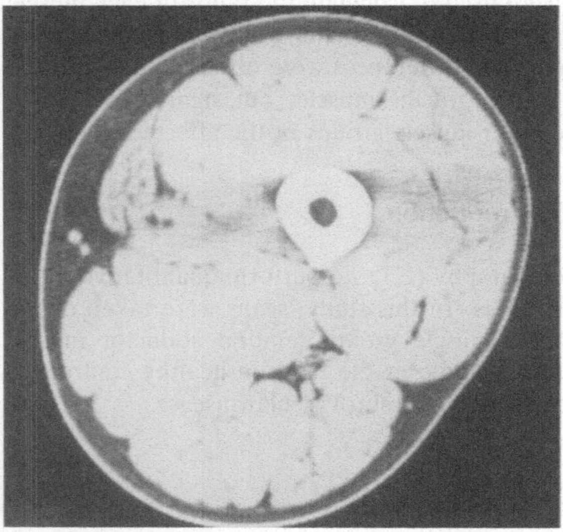

1

FIG. 1. A typical computed tomography (CT) image of the central region of the thigh taken from a group of healthy subjects

FIG. 2. A sample CT image of the central region of the thigh taken from a group of subjects with hemiplegia. *Right*, affected side; *left*, unaffected side

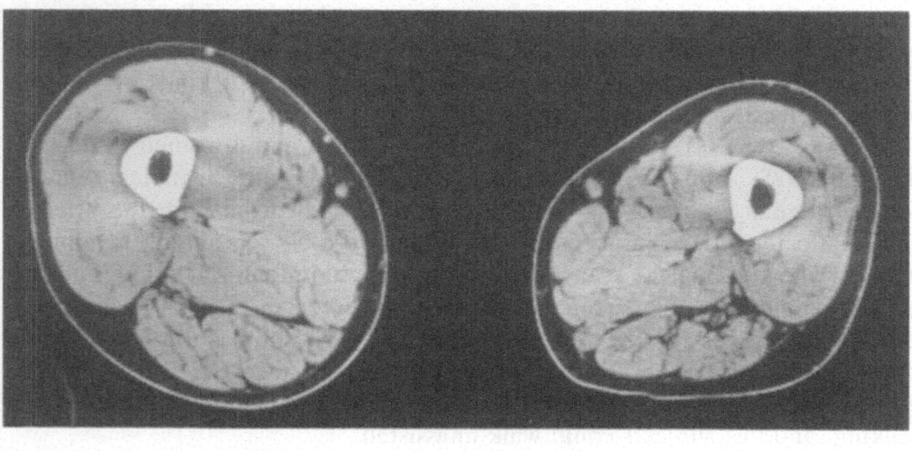

2

the area of each muscle group determined. The following muscle groups were measured in both groups: quadriceps femoris, femoral adductor muscle group, femoral flexor muscle group, and the sartorius and the gracilis muscles (Figs. 1, 2). In group 1, one scan of the targeted regions was made in each of 14 subjects, and the mean ratios for each muscle group area were then determined. In group 2, a total of 34 scans were taken of the affected and unaffected areas in 17 subjects with hemiplegia, and mean ratios for each muscle group area were determined. Comparisons between the affected and unaffected areas were made.

Results

Group 1

The mean ratios for each muscle group area are shown in Table 1; the area of the gracilis was given a value of 1.

Group 2

The mean ratios for each muscle group area are shown in Table 2; the area of the gracilis of the unaffected side has been given a value of 1.

TABLE 1. The mean ratios of the transverse section of each muscle group of the thigh region in healthy subjects. A value of 1 has been assigned to the transverse section of the gracilis.

Muscles	Transverse section ratio
Quadriceps femoris	16.6
Femoral adductor muscle	7.8
Femoral flexor muscle	6.5
Sartorius	0.9
Gracilis	1.0

TABLE 2. Comparison of affected and unaffected sides in the hemiplegic group. A value of 1 has been assigned to the area of the gracilis of the unaffected side.

Muscles	Affected side	Unaffected side	Studient's t-test
Quadriceps femoris	10.6	14.2	*
Femoral adductor muscle	6.7	8.3	*
Femoral flexor muscle	4.5	5.5	*
Sartorius	0.7	1.0	*
Gracilis	1.0	1.0	NS

NS, not significant.
* $P < 0.001$.

Discussion

Qualitative and quantitative variations in skeletal muscle differ according to individuals, but the results of our group 1 study revealed that mean ratios for each muscle group area could be approximated. In group 2, study results showed significant muscle atrophy in the quadriceps femoris, femoral adductor muscles, femoral flexor muscles, and the sartorius in the affected side of subjects with hemiplegia. There are various explanations, however, to account for muscle atrophy on the unaffected side [1, 2], and recent studies have shown this phenomenon to be most closely associated with disuse [3].

Only in the gracilis was no significant difference in the level of muscular atrophy observed between the affected and unaffected sides of group 2 subjects. Similar reports have been cited from studies of other cerebrovascular diseases. According to a study of patients with Duchenne's muscular dystrophy (DMD), for example, a slower progression of damage in the gracilis compared with the other muscle groups of the thigh was reported [4–6].

It is apparent, then, that a significantly lower proportion of atrophy of the gracilis is not unique to hemiplegia. These lower proportions can be easily explained if it can be shown that the gracilis is less susceptible to atrophy as a result of disuse in comparison to other muscles. Further research is indicated, however, to clarify this phenomenon.

Conclusion

Transverse CT scans were used to calculate the ratios of each muscle group in the thighs of healthy subjects (group 1). Ratios were then calculated for the same muscle groups in patients with hemiplegia due to cerebrovascular diseases (group 2). Comparisons were also made among group 2 subjects of affected and unaffected sides. No significant difference was observed between the affected and unaffected sides in the gracilis muscle, but significantly lower ratios were observed among the other muscle groups of the affected side.

References

1. Slager UT, et al. (1985) Histochemical and morphometric changes in muscles of stroke patients. Clin Orthop 119:159–168
2. Edström L (1970) Selective changes in the sizes of red and white muscle fibers in upper motor lesions and parkinsonism. J Neurol Sci 11:537–550
3. Okawa Y, et al. (1988) Disuse muscle atrophy in hemiplegic patients: muscle weakness in the unaffected extremities (in Japanese). Rehabiriteshon Igaku (Jpn J Rehab Med) 25:143–147
4. Hawley RJ Jr, et al. (1984) Computed tomographic patterns of muscles in neuromuscular diseases. Arch Neurol 41:383–387
5. Stern LM, et al. (1984) Progression of muscular dystrophy assessed by computed tomography. Dev Med Child Neurol 26:569–573
6. Liu M (1989) The progression of muscle damage in Duchenne's muscular dystrophy (in Japanese). Rehabiriteshon Igaku (Jpn J Rehab Med) 26:159–171

—Part III—

Motor Control

—Keynote Speech—

Normal and Abnormal Development of Posture Control in Children

MARJORIE H. WOOLLACOTT

Abstract. The development of balance control in children is approached from a systems perspective in which balance is seen as an emergent skill, with critical neural or musculoskeletal components identified as rate-limiting and thus pushing the system to a new control level when these components mature. The emergence of postural control is characterized by the development of rules which relate sensory inputs reporting the body's position in space to motor actions which control the body's position. Adaptive capabilities, which allow the child to modify sensory and motor strategies to changing task and environmental conditions, appear to develop later. Children with developmental delays and dysfunctions, such as Down syndrome and cerebral palsy, show delayed development of postural responses and additional problems associated with muscle response timing, organization (including onset latency delays), and sensory organization capabilities. Each disorder shows a specific constellation of motor problems.

Introduction

During the early years of life, the child develops an incredible repertoire of skills including crawling, independent walking and running, climbing, eye-hand coordination, and the manipulation of objects in a variety of ways. The emergence of all of these skills requires the development of postural activity which supports the primary movement. How does postural control emerge during development, and how is it integrated into skills such as walking and reaching? The purpose of this paper is to discuss the development of postural control underlying the emergence of stability and mobility skills.

Child Development Theory

There are several theories of child development regarding the relation of nervous system development and the emergence of different behaviors in infants. Classical theories of child development suggest that the emergence of posture and movement control depends on the appearance and subsequent integration of reflexes. The appearance and disappearance of these reflexes reflect the increasing maturity of cortical structures which inhibit and integrate reflexes controlled at lower levels within the CNS into more functional postural and voluntary motor responses. This classical theory has been referred to as a reflex/hierarchy theory.

More recent theories of motor control, such as the systems theory, have suggested that posture control emerges from a complex interaction during development of the musculoskeletal and neural systems. The systems which have been considered important for the emergence of postural control include (1) changes in the musculoskeletal system including the development of muscle strength and changes in relative mass of the different body segments; (2) development of neuromuscular response synergies used in maintaining balance; (3) the development of individual sensory systems including somatosensory, visual, or vestibular systems; and (4) development of adaptive and anticipatory mechanisms which allow the child to modify the way they sense and move for postural control [1].

Consistent with Gesell's developmental principles, postural development appears to be characterized by a cephalocaudal progression of control, beginning with head, then trunk, and finally the entire body. Prechtl [2] has noted that infants have very poor postural or antigravity control at birth. He has hypothesized that this could be due either to lack of muscle tone or lack of maturity of the motor processes controlling posture of the head at this age. To determine which of these possibilities was the cause of their poor head control, he attempted to determine if neonates and young infants would show any antigravity responses to a tilting surface. Infants up to 8–10 weeks old did not respond either to head downwards or upwards tilts. However, at 8–10 weeks, with the onset of spontaneous head control, the infants showed distinctive EMG patterns in response to the tilting surface. Thus Prechtl's research suggests that the emergence of coordinated postural responses in the neck muscles occurs at about 2 months of age.

As infants begin to sit independently, and thus develop trunk control, they must learn to coordinate sensory-motor information relating two body segments together in the control of posture. To do this, they need to extend the rules they learned for sensory-motor relationships for head postural control to the new set of muscles controlling the trunk. It is possible that once these rules have been established for the neck muscles, they could be readily extended to control of the trunk muscles.

How do the muscles which coordinate sway responses develop in the neck and trunk? In our lab, both cross-sectional and longitudinal studies have been used to explore the gradual development of muscle coordination underlying neck and trunk control in infants 2 months to 8 months of age [3].

EMG's are used to record muscles in the neck and trunk in infants seated in an infant seat on a moveable platform, shown in Fig. 1. Motion of the platform

FIG. 1. Moveable platform used to record EMGs

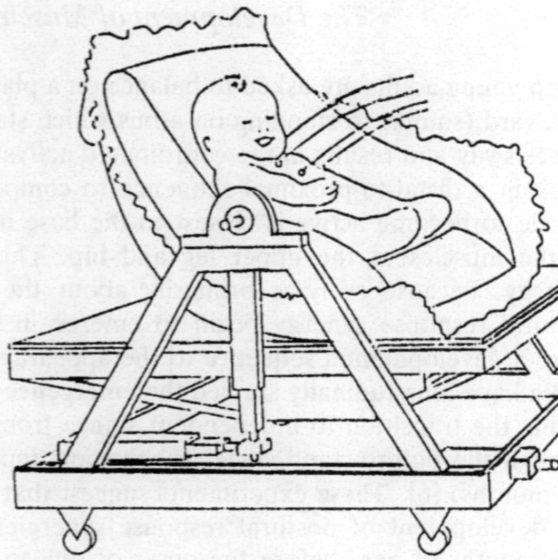

forward or backward caused a disturbance of the infant's head and trunk posture requiring a subsequent compensatory adjustment to regain balance.

Results from these studies suggest that 2-month-olds did not show consistent, directionally appropriate responses to the platform perturbations. By 3 to 4 months, infants showed directionally specific responses in the neck muscles 40% to 60% of the time. By 5 months, as infants were beginning to sit independently, activity in the trunk muscles occurred 40% of the time and by 8 months of age, muscles in the neck and trunk were well-coordinated. Taking away visual stimuli did not cause a disruption in muscle response organization in any of the infants studied. Thus somatosensory and vestibular systems are capable of activating postural actions as early as 3 to 4 months.

The Role of Strength

Researchers have suggested that a rate-limiting factor for the emergence of independent walking may be the development of sufficient muscle strength to hold the child's own weight. In a recent study [4] muscle strength of developing infants (2–8 months of age) was evaluated by measuring the changing forces they use to bounce on a force plate. It was noted that, by 6 months of age, children are producing forces well beyond their own body weight. What other factors could play a rate-limiting role in stance postural control?

The Development of Muscle Synergies

When young adults are asked to balance on a platform which moves forward or backward (similar to standing on a bus which starts to move) platform motion causes sway and results in the coordinated activation of muscles in the legs and trunk in a distal-to-proximal sequence to compensate for the sway. The first muscle to become active is closest to the base of support (at 90 ms), followed by the muscles of the upper leg and hip. This strategy is called the ankle strategy, because sway is primarily about the ankle joint. How does this postural response synergy begin to emerge in the newly standing infant? Is there a developmental sequence to the appearance of this synergy?

We have longitudinally studied the emergence of postural response synergies during the transition to independent stance from 2 months of age (pre-sitting) through the pull-to-stand stage of behavior, independent stance, and walking (18 months) [6]. These experiments suggest that a sequential process occurs in the development of postural response synergies. Infants who were tested at 2–6 months of age, before the onset of pull-to-stand behavior, did not show coordinated muscle response organization in response to threats to their balance. During early pull-to-stand behavior (7 to 9 months) the infants began to show directionally appropriate responses in their ankle muscles. Over the next weeks of pull-to-stand behavior, muscles in the thigh segment were added and a consistent distal-to-proximal sequence began to emerge. Finally, by the late pull-to-stand stage, (9 to 11 months) the trunk muscles were consistently added to the synergy. Thus, by late pull-to-stand behavior, the infants begin to organize the muscles within the leg into appropriate synergies, with the ankle muscles being consistently activated first, followed by the upper leg and hip muscles.

Refinement of stance balance control in children 15 months to 10 years of age has been studied by several researchers [7, 8]. Children from 15 months to 3 years of age produced well-organized muscle responses to postural perturbations while standing. However, the amplitudes of these responses were consistently greater, and the latencies and durations of these responses longer, than those of adults.

There was also an unusual change in the muscle response characteristics of 4- to 6-year-old children. They apparently "regressed" in their postural response organization. In this age group, postural responses were more variable and longer in latency than those found in any other age group. In addition, activation of the proximal leg muscle synergists in the 4- to 6-year-olds was significantly delayed. These longer delays caused more movement at the knee joint during compensatory body sway. In contrast, the 7- to 10-year-old age group's postural responses were basically like those of the adult.

Adaptation

Postural control is characterized by the ability to adapt our use of sensory information to changing tasks and environmental conditions. This process involves (1) determining the accuracy of incoming sensory inputs and selecting the most appropriate sense for the context; and (2) changing the relative weighting of sensory inputs for postural control depending on their accuracy for orientation. How does the CNS learn to adapt the use of sensory information?

Sensory organization tests have been used to examine the development of intersensory integration for postural control. In these tests, body sway is measured during quiet stance under six different conditions. These include (1) somatosensory ankle joint, visual, and vestibular inputs normal; (2) somatosensory ankle joint inputs and vestibular inputs normal, eyes closed; (3) ankle joint inputs normal but visual room moves in direct relation to sway; (4) ankle joint inputs made incongruent with sway (by rotating the platform in the same direction relative to body sway), but vision and vestibular inputs normal; (5) ankle joint inputs incongruent with sway (as above), eyes closed, vestibular system normal; and (6) ankle inputs and visual inputs both incongruent with body sway. Using these tests, studies have shown that adults are able to maintain balance under all six conditions, but gradually show increasing sway over the six conditions with greatest sway in conditions 5 and 6, in which vestibular inputs primarily control posture.

We examined the development of intersensory integration in children 4 to 10 years of age using four of the six sensory conditions described in Nashner's protocols [8]. Even under normal stance conditions (condition 1), the 4- to 6-year-olds swayed significantly more than the older children or adults. With eyes closed (condition 2) their stability decreased further, but they retained balance. When somatosensory information about the body's position with reference to the surface was made inaccurate by rotating the surface and keeping the ankle joint at approximately 90° (condition 3), the 4- to 6-year-olds were greatly destabilized and lost balance. In the final condition somatosensory inputs were minimized through platform rotation and eyes were closed, leaving only vestibular cues to aid in balance. Four of the five children in this age group lost balance while none of the older children or adults needed assistance to maintain their stability.

These results suggest that children under 7 years of age are unable to balance efficiently when both somatosensory and visual cues are removed, leaving only vestibular cues to control stability. It also suggests that children under 7 show a reduced ability to resolve intersensory conflict during postural control.

Abnormal Postural Development

Much research has been performed on the neurologically impaired child and results are consistent in showing that these children achieve sensory-motor milestones at a much later chronological age than their normal peers. As was mentioned above, postural development is an essential element in normal voluntary development. Thus, postural abnormalities could account for some of the delays seen in the neurologically impaired child. In the following section, we will discuss the development of balance control in children with motor delays.

Cerebral Palsy

The incidence of connective tissue and muscle contractures is high in children with cerebral palsy (CP) [9], and clinical studies show increased muscle tone in muscles of the involved leg. However, in a study on dynamic postural control in these children [10] the passive stiffness of the ankle joint was observed to be the same in both legs of the child. There was almost a complete lack of stretch reflexes in response to platform perturbations, despite the presence of enhanced deep tendon reflexes on the clinical exam.

Spastic hemiplegics also had problems with response timing. Normal children responded to perturbations with latencies that were about 95–110 ms but spastic hemiplegics showed delayed onset latencies in the involved leg [10]. Children with ataxic cerebral palsy showed not only delays in onset latency but considerable trial-to-trial variability.

In addition, children with CP showed intermuscle timing problems. Normal adults show a tight coupling of muscles of the leg: distal muscles are activated first, followed 20–45 ms later by the proximal muscles. In spastic hemiplegics, proximal muscles were activated before distal muscles. Because of these problems, the involved leg did not generate enough torque to help compensate for the perturbation.

Surprisingly, these postural response characteristics did not correlate well with the clinical diagnosis of abnormal muscle tone. The muscles identified as spastic showed a delayed response onset even to direct stretch input by the platform perturbations [9]. In contrast to spastic hemiplegic children, ataxic children did not show inter-muscle timing problems.

The ability of children with CP to balance under changing sensory conditions was also examined. Ataxic children with CP were unable to balance under conditions with conflicting sensory inputs. These data are similar to those of adults with cerebellar pathology. Thus these children do not have problems with motor coordination, but with sensory integration. Interestingly, the spastic hemiplegics did not have this problem.

Down Syndrome

Shumway-Cook and Woollacott [12] examined 4- to 6-year-old Down syndrome children in similar test paradigms and showed that they have significant delays in muscle activation in response to postural perturbations, so their response onsets were 26–78 ms later than those found in normal children. This delay in response onset was accompanied by greater sway. The children were also unable to adapt responses to changing task conditions.

In addition, they looked at younger Down syndrome children and found that the youngest one tested (22 months) also showed highly variable responses, with only distal muscles being activated or no response in many trials. This response organization was similar to that seen in the normal 8- to 10-month-old child. Since responses were normally organized in the 4- to 6-year-old child with Down syndrome, a developmental delay may contribute to the motor control problems in these children.

Clumsy Children

Research on posture control in clumsy children [13] has shown some response characteristics similar to those found in children with cerebral palsy, including a slight response slowing, increased response variability, and inefficient sequencing of muscles responses. Williams and Woollacott [13] examined children 6–7 and 9–10 years of age. Each group was more variable than their normal counterparts. Since in normal children, response variability drops to low levels by 6–7 years of age, one would expect that if clumsy children were developmentally delayed, the responses would be less variable in the 9–10 year range. In fact, there was a drop in variability in the older clumsy children compared to the younger. There was also an increased number of reversals of response sequence in the clumsy child. This may indicate that motor control problems in the clumsy child are due to undiagnosed nervous system dysfunction in addition to slow maturation.

References

1. Woollacott M, Shumway-Cook A, Williams H (1989) The development of posture and balance control. In: Woollacott MH, Shumway-Cook A (eds) Development of posture and gait across the life span. University of South Carolina Press, Columbia, pp 77–96
2. Prechtl HFR (1986) Prenatal motor development. In: Wade MC, Whiting HTA (eds) Motor development in children: aspects of coordination and control. Martinus Nighoff, Dordrecht, pp 53–64
3. Woollacott M, Debu B, Mowatt M (1987) Neuromuscular control of posture in the infant and child: is vision dominant? J Motor Behav 19:167–186
4. Roncesvalles NC, Jensen J (1993) The expression of weight-bearing ability in infants between four and seven months of age. NASPSPA Society Abstracts
5. Nashner LM, Woollacott MH (1979) The organization of rapid postural adjustments of standing humans: an experimental-conceptual model. In: Talbot RE, Humphrey DR (eds) Posture and movement. Raven, New York, pp 243–257
6. Woollacott MH, Sveistrup H (1992) Changes in the sequencing and timing of muscle response coordination associated with developmental transitions in balance abilities. Hum Movement Sci 11:23–36

7. Forssberg H, Nashner L (1982) Ontogenetic development of postural control in man: adaptation to altered support and visual conditions during stance. J Neurosci 2:545–552
8. Shumway-Cook A, Woollacott M (1985) The growth of stability: postural control from a developmental perspective, J Motor Behav 17:13–147
9. Shunway-Cook A (1989) Equilibrium deficits in children. In: Woollacott M, Shumway-Cook A (eds) The development of posture and gait across the lifespan. University of South Carolina Press, Columbia
10. Nashner L, Shumway-Cook A, Marin O (1983) Stance posture control in selected groups of children with cerebral palsy: Deficits in sensory organization and muscular coordination. Exp Brain Res 49:393–409
11. Shumway-Cook A, Woollacott M (1985) Dynamics of postural control in the child with Down syndrome. Physical Therapy 65:1315–1322
12. Williams H, Woollacott MH (1993) Speed, consistency, and organization of automatic postural responses in clumsy and normal children. J Motor Behav (in press)

—Tutorial Lecture—

A Psychophysiological Approach to Physical Activity

MICHEL BONNET

Abstract. When they work under temporal constraints, implying attention control, human subjects can be considered as information processing systems that fulfill a succession of sequential operations where sensory messages are progressively transformed into motor messages. Within this framework of an information-processing view of motor control, the experimental evidence for the motor program to be formed by a set of instructions that correspond to different parameters is provided by using the advance information paradigm about an upcoming movement. Partial advance information is sufficient to trigger preparatory activities specific for the revealed dimension of the ensuing movement. The neurophysiological mechanisms which underlie the preparatory processes for action were studied by recording either the variations in excitability of the spinal and transcortical loops of the stretch reflex, or the scalp Contingent Negative Variation, using laplacian derivations. Different sensorimotor networks appeared to be engaged by preparation of movement according to the parameters involved. This provides evidence in favor of a parametric organization of motor programming.

Introduction

In the field of physical activity, the psychophysiological approach assumes that movement execution results from the activation of a mental representation. Such a representation contains the broad outlines of the schema of gestures and learned skills. When a particular movement execution takes place, the corresponding mental representation is activated and specified according to the current goal.

Motor representations are comparable in many aspects to perceptual representations. They are stored in brain structures, mainly in the cerebral cortex; they are improved by repetition and lost after brain lesions; and a conscious access to mental motor representations is generally possible. As we have access consciously to the auditory representation of our first name, we can activate the motor representation of our signature, with its specific dynamics, without any visible cues.

The mental motor representation, which is an operational plan of action, is often called a motor program. This brain product must be directly usable by the executive motor system. However, due to the hierarchical organization of the motor system, the concept of motor program is used to describe a variety of phenomena in the literature.

As for the different visual features (primitives) of an object, the motor program seems to consist of the association of several elementary components. There is general agreement concerning the fact that when we look at a scene, we do not perceive a patchwork of elementary features; rather we perceive the diverse perceptual objects independently which form that scene. Likewise, when we intend to do something, we do not turn our attention to the elementary features, whether they are spatial, temporal, or intensive. Instead, we decide to reach some goal. Consequently, in terms of processing level, the motor program concept corresponds to the object level on the perceptual side.

Information Processing View of Motor Control

When humans work under temporal constraints demanding attention control, they may be considered as information processing systems that fulfill a succession of sequential operations during which sensory messages are progressively transformed into motor messages.

Five successive processing stages are currently distinguished between a triggering stimulus and the onset of the response. They are: (1) sensory feature extraction; (2) stimulus identification; (3) response selection; (4) motor programming; and (5) response execution (see Sanders [1] for a review). Those mental operations are not directly observable but can be inferred from reaction time (RT) measurements.

Mental chronometry is the most popular method to analyze mental activity. In typical experimental tasks, the subject is given temporal constraints; the attention control which is hence required is a fundamental aspect of the task. With preliminary hypotheses about the processing system features, the relevance of comparisons between simple and choice RT may be considered. When a simple RT is involved, the stage numbers 2, 3, and 4 are assumed to be executed mainly before the response signal, on the basis of conditioning in animals or of instructions in humans. In contrast, when a choice RT is involved, the response is selected and programmed only after the response signal. Therefore the programming time is a necessary component of the choice RT.

In this serial model of information processing, the time necessary to process a given stage depends on the operation complexity, and the sum of all the elementary durations constitutes the RT. This model is the object of an important debate between the experimental psychologists, most of whom are in favor of it, and the neuroscientists, who question it because of the obvious structural parallelism of the central nervous system. Nevertheless, this model is currently dominant in the field of information processing for voluntary movements, since the numerous attempts that have been done to invalidate it have not been successful.

Motor Program

The motor program which is assumed to control the production of an intentional movement specifies various parameters such as direction, amplitude, force, or duration, depending on the relations between the goal and the starting conditions. For instance, the role of the handwriting program, once it is learned, is to prescribe values on certain kinematic parameters that are under program control.

It is possible to detect those parameters and to study their rules of specification in the frame of mental chronometry, that is, in RT tasks. One of the first detailed experimental investigations of this parametric model of motor programming was carried out by Rosenbaum [2], at the behavioral level only. The major question addressed was how response dimensions, such as the arm involved, the direction and the extent of the movement, are specified.

In an RT task, Rosenbaum used the "partial advance information" method, providing a cue, called a precue, a few seconds before the response signal. Subjects were required to execute simple limb movements that varied in three dimensions (arm, direction, and extent). The precue signalled total, partial, or no information about the intended movement. By comparing the possible combinations of precues, inferences were made about the independent and interactive roles of each movement parameter in motor program construction. From his data, Rosenbaum concluded that the specification of the various movement dimensions consists of serially organized operations, but without a fixed order, and that programming times are longer for specifying the choice of arm than the direction of the movement, and are longer for specifying direction than extent.

The results and their general interpretation were first criticized, but the results were repeated by several different authors under many different experimental conditions with various parameters and different primate species, thus providing firm support for the parametric model of motor programming [3–8].

Experimental Studies

In studies on motor program using the precueing methodology, the questions to be asked are the following. First, which movement dimensions can be submitted to this kind of abstract prespecification and which cannot? Secondly, is there a hierarchical dependence between the movement dimensions, for instance between direction and extent, and, if so, what is the processing order? At the present time, the elementary processing operations seem to be independent, but it is an important point of debate especially if one considers the neural mechanisms involved [5, 7]. Thirdly, is it possible to localize the nervous structures specifically involved in the programming of elementary parameters? Since the study by Tanji and Evarts [9] concerning the direction of an intended movement, numerous experiments in monkeys have demonstrated that neuron discharges are modulated in relation to the advance information concerning a movement parameter [4]. While these studies were mainly concerned with the cortical motor areas, this is now a fast expanding field of research in cognitive neurosciences. EEG investigations in humans have also developed rapidly since the implementation of methods for spatial localization of cerebral activity.

The psychophysiological studies presented below are composed of two steps. The first is to infer from the chronometric data the presence of a programming operation, and the second is to localize and to describe the activity of the assumed neuronal networks activated when this operation is executed.

Programming the Hand, Direction or Extent

The rationale underlying this experiment [10] was to combine the muscle stretch and the movement precueing techniques so as to examine differential changes in EMG response components (M1, M2, and M3) during the preparation period of an RT task. Subjects moved handles to control the vertical displacements of oscilloscope beams, to point to eight targets. Advance information about the hand to be moved, the movement direction, or the movement extent was provided.

Providing advance information about any movement parameter significantly shortened the RT, although the extent of shortening differed according to the precued movement parameter; it was larger for direction than for choice of hand and larger for hand than for extent. For movement direction, the difference in RT between parameter values (flexion versus extension) which was found when this parameter remained to be specified disappeared when movement direction was specified in advance. This finding is a strong argument for the hypothesis that precued parameters are programmed before the imperative signal occurs.

The latest stretch reflex component (M3) was selectively modulated when movement direction was precued. These changes were symmetrical in extensor and flexor muscles. Their functional significance can be viewed as a tuning process adapting the gain of the reflex loop involved. When the muscle to be activated is an agonist, the gain increase would make the transcortical reflex pathways assist movement execution. In contrast, the relaxation of an antagonist muscle would be facilitated by a decrease in its reflex loop gain.

Programming the Direction or Force of a Forearm Movement

This study was undertaken to determine if preparation of direction (elbow flexion or extension) or force (two levels) could be distinguished on the basis of the slow brain potential change called the Contingent Negative Variation (CNV).

The locus of the maximal rate of increase in scalp negativity migrated from the frontal lobe to the parietal lobe during the preparatory period, under all advance information conditions. The CNV over the somatosensory arm area was greatest when information on direction was given in advance. The CNV over the arm motor region was greatest when information on force was available. These data support a parametric model of motor preparation, with direction and force being processed by at least partially independent networks.

Programming the Duration of a Motor Sequence

Slow brain potentials were recorded before and during a motor timing task as a function of advance information conditions. Subjects had to trigger, as fast as possible, an interval delimited by two brief button presses. Depending on the trial, the response duration could be either 0.7 or 2.5 s. A warning signal sometimes indicated (condition Duration) or not (condition No) which duration to prepare for.

Reaction times were longer in condition No than when the precue was present, and were longer before a long than a short interval (0.7 s) but only in condition No. We concluded, therefore, that the duration of the response can be programmed and that the programming time is longer for a long interval than for a short one.

In addition, the early CNV over the supplementary motor area was larger when the duration was precued than when it was not, and was larger for the short interval. While this specificity vanished over the supplementary motor area at the end of the preparatory period, it appeared over the primary motor cortex. This suggests that information was transferred from one area to the other and that a hierarchy exists between the supplementary and the primary motor areas. The supplementary motor area seems to be particularly involved in programming processes when the timing features of a response are specified.

In conclusion, it seems necessary to stress the importance of studies concerning the parametric organization of motor programming so as to understand the modularity of the motor system.

References

1. Sanders AF (1990) Issues and trends in the debate on discrete vs. continuous processing of information. Acta Psychol 74:123–167
2. Rosenbaum DA (1980) Human movement initiation: specification of arm direction and extent. J Exp Psychol Gen 109:444–474
3. Favilla M, Hening W, Ghez C (1989) Trajectory control in targeted forces impulses. VI: Independent specification of response amplitude and direction. Exp Brain Res 75:280–294

4. Kurata K (1993) Premotor cortex of monkeys: Set- and movement-related activity reflecting amplitude and direction of wrist movements. J Neurophysiol 69:187–200
5. Lepine D, Glencross D, Requin J (1989) Some experimental evidence for and against a parametric conception of movement programming. J Exp Psychol Hum Percept Perform 15:347–362
6. MacKay WA, Bonnet M (1990) CNV, stretch reflex and reaction time correlates of preparation for movement direction and force. Electroencephalogr Clin Neurophysiol 76:47–62
7. Riehle A, Requin J (1989) Monkey primary motor and premotor cortex: Single-cell activity related to prior information about direction and extent of an intended movement. J Neurophysiol 61:534–549
8. Zelaznik HN, Hahn R (1985) Reaction time methods in the study of motor programming: the precueing of hand, digit, and duration. J Motor Behav 17: 190–218
9. Tanji J, Evarts EV (1976) Anticipatory activity of motor cortex neurons in relation to direction of an intended movement. J Neurophysiol 39:1062–1068
10. Bonnet M, Requin J, Stelmach GE (1991) Changes in electromyographic responses to muscle stretch, related to the programming of movements parameters. Electroencephalogr Clin Neurophysiol 81:135–151

Postural Sway Biofeedback Training in Congenitally Blind Children

HIDEO NAKATA, YUKO ENZAKI, and KYONOSUKE YABE

Abstract. The aim of this experiment was to determine whether or not congenitally blind children were able to control postural sway under auditory feedback and to examine the effect of such training in congenitally blind children. To assess postural control, a newly developed apparatus was used. Seven untrained congenitally blind children, aged 6 to 10 years, were tested on a force plate. When anteroposterior sway stayed within 10 mm in the sagittal plane, no auditory feedback was given. If anteroposterior sway was more than 10 mm, they were presented with a 500-Hz pure tone with a speaker. The width of 10 mm corresponded to approximately 80% of the amplitude of anteroposterior sway in each subject. Information about lateral sway was not provided. Time taken while anteroposterior sway exceeded and returned to the width of 10 mm was defined as the response time to a 500-Hz pure tone. Subjects stood for 60 s on a force plate with arms held at the sides and feet together, and performed three trials for each training session. Training sessions were done once a week for five consecutive weeks. The results showed that the total time for which postural sway deviated from the width of 10 mm decreased as training continued. The results also indicated that the response time to the 500-Hz pure tone became shorter as training progressed. It is apparent that congenitally blind children changed their pattern of posture movements for postural correction; it may be associated with changes in postural strategy. Congenitally blind children may be refining their interpretation of auditory feedback and learning to integrate it in the control of posture. We will call the ability of the remaining sensory systems to control posture "nonvisual postural control systems". In conclusion, it was found that postural sway biofeedback training was effective for the assessment of postural control in congenitally blind children.

Introduction

Most of the studies on postural control have reported that vision plays an important role in postural control. Congenitally blind children have never received any visual stimulation nor presumably have had any visual storage capacity. Blind children, therefore, must control postural sway with nonvisual input while standing, and they may be more destabilized than sighted children. Edwards [1] found that blind subjects had reduced stability during quiet stance. Leonard [2], Gipsman [3], and Ribadi et al. [4] showed poor balancing ability in blind and visually impaired children. Nakata [5] reported that out of all the subjects in congenitally totally blind adults, the power spectra of body sway were similar to those found in the sighted with eyes open while maintaining an upright stance. Ribadi et al. [4] pointed out the importance of balance training for visually impaired and blind individuals, and emphasized that this training should be initiated early in life to facilitate the development of adaptation to the nonvisual environment and mediate any learning that will take place.

However, little research has been reported on the effects of training on the balancing ability in blind children. The present study was designed to determine whether or not congenitally blind children were able to control postural sway under auditory feedback. A second purpose was to examine the influence of such training on postural control in congenitally blind children.

Methods

Subjects

The subjects of this study were seven congenitally blind pupils from a school for the blind in Tokyo, who were selected by classroom teachers. They were four boys and three girls 6 to 10 years of age (mean age = 8.3 years, SD = 1.4) and had no other identified disabilities. Two of the subjects could perceive either light or finger movement in vision and five had no vision.

Apparatus

The apparatus used for measuring postural sway is illustrated in Fig. 1. The center of the force plate was 9 cm from the heel. When anteroposterior sway stayed within 10 mm in the sagittal plane, no auditory feedback was given. If postural sway exceeded 10 mm, the subject was given a 500-Hz pure tone with a speaker placed 1 m aways from the subject at eye level. The anteroposterior sway provided the subject with information about body position. About 80% of the amplitude of anteroposterior sway in each subject was within the 10 mm width. Information about lateral sway was not provided. Time spent in the anteroposterior sway area beyond 10 mm was calculated in the trials with auditory feedback. Because a 500-Hz pure tone was presented as soon as anteroposterior sway exceeded the width of 100 mm, the subjects had to respond to the tone and control anteroposterior sway to bring it back to within 10 mm. The time taken while the sway deviated from and returned to the 10-mm width was defined as the response time to the 500-Hz pure tone. The subjects stood for 60 s on a force plate with arms held at the sides and the feet together. They

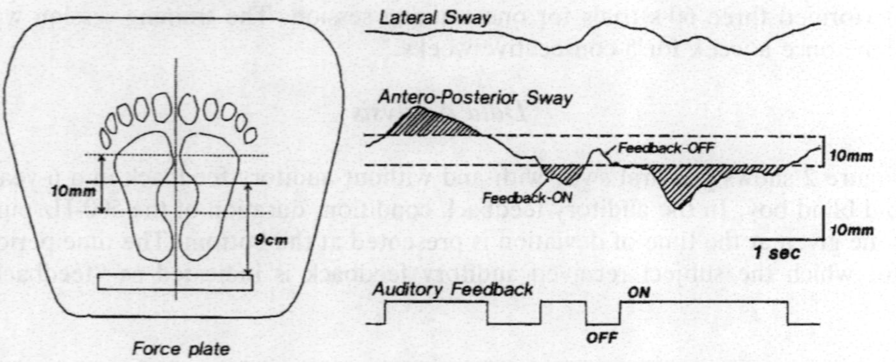

FIG. 1. Diagram of the experiment

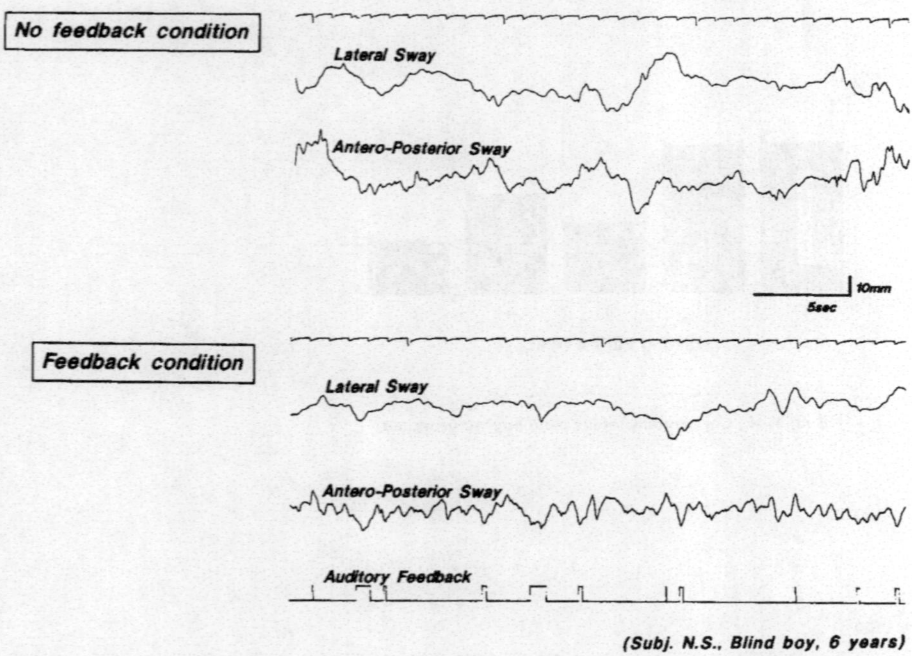

FIG. 2. Anteroposterior sway with and without auditory feedback and lateral sway in a congenitally blind boy (6 years of age). Subjects were provided auditory feedback on anteroposterior sway

performed three 60-s trials for one training session. The training session was done once a week for 5 consecutive weeks.

Data Analysis

Figure 2 shows postural sway with and without auditory feedback in a 6-year-old blind boy. In the auditory feedback condition, duration of the 500-Hz pure tone given at the time of deviation is presented at the bottom. The time period for which the subject received auditory feedback is indicated as "feedback-

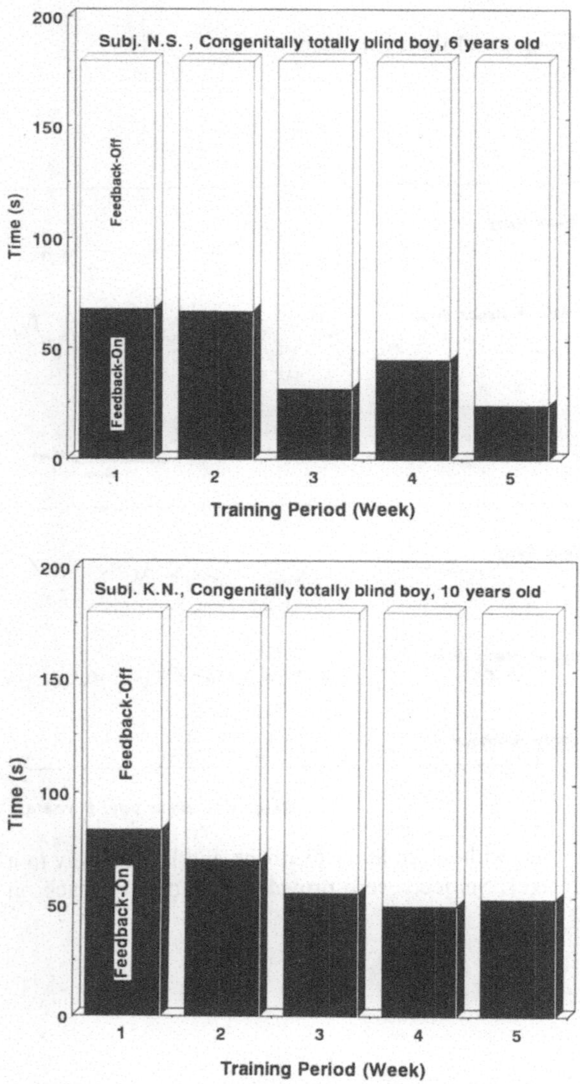

FIG. 3. Effect of feedback training in 6- and 10-year-old blind boys

ON" in Fig. 1. The sum and relative frequencies of "feedback-ON" or response time were calculated for three trials.

Results and Discussion

Figures 3 and 4 indicate that total time in which postural sway exceeded the 10-mm width decreased as training progressed. In response to auditory informa-

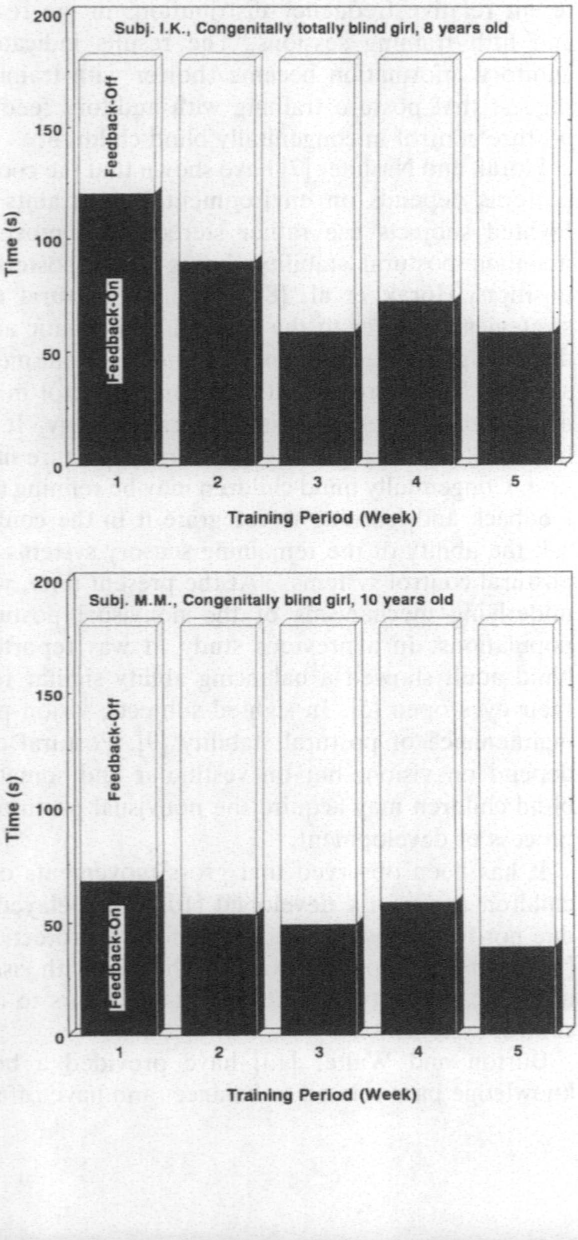

FIG. 4. Effect of feedback training in 8- and 10-year-old blind girls

tion, congenitally blind children made adequate adjustments of posture and became capable of controlling postural sway within the 10-mm area. This means that when congenitally blind children without any visual experience were given appropriate information about the position of their body, they were able to control postural sway. In addition to motor strategies for posture control, a number of sensory strategies are available to aid in balancing [6]. Congenitally blind children also may create a certain rule for combining the use of the available sensory input depending on the environmental circumstances.

Figure 5 shows the relative frequency of response time for anteroposterior sway in a 7-year-old blind girl and a 10-year-old blind boy. There were different relative frequency distributions in the response time between the first and fifth training sessions. The results indicate that the response time to auditory information became shorter with training. Our experimental results suggest that posture training with auditory feedback has a positive effect on posture control in congenitally blind children.

Horak and Nashner [7] have shown that the coordination of postural response patterns depends on environmental constraints imposed by task conditions. Sighted subjects use rather stereotypical movement patterns to achieve or maintain postural stability during anteroposterior sway with a fixed stance position. Horak et al. [8] call these postural movement patterns "postural strategies" to refer to the particular kinematic and dynamic parameters which describe goal-directed behavior under certain mechanical conditions. It is considered that improvement of posture control in congenitally blind children is associated with changes in postural strategy. It is apparent that congenitally blind children changed their pattern of posture movements for postural correction. Congenitally blind children may be refining their interpretation of auditory feedback and learning to integrate it in the control of posture. Thus, we will call the ability of the remaining sensory systems to control posture "nonvisual postural control systems". At the present time, we do not understand fully the underlying mechanisms of the nonvisual postural control systems in blind populations. In a previous study, it was reported that a congenitally totally blind adult showed a balancing ability similar to that in sighted people with their eyes open [5]. In sighted subjects, vision plays an important role in the maintenance of postural stability [9]. Postural control of the blind does not depend on vision, but on vestibular and somatosensory input. Congenitally blind children may acquire the nonvisual postural control systems through the process of development.

It has been observed that gross movements of visually impaired and blind children are poorly developed [10, 11]. Delayed gross motor development is due not to the loss of vision, but to overprotection by parents and/or teachers [12]. Increased opportunities for children with visual impairments to participate in physical activity may be important factors to refine their nonvisual postural control systems.

Burton and Walter [13] have provided a brief overview of the current knowledge base related to balance, and have offered some suggestions on how

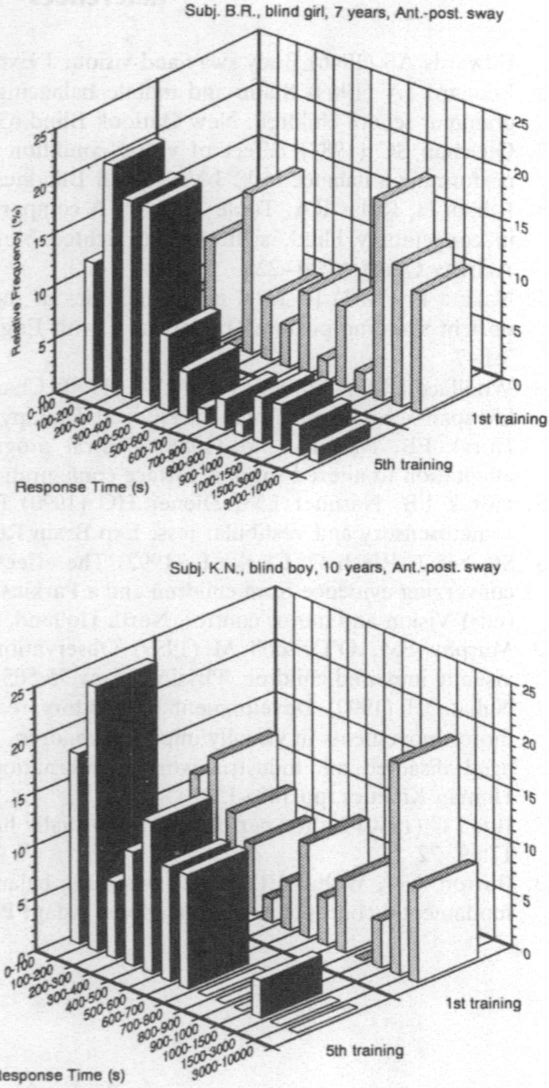

FIG. 5. Relative frequency distributions of response times for a 7-year-old blind girl and a 10-year-old blind boy in the first and fifth training periods

to improve balance assessment procedures in adapted physical education. Eight problems or limitations in traditional tasks used to assess balance in adapted physical education were identified. Suggested modifications in the traditional tasks include adding or modifying items to require some feedback-based movements, and using more process-oriented measures of balance competency. In our study, a new method to assess balancing ability was used, and the results of the experiment showed that postural sway biofeedback training was effective for the assessment of postural control in congenitally blind children.

References

1. Edwards AS (1946) Body sway and vision. J Exp Psychol 36:526–536
2. Leonard JA (1969) Static and mobile balancing performance of blind adolescent grammar school children. New Outlook Blind 63:65–72
3. Gipsman SC (1981) Effect of visual condition on use of proprioceptive cues in performing a balance task. J Vis Impair Blindness 75(2):50–54
4. Ribadi H, Rider RA, Toole T (1987) A comparison of static and dynamic balance in congenitally blind, sighted, and sighted blindfolded adolescents. Adapt Phys Activity Quart 4:220–225
5. Nakata H (1983) Postural controllabilities of the visually impaired in maintaining upright standing posture (In Japanese with English abstract). Jpn J Hum Posture 3:1–7
6. Woollacott MH, Shumway-Cook A (1990) Changes in posture control across the life span—A system approach. Physical Therapy 70:799–807
7. Horak FB, Nashner LM (1986) Central programming of postural movements: adaptation to altered support surface configurations. J Neurophysiol 55:1369–1381
8. Horak FB, Nashner LM, Diener HC (1990) Postural strategies associated with somatosensory and vestibular loss. Exp Brain Res 82:167–177
9. Starkes J, Riach C, Clarke B (1992) The effect of eye closure on postural sway: converging evidence from children and a Parkinson patient. In: Proteau L, Elliot D (eds) Vision and motor control. North-Holland, pp 353–373
10. Murphy FM, O'Driscoll M (1989) Observations on the motor development of visually impaired children. Physiotherapy 75:505–508
11. Nakata H (1990) Development of auditory reaction times, using fine and gross motor movements in visually impaired children. In: Kaneko M (ed) Fitness for the aged, disabled, and industrial worker. International series on sport sciences, vol 20. Human Kinetics, pp 148–153
12. Buell C (1950) Motor performance of visually handicapped children. Except Child 17:69–72
13. Burton AW, Walter ED (1992) Assessing balance in adapted physical education: fundamental concepts and applications. Adapt Phys Activity Quart 9:14–46

Motor Pattern During the Standing Long Jump in Individuals with Mental Retardation

Yasuhiro Matsuzaki and Tatsuko Hentona

Abstract. The aim of this study was to investigate the motor pattern during the standing long jump in the mentally retarded. The subjects included 34 elementary pupils and 16 upper secondary students in a school for the mentally retarded, aged 6–12 and 17–18 years, respectively. Their form in the standing long jump was shot with a video camera, and every frame was analyzed with reference to the developmental sequence for the standing long jump proposed by Clark et al. (1985) and Miyamaru (1973). The results showed that the development of arm action while performing the jump tended to occur behind that of leg action. In 10 elementary pupils, practicing the long jump facilitated differentiation between development of arm pattern and leg pattern. In flight, some of the upper secondary students showed a sideward-upward action of the arms although the backward movement of the swung arm was complete at takeoff. The results are discussed in terms of the poor balance of the mentally retarded.

Introduction

Most persons with mental retardation show a reduced ability to perform as instructed compared with normal students on various tests of motor ability. Many school teachers of students with mental retardation regard physical fitness development programs as an important part of the curriculum for the retarded. We have emphasized providing as much opportunity as possible to evaluate the effectiveness of the instruction.

Recently, some schools in Japan for children with mental retardation have introduced a physical coordination pattern (a special jumping pattern) to evaluate the motor ability of the children. It was determined that the pattern was useful to improve instruction and to adapt the evaluation of coordination skills in individuals with mental retardation to comparisons with scores on motor performance tests.

There have been a few studies done on the motor pattern during the standing long jump in children with mental retardation. DiRocco et al. [1] showed that subjects with mental retardation tend to exhibit a less developed coordination pattern. They exhibit more arm action than leg action. However, the study did not address two aspects, that is, practice and growth. The investigation and observation of changes in coordination pattern with practice and growth might provide a more in-depth understanding of the effect of instruction on the motor ability of children with mental retardation. The aim of this study was to clearly define the characteristics of jumping patterns in individuals with mental retardation based on the data obtained to evaluate motor ability.

Subjects and Methods

Subjects

For this study, 34 elementary school (20 boys and 14 girls) and 16 high school students (12 boys and 4 girls) in a school for the mentally retarded were selected. The younger subjects were 6–12 years of age and their IQs ranged from 16 to 64 (mean 34.48, SD 9.13). The older subjects were 17–18 years of age, and their IQs ranged from 33 to 66 (mean 47.25, SD 8.91). All of the older subjects were members of a basketball club in school.

Procedure

All subjects were tested at their school. Elementary school participants were instructed to jump as far forward as possible from a standing position by the teachers in charge of each subject's class. High school participants were instructed by the investigators. A video camera was used to record the side view of all jumps. The older subjects were later shot from the front. The camera-to-subject distance was about 4 m. Each video frame was analyzed by an editing controller.

Developmental Sequence for the Standing Long Jump

The arm and leg actions in the standing long jump were evaluated by use of the Developmental Sequence of the Standing Long Jump by Clark and Phillips [2] and Miyamaru [3]. Both developmental sequences consisted of two components, arm action and leg action, respectively (Table 1).

Results

Takeoff Pattern of Jumping

A typical takeoff pattern of the standing long jump is shown in Fig. 1. The arm action of subject S was judged to be Level 1 of the development sequence and

TABLE 1. Developmental sequence of the standing long jump by Clark and Phillips.

Level	Arm action	Leg action
1	No arm action. May exhibit "winging".	One-footed takeoff.
2	Shoulder flexion only, occurs during lower extremity extension. Some shoulder abduction may be present.	Knee extension precedes heel up.
3	Incomplete biphasic arm action. Shoulder hyperextension occurs during lower extremity extension. Shoulder flexion is incomplete at takeoff.	Knee extension and heel up simultaneous.
4	Complete biphasic arm action. Biphasic action similar to Level 3 except shoulder flexion is complete at takeoff.	Knee extension follows heel up.

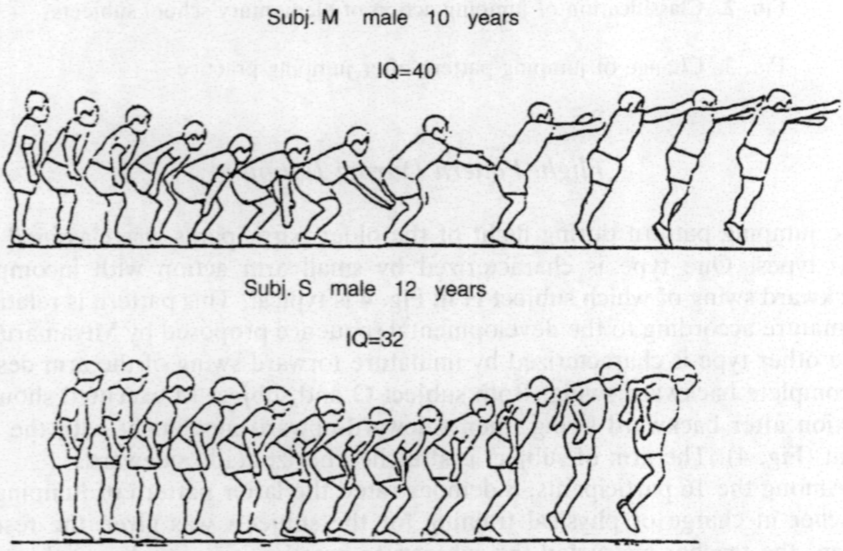

FIG. 1. Takeoff pattern of standing long jump in elementary school students

the leg action was judged to be Level 2. Both the arm and the leg action of subject M was judged to be Level 2.

Figure 2 illustrates the classification of the jumping action of all subjects individually. For arm action, Level 1 was the most prevalent, and for leg action Level 2 was the most frequent.

Ten elementary school participants practiced jumping to increase their distance (Fig. 3). Among the ten subjects, six improved leg development level by the training. For arm action, two participants improved while one regressed.

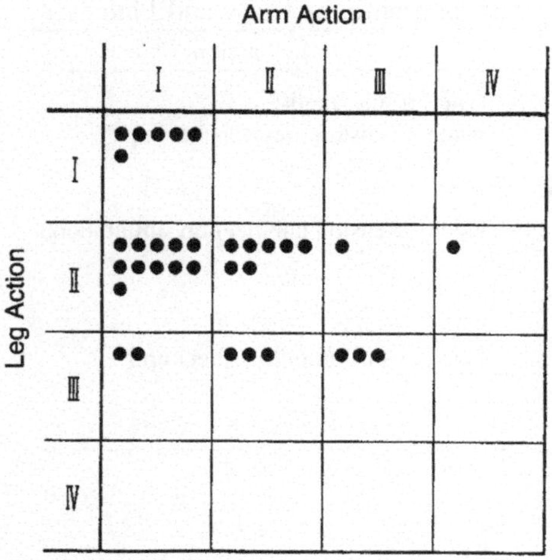

2

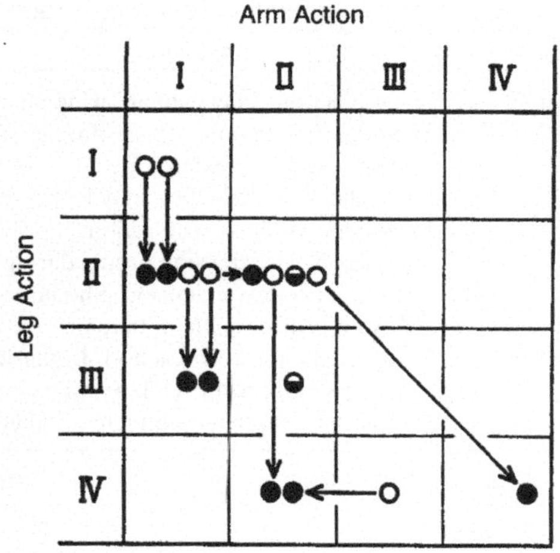

3

FIG. 2. Classification of jumping action of elementary school subjects

FIG. 3. Change of jumping pattern after jumping practice

Flight Pattern During Jumping

The jumping pattern during flight of the older participants was classified into two types. One type is characterized by small arm action with incomplete backward swing of which subject H in Fig. 4 is typical. This pattern is relatively immature according to the developmental sequence proposed by Miyamaru [3]. The other type is characterized by immature forward swing of the arm despite a complete backward swing. Both subject O and subject M executed shoulder flexion after backward swing, then sideward-upward movement with the arm bent (Fig. 4). The arm of subject is stretched horizontally sideward.

Among the 16 participants, 8 demonstrated the latter pattern of jumping. A teacher in charge of physical training for the subjects was given the results. Then, the teacher instructed the subjects to practice jumping during the physical education class for about 4 months. The result of the retest was that five of the 8 participants executed a more mature (larger) forward swing.

Discussion

In the standing long jump performed by children with mental retardation, the sequence of arm action is more behind developmentally than that of leg action. This developmental retardation was improved by practice. The immature arm action even appeared in the high school participants. Balance ability of persons with mental retardation was inferior in comparison with nonretarded [4–6]. The result of this study supports DiRocco et al. [1]; children with mental

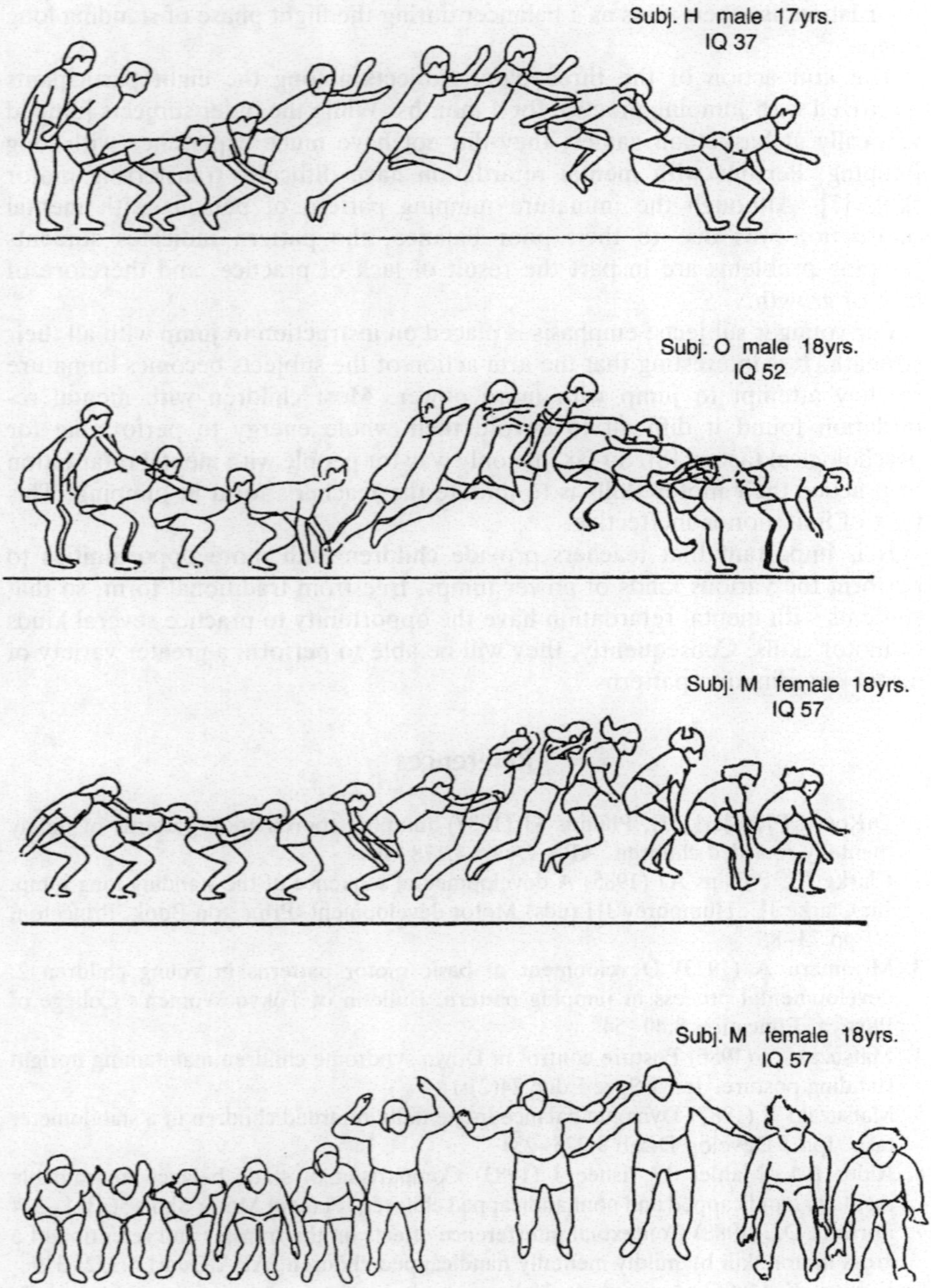

FIG. 4. The jumping pattern of high school students. *Row 1*, jumping pattern of small arm action with incomplete backward swing; *Rows 2 and 3*, the arm stretched horizontally sideward; *Row 4*, front view of the jumping pattern

retardation use their arms as a balancer during the flight phase of standing long jump.

The arm action of the three older subjects among the eight participants improved with jumping practice for 4 months. While the older subjects jumped vertically at basketball games, they did not have much experience with long jumping. Persons with mental retardation have difficulty transferring motor skills [7]. Although the immature jumping pattern of persons with mental retardation was due to their poor balance, the pattern indicates students jumping problems are in part the result of lack of practice, and therefore of lack of growth.

For younger subjects, emphasis is placed on instruction to jump with all their strength. It is interesting that the arm action of the subjects becomes immature as they attempt to jump with more power. Most children with mental retardation found it difficult to devote their whole energy to performing for psychological factors [8]. So far, the only way for people with mental retardation to practice their motor skills is to imitate the teacher's form in jumping. This type of imitation is ineffective.

It is important that teachers provide children with more opportunities to perform the various kinds of power jumps, free from traditional form, so that students with mental retardation have the opportunity to practice several kinds of motor skills. Consequently, they will be able to perform a greater variety of motor coordination patterns.

References

1. DiRocco PJ, Clark JE, Phillips SJ (1987) Jumping coordination patterns of mildly mentally retarded children. APA Quart 4:178–191
2. Clarke JE, Phillips AJ (1985) A developmental sequence of the standing long jump. In: Clarke JE, Humphrey JH (eds) Motor development. Princeton Book, Princeton, NJ pp 73–85
3. Miyamaru A (1973) Development of basic motor patterns in young children 2: developmental process in jumping pattern. Bulletin of Tokyo Women's College of Physical Education 8:40–54
4. Matsuzaki Y (1986) Posture control in Down syndrome children maintaining upright standing posture. Jpn J Spec Educ 24(2):1–9
5. Matsuzaki Y (1987) Dynamic balance in mentally retarded children in a stabilometer task. Jpn J Develop Disab 9:225–231
6. Rider RA, Mahler TJ, Ishee J (1983) Comparison of static balance in trainable mentally handicapped and nonhandicapped children. Percept Motor Skills 56:311–314
7. Porretta DL (1988) Contextual interference effects on the transfer and retention of a gross motor skill by mildly mentally handicapped children. APA Quart 5:332–339
8. Kusano K (1986) A psychological approach to the motor training of mentally retarded children. Asian Scientific Congress Proceedings—Better life through sports, pp 506–511

Electromyographic Characteristics of the Learning Process of Walking in Normal Infants and Children

Kayoko Okamoto, Tsutomu Okamoto, Hideaki Yamashita, Ryokei Ogawa, Hiromi Tsutsumi, Emi Okamoto, Hirotake Maruyama, Yasuhiko Tokuhara, Nobuyuki Kazai, and Yukihiro Goto

Abstract. To determine the electromyographic characteristrics of normal infant walking, we studied 10 approximately one-year-old infants who were learning to walk. We examined the functional mechanisms of their leg muscles from the initial period of learning to walk through the transitional period to the adult walking pattern. The co-contraction of the antagonistic leg muscles, which indicated a lack of stable equilibrium, seemed to characterize the onset of independent walking around 12 months after birth. The period of transition to the child walking pattern, i.e., comparatively stable walking with the body inclined forward, seemed to take place around 2 or 3 months after the infant had learned to walk. The period of transition to the adult walking pattern, characterized by active motions of lifting the heel with the body erect, appeared to start around the end of the child's second year of life.

Introduction

We frequently noted co-contraction of mutual antagonists among leg muscles as the child first began to walk, and we interpreted this to indicate a lack of stable equilibrium. A very few cases, however, displayed adult-like patterns from the very beginning of independent walking, suggesting that the pattern adults use may already be inherent in a baby who is just starting to walk for the first time.

In the present study, we followed EMG activity in ten children from the time they first walked independently until they displayed adult-like patterns, usually until 3 or 4 years of age. We sought evidence to further clarify whether or not babies beginning to walk already have the basic mechanism to generate an adult-like pattern, and we also wished to reconfirm our previous observations on normal infant walking [1, 2].

Methods

The EMGs of all the subjects were recorded from the right leg muscles: tibialis anterior, gastrocnemius (lateral head), vastus medialis, rectus femoris, biceps femoris (long head), and gluteus maximus (upper part), using surface electrodes 5 mm in diameter. For some of the subjects, EMGs of the semimembranosus, rectus abdominis, and sacrospinalis muscles were recorded. The EMG recordings were made with an 18-channel penwriting "electroencephalograph" (recording speed: 60 mm/s) and a 12-channel electromagnetic oscillograph (recording speed: 200 mm/s). Simultaneous with the EMGs, we took video recordings (at 60 frames/sec) of: heel and toe contacts of both feet with the floor (electrobasograms); and angular changes of the ankle, knee, and hip joints (electrogoniograms).

Results and Discussion

Swing Phase in First Steps

We noted the strong burst from the rectus femoris as the hip began to flex. In most cases, we saw the vastus medialis active at this time, as well as the gastrocnemius and the biceps femoris. A look at the gait pattern shows that the biceps femoris appeared to be flexing the knee. The gastrocnemius may have contributed to the knee flexion as well, but it may instead have been restraining the active dorsiflexion that was taking place. The vastus medialis may have been activated by a stretch reflex mechanism during this knee flexion.

In the latter half of the swing phase, the vastus medialis and gastrocnemius showed strong activity with the knee extending and the ankle plantarflexing. All of this activity in the swing phase resembled the pattern of muscle activation seen when an older child or an adult runs fast.

Stance Phase in First Steps

As the foot contacted the floor, the tibialis anterior and gastrocnemius continued a strong co-contraction pattern that began during the swing. This co-contraction may help stabilize the ankle to compensate for inadequately developed balance function. Meanwhile, at the hip and knee, the vastus medialis, rectus femoris, biceps femoris, and gluteus maximus contracted together if the baby took only two or three steps, but the activity of the rectus femoris died out as the baby learned to take more steps. Activity of the rectus femoris was associated with holding the trunk upright over slightly flexed legs, whereas this muscle displayed less or no activity as the baby began to lean the upper body forward over the slightly flexed legs. The rectus abdominis, inactive in adult gait, also displayed bursts not only in the swing phase but also in stance.

Adult Pattern Present from Start?

Even at such an early stage, signs of decreasing co-contraction in conjunction with a forward migration of the originally upright trunk were associated with a more adult-like pattern. This suggests that elements of the adult pattern already reside in the baby who is just beginning to walk independently. Most novice walkers fail to display an adult pattern at the beginning because of poorly developed muscle strength and equilibrium function. These deficiencies give rise to instability, and so excessive muscular activity results in a pattern that looks more like an adult running fast than walking.

The First Few Weeks

Figure 1 shows representative EMGs for an infant that could walk more than 10 steps on the 7th day after walking for the first time. One week after independent gait began, activities of the tibialis anterior and rectus femoris diminished during stance, the strong bracing action at the ankle apparently decreasing, and the upper body began to lean forward over still slightly flexed legs. A few babies, presumably because of the posture assumed and the speed of walking employed, showed adult-like patterns.

After walking for 2–4 weeks, the baby could generally take 20 steps and used a reciprocal pattern between the tibialis anterior and gastrocnemius. The vastus medialis showed less activity during stance phase, associated with a straightening of the legs and thus less load on the knee. The tibialis anterior failed to show any burst of activity just prior to foot contact in some cases, unlike the adult pattern. In these instances, the foot was not inverting during plantarflexion as it had been before when the tibialis anterior had been active.

Subsequent Development

The "unstable infant walking pattern—the discharge pattern of gastrocnemius prior to foot contact" that originally characterized the swing phase began to disappear between 1 and 2 months of independent walking [2].

Between 2 and 3 months, the "unstable infant walking pattern" and activity of the rectus abdominis went away completely, suggesting a considerably more stable equilibrium. The lack of activity in the tibialis anterior just prior to foot contact continued to be seen in a number of babies, so this feature may be considered one pattern peculiar to early walking in babies. During stance, the biceps femoris and gluteus maximus exhibited continuous discharge patterns associated with a forward-leaning trunk.

Until about the end of 2 years of age, the baby propelled itself forward with a pumping action of the thigh as the trunk leaned forward, rather than by a strong push-off at the ankle as seen in the adult gait. After the foot contacted the ground, a quick shift of the body to the forefoot, a subsequent pattern characteristic of gait in small children appeared. At about 3 years of age, however, the continuous activity of the biceps femoris and gluteus maximus, associated with forward inclination of the trunk, began to dwindle as the trunk started to assume a more upright position. Activity of the gastrocnemius in the first half of the stance phase disappeared, but condensed into a strong burst

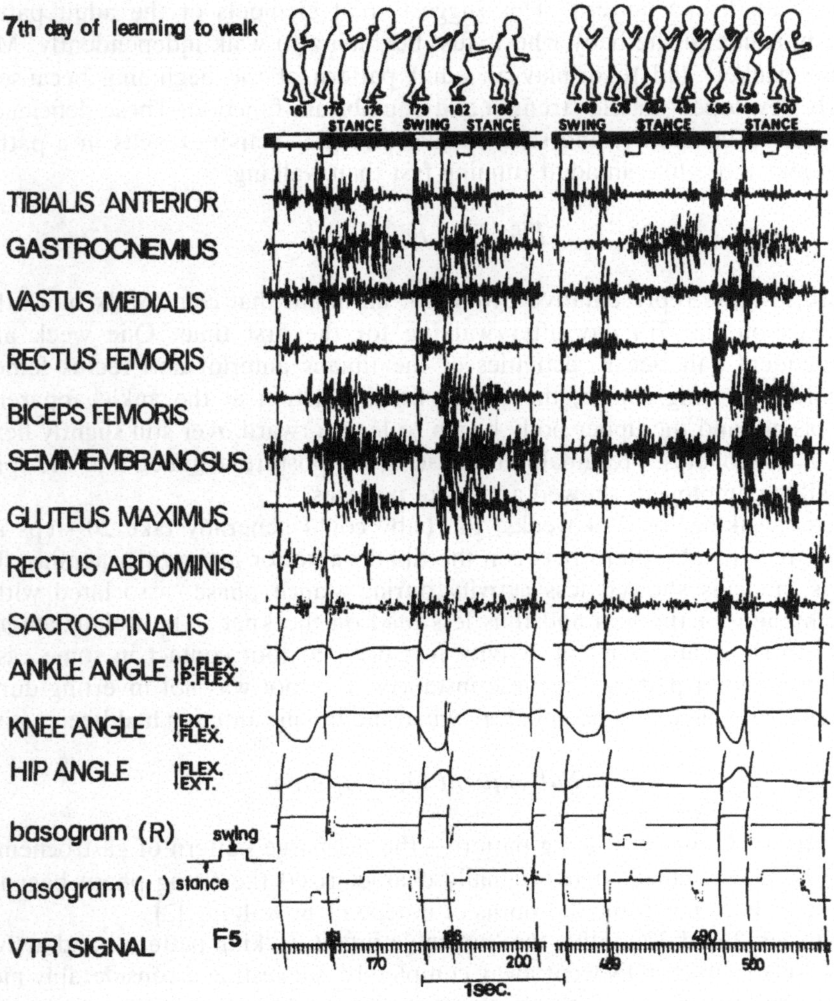

FIG. 1. EMGs of a 12-month-old infant on the 7th day after learning to walk. *swing*, swing phase; *stance*, stance phase

during the latter half of stance, similar to the adult pattern, to effect a strong push off by the foot. These findings enabled us to reconfirm one idea drawn from our previous work, namely that at about 3 years of age, the child walks with a muscle activation pattern that begins to look similar to the pattern seen in adults.

Summary

To reconfirm the electromyographic characteristics of normal infant walking, the learning process of walking in ten infants was studied. We examined the functional mechanisms of leg muscles from the initial period of learning to walk until the transition to an adult pattern.

1. The co-contraction of mutual antagonists among leg muscles, which indicate a lack of stable equilibrium, seems to be characteristic of the onset of independent walking around 12 months after birth.
2. The period of the transition to the child walking pattern indicating a comparatively stable walking with forward body incline seems to be about 2–3 months after learning to walk.
3. The period of the transition to the adult walking pattern, which indicates strong pushing-off motions of the foot, with the body erect appears to take place around the end of 2 years of age.
4. We reconfirmed the unstable period in the onset of independent walking and the period of the transition to the child and adult walking pattern.

References

1. Okamoto T, Kumamoto M (1972) Electromyographic study of the learning process of walking in infants. Electromyography 12:149–158
2. Okamoto T, Goto Y (1985) Human infant pre-independent and independent walking. In: Kondo S (ed) Primate morphophysiology, locomotor analyses and human bipedalism. University of Tokyo Press, Tokyo, pp 59–79

Postural Sway in Normal and Mentally Retarded Persons

Hideyuki Okuzumi, Kouichi Haishi, and Mitsuru Kokubun

Abstract. The purpose of this study was: (1) to examine the magnitude of postural sway in persons with mental retardation (PMR) according to clinical types of retardation in comparison with non-handicapped persons, and (2) to investigate the relation between magnitude of sway (MS) and body balance exercises (beam walking and one-foot balance) according to clinical types. The subjects were 134 non-handicapped persons and 45 PMR. The results were as follows: (1) The average MS of autistic persons and other PMR was about the same as that of non-handicapped children aged 4 or 5 years. Among other PMR, however, the MS distribution was relatively large. On the other hand, MS in persons with Down syndrome was generally small, and was similar to that of nonhandicapped children aged 6 years; this small MS appeared to be characteristic of the syndrome. (2) With regard to MS and body balance exercise performance, all subjects in the small magnitude group belonged to the high-performance group except for the persons with Down syndrome.

Introduction

Postural sway has been taken to be an index of body balance; in general, the larger the magnitude of sway (MS), the more unstable the balance. There is still little agreement among researchers as to the evaluation of MS in persons with mental retardation (PMR). Matsuzaki et al. [1] reported that MS in PMR was larger than that in normal persons (non-handicapped persons) and that their balance was unstable, whereas Wade [2] reported it was smaller and their balance was stable. Moreover, little is known about the relationship between MS and body balance exercise performance in PMR. On the other hand, body balance exercise performance (e.g., beam walking, one-foot balance) has been considered to differ according to the clinical types of mental retardation (i.e., autism, Down syndrome, and other PMR). This suggests that the disagreement over MS in PMR may be due to different clinical types studied. The purposes of this study are: (1) to examine MS in PMR according to clinical types in comparison with non-handicapped persons, and (2) to investigate the relation between MS and body balance exercise performance by these types.

Method

Subjects

A total of 134 non-handicapped persons and 45 clinically diagnosed PMR, without visual or motor impairment, participated in this study. The 134 non-handicapped persons consisted of 67 children (15 aged 3–4 years, 39 aged 5 years, and 13 aged 6 years), 50 adults aged 18–24 years, and 17 elderly persons aged 61–93 years. The average chronological and mental ages of PMR were 17.3 ± 3.0 and 6.5 ± 2.4 years, respectively. Clinically, 9 persons were autistic, 9 had Down syndrome, and 27 had other types of mental retardation.

Measurement of Magnitude of Sway

The sway of "center of foot pressure" was measured as postural sway by a strain-gauge force platform (1G06 NEC-Sanei, Tokyo, Japan). Subjects stood stationary and upright on the force platform with Romberg's stance for about 60 s. In measuring all but elderly subjects, the "Visual Information Presentation Board" (Kawamura Ironworks, Sendai, Japan), which we designed, was used to control visual information (Fig. 1). The presented visual information was a fixation point 30 cm in front of the subject (foveal information) and cross-shaped vertical and horizontal lines stretching to the limits of the subject's viewing range (peripheral information). Elderly subjects stood in front of a white wall 1 m apart and fixated a small object. Lateral and fore-aft sway were

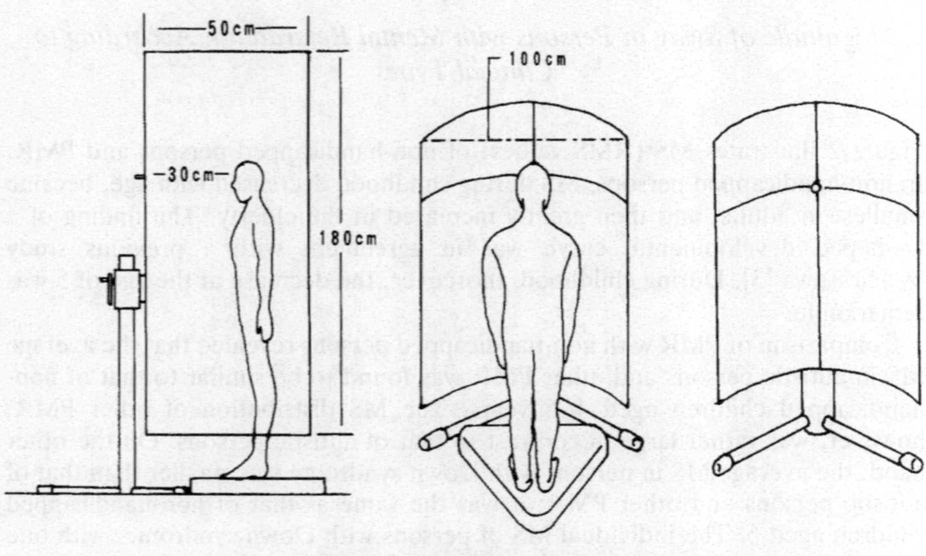

FIG. 1. The visual information presenting board

recorded with a data recorder (XR-710 TEAC, Tokyo, Japan) from the force platform. The most stable sway for 25.6 s was analyzed. These two signals (sway) were conditioned [low-pass 10 Hz filter (P83, NF Electronic Instruments, Yokohama, Japan)] prior to analog-to-digital conversion at a sampling frequency of 20 Hz. Root mean square (RMS) values were determined as the MS. RMS value was calculated as follows: RMS = $\sqrt{X^2 + Y^2}$ where X = standard deviation of lateral sway and Y = standard deviation of fore-aft sway.

Measurement of Body Balance Exercise Performance

Beam Walking. The apparatus consisted of 5 beams of equal length (3 m) and height from the ground (5 cm) with varying widths of walking surface (12.5 cm, 10 cm, 7.5 cm, 5 cm, and 2.5 cm). The subjects were instructed to walk forward on each of these progressively narrow beams without falling off. A maximum of three trials were allowed per beam. Performance was classified into 6 stages (I–VI).

One-foot Balance (Eyes Open). Subjects were given a total of 6 trials: 3 on the right foot, and 3 on the left. The time was recorded either for 60 s, until either the subject's lifted foot touched the ground or the supporting foot moved. The longest of the 6 trials was recorded and transformed into log-value (from log 1 to log 59). The results were classified into five groups as follows: A, 60 s; B, 59–26 s; C, 25–11 s; D, 10–6 s; E, 5–3 s; and F, 2–1 s).

Results and Discussion

Magnitude of Sway in Persons with Mental Retardation According to Clinical Types

Figure 2 illustrates MS (RMS values) of non-handicapped persons and PMR. In non-handicapped persons, MS during childhood decreased with age, became smallest in adults, and then greatly increased in the elderly. The finding of a U-shaped developmental curve was in agreement with a previous study by Hirasawa [3]. During childhood, moreover, the decrease at the age of 5 was remarkable.

Comparison of PMR with non-handicapped persons revealed that the average MS in autistic persons and other PMR was found to be similar to that of non-handicapped children aged 4–5 years. The MS distribution of other PMR, however, was rather large in contrast to that of autistic persons. On the other hand, the average MS in persons with Down syndrome was smaller than that of autistic persons and other PMR; it was the same as that of non-handicapped children aged 6. The individual MS of persons with Down syndrome, with one exception, was also comparatively small.

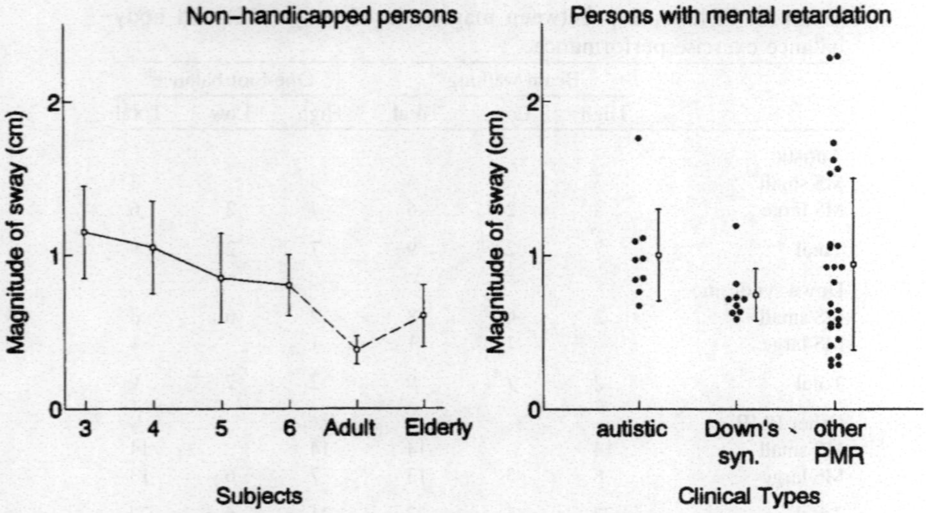

FIG. 2. Magnitude of sway of non-handicapped persons and persons with mental retardation (*PMR*)

Relationship Between Magnitude of Sway and Body Balance Exercise Performance in Persons with Mental Retardation

In order to examine the relationship between MS and body balance exercise performance, subjects were classified into 2 groups for the respective measurements (Table 1). For body balance exercises, subjects were divided into high- and low-performance groups according to Kokubun and Koike [4]. For MS, they were divided into large- and small-magnitude groups based on the average MS of children aged 5 years (0.85 cm). Among autistic persons and other PMR, in the large-magnitude group some belonged to the high-performance and others to the low-performance group. The relationship between performance and MS was not clear. In the small-magnitude group, however, all belonged to the high-performance group in terms of body balance. On the other hand, most persons with Down syndrome belonged to the small-magnitude group whether their exercise performance was high or low. And their performance was generally low. This small MS in persons with Down syndrome appeared to be peculiar to their syndrome. Further research is necessary to determine whether any relationship exists between such small MS and low muscle tone. Low muscle tone has often been pointed out as a characteristic of Down syndrome. We propose that measurement of the frequency of postural sway is a valid approach, since muscle afferentation has been related to high frequency of postural sway [5]. The characteristic of postural sway frequency of persons with Down syndrome should thus be investigated.

TABLE 1. Relationship between magnitude of sway (MS) and body balance exercise performance.

	Beam walking[a]			One-foot balance[b]		
	High	Low	Total	High	Low	Total
Autistic						
MS small	3		3	3		3
MS large	4	2	6	4	2	6
Total	7	2	9	7	2	9
Down syndrome						
MS small	2	6	8	2	6	8
MS large		1	1	1		1
Total	2	7	9	2	7	9
Other PMR						
MS small	14		14	14		14
MS large	8	5	13	7	6	13
Total	22	5	27	21	6	27

[a] Beam walking: high-performance group (I–III), low-performance group (IV–VI).

[b] One-foot balance: high-performance group (A–D), low-performance group (E–F).

Acknowledgement. This research was supported in part by a Grant-in-Aid for JSPS Fellows (No. 0050640), from the Ministry of Education, Science and Culture of Japan.

References

1. Matsuzaki Y, Nakata H, Saito Y (1982) Postural control abilities of mentally retarded children (in Japanese with English abstract). Bull Defectol 6(1):79–87
2. Wade MG (1990) Impact of optical flow on postural control in normal and mentally handicapped persons. In: Vermeer A (ed) Motor development, adapted physical activity and mental retardation. Med Sport Sci 30:21–29
3. Hirasawa Y (1979) An observation on standing ability of Japanese males and females (in Japanese with English abstract). J Anthrop Soc Nippon 87(2):81–92
4. Kokubun M, Koike T (to be published) Problem in balance performance of persons with mental retardation. In: Vermeer A (ed) Aspects of gross and sensory motor development in mental retardation. Med Sport Sci
5. Aggashyan RV, Gurfinkel VS, Mamasakhlisov GV, Elner AM (1973) Changes in spectral and correlation characteristics of human stabilograms at muscle afferentation disturbance. Agressologie 14(D):5–9

Gaze Control in Children with High Versus Low Motor Proficiency

CLAUDIA EMES, JOAN VICKERS, and LORI LIVINGSTON

Abstract. Gaze control was compared between children demonstrating high *vs* low motor proficiency on the Bruininks-Oseretsky Test of Motor Proficiency. Gaze during the response speed task, which measures reaction to a moving visual stimulus, was observed. Eye events were coded just prior, during, and after the release of the stick in the response speed task. A set of six gazes across seven trials of the task was recorded for all subjects. Low proficiency children were slower to respond to the falling stick than the high proficiency group. High performers tended to use a higher percentage of fixations across all trials. Most noticeble were differences between the groups at the moment of release. For high performers, fixations tended to be much longer, indicating the use of a steady gaze through to the final clamping motion of the thumb on the stick. Additionally, the location of gaze at the moment of release differed noticeably. High performers sustained their gaze on the stick while the low performers were as likely to focus on the stick, off the stick or at their own thumb. This study describes the role of gaze in the performance of tasks requiring a quick response to visual stimuli. The results suggest that differences between between proficient and clumsy motor responses in children may be associated with gaze control.

Gaze Control in Children with High Versus Low Motor Proficiency

The role of eye movement in relation to activity is an established field of study, emerging from investigations which observe various behaviors and how they relate to a subject's gaze control. For example, research consisting of the observation of eye movement while reading is readily available [1, 2]. More specifically, research on children with dyslexia is abundant [3–6]. However, these studies have used eye monitoring equipment which required that the subject remain stationary, head fixed. This study was designed to observe gaze control in children participating in a motor proficiency test with normal head and eye motion. The purpose was to compare gaze control in children with high *vs* low motor proficiency as determined by the results of the Bruininks-Oseretsky Test of Motor Proficiency.

The task of controlling gaze is explained through a two-part hierarchical model proposed by Schmid and Zambarbieri [7]. According to their definition, gaze is "the absolute position of the eyes in space and depends on both eye position in the orbit and head position in space" (p 229). At the highest level in their model, sensory information is received from the environment with voluntary generation of commands that direct gaze according to the goals and intentions of the subject. At the lower levels, the head, body, and oculomotor control systems act as one closely coupled system [8, 9].

During the normal scanning of a visual scene, two types of gaze control, known as fixations and saccades, are typically observed. Fixations are those instances in which the eye is fixated or stopped for a period of 100 to 150 ms [10]. It is during these fixations that most visual information is acquired and processed. Saccades represent the shift in gaze from one fixation location to another. Their duration ranges from 30 to 120 ms, and they determine the duration between fixations [11].

Method

Sample

Based on their performance on the Bruininks-Oseretsky Test of Motor Proficiency—Short Form ($n = 234$) eight young females, ages 7 and 8 years (mean 7.7) were selected to participate in the study. The Bruininks-Oseretsky Test of Motor Proficiency—Short Form (8 subtests and 14 motor skill activities) is one of the most widely used tests of motor development in children and may be of further use as a diagnostic tool [12]. Therefore, this test was chosen to distinguish children based on motor proficiency. The subjects were classified as being either high ($n = 5$) or low ($n = 3$) in motor proficiency. The mean percentile rankings for high motor proficiency ranged from 98 to 100 (mean 99.4) and low from 12 to 31 (mean 22.0).

Apparatus and Procedure

Prior to beginning the task, the subjects were fitted with the Applied Science Laboratories Series (ASL) 3100H helmet-mounted gaze control monitoring system.

Gaze data were collected with a mobile ASL 3100H Eye View monitor, a monocular corneal reflection system that measures eye line-of-gaze with respect to the helmet. A 30-m cord connected the optics of the helmet to the main computer yet allowed normal mobility of the subjects. Miniaturized optics, an illuminator, a solid-state sensor, relay lens, and a visor were mounted on the helmet, the total weight of which was 700 g. The eye was illuminated by a near-infrared light source, beamed coaxially with the optical axis of a solid-state camera (pupil camera). The result was a backlighted bright, rather than dark, pupil image. Both paths (illuminator and camera) were reflected from the visor, which was coated so as to be transparent in the visible spectrum but reflective in the near infrared.

The system measures eye line-of-gaze by using a miniature scene-camera mounted on the helmet; thus the measurable field of view is virtually unlimited. A cursor was superimposed on the scene-camera image to show the precise point of gaze. The measurement update rate was 60 Hz and the video rate was 30 Hz. The system had an accuracy of $\pm 1°$ visual angle and a precision of 1/2°. The transport delay was 3 fields of video or 49.45 ms. Following a brief calibration process of the gaze control apparatus, the response speed task was administered according to the procedure outlined in the Bruininks-Oseretsky Examiner's Manual [13]. Response Speed (subtest 6) assesses the ability to respond quickly to a moving stimulus. The subject places the preferred hand flat on the wall, next to the response speed stick. The tester holds the stick vertically against the wall and then drops the stick. The subject stops the stick as it drops, with the thumb of the preferred hand. The test score is the number that is at or above the tape strip when the stick is stopped. A point score is derived from 7 trials. One examiner administered the test to all subjects and each subject was tested on an individual basis.

Data Coding and Analysis

Six gazes per trial were coded: two just prior, one during, and three immediately following release of the response speed stick. All gazes were coded with reference to the initial movement of the stick. The release of the stick was easily determined from the videotape. All coding was derived from the video data, with one frame equal to 33.3 ms. A fixation was coded when the gaze was steady for 3 frames or more, or a minimum of 99.9 ms. A saccade was coded when an overt shift in gaze was observed from one fixation location to another.

Data were labelled as follows: gaze 1 and 2 occurred prior to stick release, 3 during release, and 4–6 inclusive were immediately following release of the stick. Each gaze was evaluated according to its type (fixation, saccade, other), duration (ms), and location (on stick, off stick, on thumb, or other).

Results

Response Speed Scores

The results of the response speed stick test were as expected, with high performers achieving a higher median score (10.2), than did their lower performing counterparts (4.3). The point score was obtained by ranking the scores for the complete seven trials from highest to lowest and recording the median score.

TABLE 1. Type and frequency of gazes observed.

Subjects	Trials coded	Type of gaze	Eye event[a] 1	2	3	4	5	6
High	34	Fixations	66.7	04.5	97.1	82.4	—	—
($n = 5$)		Saccades	19.0	90.9	02.9	08.8	92.3	40.0
		Other	14.3	04.6	00.0	08.8	07.7	60.0
Low	18	Fixations	56.3	12.5	77.8	66.7	18.8	—
($n = 3$)		Saccades	31.3	75.0	22.2	16.6	62.5	100.0
		Other	12.4	12.5	00.0	16.7	18.7	—

[a] All values are reported as percentages.

Type of Gaze Control

Table 1 summarizes the percentages of gaze observed across 34 (high) trials and 18 (low) trials. Whereas the complete data set would have been 49 (high) and 21 (low) trials, some trials were not codeable. Across all six eye events, fixations and saccades accounted for 81.3% to 100% of all gazes monitored. The term "other" referred to instances when the cursor disappeared from the videotape as the subjects blinked or when subjects shifted their gaze out of range.

The sequence of gaze saw fixations interconnected by saccades as expected. Eye events 1, 3 (release), and 4 were predominantly fixations, while 2 and 5 showed a greater percentage of saccades. This result was observed for both groups. However, Table 1 shows that the motor proficient group exhibited higher percentages of fixation than the low proficient group who tended to use a much higher percentage of saccades over the course of all trials. Consider, for example, the third eye event, which occurred as the stick was released, where 97.1% of all eye events for the high group were fixations. In contrast, fixations for the low performers occurred with a frequency of 77.8%. Similar differences were noted for the fourth eye event, immediately following the experimenter's release of the response speed stick. From this, it is clear that the high performers preferred to hold their gaze still at the moment of release and immediately after while the lower performers showed a greater tendency to shift the gaze just as the stick dropped.

Mean Duration of Gaze

Table 2 presents the mean duration (ms) observed per eye event, for each group. The largest difference in the mean duration per eye event between the two groups was observed for event three (at release) where the mean duration observed for the high performers (1027.9 ms) was almost three times greater than that of the low performers (390.5 ms). This high overall mean of the

TABLE 2. Duration of gaze per eye event.

Subjects	Trials coded	Type of gaze	Eye event[a] 1	2	3	4	5	6
High	34	Fixations	608.1	198.0	1057.0	254.6	—	—
(n = 5)		Saccades	82.5	90.8	66.0	99.0	75.0	82.5
Low	18	Fixations	403.3	495.0	572.8	203.5	132.0	—
(n = 3)		Saccades	99.0	101.8	82.5	88.0	112.2	55.0

[a] All values are reported in milliseconds.

motor proficient group is a reflection of the significant period of fixation (1057.0 ms) during event three. Not only were the high performers better able to hold their gaze steady at release, but they also tended to hold the gaze still for a much longer duration while the thumb was moving to stop the movement of the stick.

Location of Gaze

A great deal of information may be obtained by identifying the location of the subjects' gaze during performance of the task. Table 3 presents the frequency with which the subjects focused upon different locations within the testing environment. The high performers tended to be primarily focused on the response speed stick throughout the course of the first four eye events while the low performers tended to distribute their attention from the stick to their thumb and other locations. This difference is most apparent during the third eye event, during the release of the response speed stick. For high performers, 82.4% of all gazes were on the stick compared to 33.3% for the low performers. From this, it can concluded that the high performers tended to identify one locus potentially for their attention. However, the low performers were unable to do this. Their attention was distributed fairly equally on the stick (33.3%), off the stick (38.9%), and their own thumb (27.8%) loci.

TABLE 3. Percentage of gaze location by event.

Subjects	Trials coded	Location	Eye event[a] 1	2	3	4	5	6
High	34	On stick	71.5	68.3	82.4	79.4	30.8	40.0
(n = 5)		Off stick	19.0	22.7	14.7	17.6	23.0	20.0
		Thumb	09.5	04.5	02.9	03.0	46.2	40.0
		Other	—	04.5	—	—	—	—
Low	18	On stick	50.0	35.3	33.3	50.0	62.5	33.3
(n = 3)		Off stick	25.5	29.4	38.9	27.8	06.3	16.7
		Thumb	25.0	23.5	27.8	05.6	18.7	16.7
		Other	—	11.8	—	16.7	12.5	—

[a] All values are reported in percentages.

Discussion

The response stick test provides a measure of the child's ability to anticipate and respond to a moving visual stimulus. Each trial began with the auditory command "Get set" from the examiner who, after a short interval, released the stick. The child then clamped their thumb down on the falling stick as quickly as possible.

Normally, it takes an adult a minimum of 180–200 ms to respond to a visual stimulus. Response latencies for children tend to fall within similar bandwidths, while those for clumsy children tend to be slower [14]. These results were confirmed in this study with the low proficiency children being slower to respond to the falling stick than the high proficiency children. The current study also determined the gaze behavior of low and high performance children during the response stick task. Two gazes were coded just prior to the stick falling, one during and three during and after its fall, resulting in a constant data set of six gazes for all subjects.

High performers tended to use a higher percentage of fixations across all trials. Most noticeable were differences between the groups at the moment of release of the stick; the high performers exhibited fixations in 97.1% of all trials, compared to 77.8% for the low performers. These fixations also tended to be much longer, 1057 ms as compared to 572.8 ms indicating the use of a steady gaze maintained through to the final clamping motion of the thumb on the stick. Finally, at the moment of release, the location of gaze was on the stick for the high performers, while the distribution of location of gaze for low performers was equally likely to be on the stick, off the stick, or on their own thumb.

These results show clearly the use of a different form of gaze control by the low and higher performers. The critical question is the extent to which gaze contributed to the overall response stick scores. Does a steady gaze of long duration on target contribute to increased performance in tasks requiring a quick response to visual stimuli? Conversely, does a mobile gaze, one that is often off target, act as a detractor? Due to the lack of gaze control research it is difficut to answer this question, especially as it relates to high *vs* low performances in children. However, the gaze utilized by each group indicated that the highly proficient subjects were more likely to be focused (i.e., fixated) and therefore more likely to be processing information critical to performance of the task. The gaze location results additionally suggest that the location where the subject is looking at the time of stick release strongly influences the location of the eye line of gaze immediately thereafter. Moreover, the high subjects appeared to be focused on the stick, while the lows tended to distribute their attention over several stimuli.

Overall, the tendency for high performers to be fixated for longer periods of time on objects relevant to the task being executed is likely responsible in part for their superior performance. Perhaps successful motor performance (i.e., proficiency in movement) requires more attention to relevant environmental information and attentional abilities than has previously been cited. For example, Smith and Glencross [15] have suggested that abnormal clumsiness is associated with an information processing dysfunction which is specific to the proprioceptive modality. Significant differences in reaction time to proprioceptive cues were evident in their study comparing clumsy and normal children. They did not demonstrate any differences in reaction time to visual information processing. The present study suggests, however, that deficits in gaze control may exist between clumsy and non-clumsy children. Furthermore, gaze may play a crucial role in determining efficient response to visual stimuli.

Based on the limited evidence provided in this study, clearly further investigation is required. Traditional response speed (reaction time) studies provide visual stimuli which are stationary. Here the moving visual stimulus could have had the effect of increasing the sensory "load" at the stimulus stage which, in turn, magnified the differences in the reaction time.

In summary, the results of the present experiment extend the questions which surround our understanding of perceptual-motor deficits in clumsy children. There would be value in extending this approach to more complex visual stimuli associated with the control of more complex motor responses such as catching.

References

1. Olson RK, Kliegl R, Davidson BJ (1983) Eye movements in reading disabilities. In: Rayner K (ed) Eye movements in reading: perceptual and language processes. Academic, London, pp 467–479
2. Rayner K (1983) The perceptual span and eye movement control during reading. (pp 97–120) In: Rayner K (ed) Eye movements in reading: perceptual and language processes. Academic, London, pp 467–479
3. Fischer B, Weber H (1990) Saccadic reaction times of dyslexic and age matched normal subjects. Perception 19:805–818
4. Raymond JE, Ogden, Fagan NA, Kaplan BJ (1988) Fixational instability and saccadic eye movements of dyslexic children with subtle cerebellar dysfunction. Am J Optom Physiol Optics 3:174–181
5. Jones A, Stark L (1983) Abnormal patterns of normal eye movements in specific dyslexia. In: Rayner K (ed) Eye movements in reading: perceptual and language processes. Academic, London, pp 491–498
6. Pavlidis GT (1981) Sequencing, eye movements and the early objective diagnosis of dyslexia. In: Pavlidis GT, Miles TR (eds) Dyslexia research and its application to education. Wiley, London, pp 99–163
7. Schmid R, Zambarbieri D (1991) Strategies of eye-hand coordination. In: Schmid R, Zambarbieri D (eds) Oculomotor control and cognitive processes. North Holland, Amsterdam, pp 229–248
8. Zangemeister WH, Stark L (1982) Gaze latency: Variable interaction of head and eye latency. Exp Neurol 75:217–136
9. Guitton D, Volle M (1987) Gaze control in humans: eye-head coordination during orienting movements to targets within and beyond the oculomotor range. J Neurophysiol 58:427–459

10. Optican LM (1985) Adaptive properties of the saccadic system. In: Berthoz A, Jones M (eds) Adaptive mechanisms in gaze control: facts and theories. Elsevier, New York, pp 71–79
11. Fischer B (1987) The preparation of visually guided saccades. Rev Physiol Biochem Pharmacol 106:2–35
12. Hattie J, Edwards H (1987) A review of the Bruininks-Oseretsky Test of Motor Proficiency. Br J Educ Psychol 57:104–113
13. Bruininks RH (1978) Test of motor proficiency manual. American Guidance Service, Circle Pines
14. van Dellen T, Geuze RH (1988) Motor response processing in clumsy children. J Child Psych 29:489–500
15. Smith TR, Glencross DJ (1986) Information processing deficits in clumsy children. Aust J Psych 38:13–22

Why Do Lower Limb-Deficient People Have Difficulty in Downhill Walking? —Kinetics of Downhill Versus Level Walking

Shinji Sakurai, Markus Kuster, and Graeme A. Wood

Abstract. Downhill walking is a very important type of movement, especially from a clinical viewpoint, because many patients with lower limb deficiency tend to have difficulty during downhill walking rather than level or uphill walking. The purpose of this study was to compare downhill with level walking from a kinetic viewpoint. A new measurement system for joint kinetics of downhill walking was developed for this purpose. Twelve healthy subjects without lower limb or back musculoskeletal pathology were studied. For downhill walking a slope 6 m in length and with a grade of 19.3% was used. Joint kinetic variables such as joint forces, torque, and power were calculated for ankle, knee, and hip joints over the stance phase by combining anthropometric, kinematic, and ground reaction force data in link-segment model for both downhill and level walking. Peak extension torque and power absorption at the knee joint during the early stance phase were 2.2 times and 5.9 times larger for downhill walking (2.60 Nm/kgBW, 7.50 W/kgBW) than for level walking (1.16 Nm/kgBW, 1.27 W/kgBW), respectively.

Introduction

Great numbers of studies have been done on gait from many points of view. Although kinematic studies of level and downhill walking have been conducted, there are no published reports of kinetic analyses of joint reactions during downhill walking.

Downhill walking is a very important type of movement, especially from a clinical viewpoint, because many patients with lower limb deficiency tend to have difficulty during downhill walking rather than level or uphill walking.

The purpose of this study was to compare downhill with level walking from a kinetic viewpoint. A new measurement system for joint kinetics of downhill walking was developed for this purpose.

Methods

Twelve healthy subjects without lower limb or back musculoskeletal pathology were studied.

Three-dimensional kinematic data were collected during downhill and level walking using a video-based motion analysis system with a sampling rate of 60 Hz (APAS, Ariel Life Systems, Calif., USA). Step frequency was governed as 120 steps/min for both downhill and level walking using a metronome. The subjects performed both the downhill and level walking trials during the same recording session and using the data collection setup.

The experimental setup used for downhill walking is shown diagrammatically in Fig. 1. A wooden sloped walkway 6-meter length and with a grade of 19.3% was used. A frame made of aluminum was bolted over a Kistler force platform fixed down on the floor. The top surface of the frame was the same size as the force platform (0.4 × 0.6 m) and was set at the same plane as the walkway. The resonance frequency of the measuring system including the frame and the force platform was 270 Hz, 130 Hz, and 75 Hz in x, y, and z directions, respectively. The walkway and the force measurement system did not touch each other. To eliminate bouncing, the slope was strongly built and reinforced.

For the calculation of joint kinetics, the location of the center of pressure of the ground reaction force is necessary as well as the magnitude of the force. The location of the center of pressure on the surface of the frame (X and Z) was obtained by calculation using the measured force and force application point data. For calibration of the accuracy of the center of pressure of the ground reaction force, a rectangular grid at 0.1-m intervals was set up on the surface of the frame to apply forces at a known position (x and z). A stick with a sharp tip was used for applying force on to the surface. Force was applied dynamically in various direction. Across positions, the errors (X-x) and (Z-z) ranged from −3.9 to 6.0 mm. The average over 24 points of the absolute errors [X-x] and [Z-z] amounted to 1.2 and 1.6 mm, respectively.

For level walking, the same camera setup was used as for the downhill walking except for the slope and frame over the force platform.

In this study, analysis was limited to two dimensions (x-y plane). Joint kinetic variables such as joint forces, torque, and power were calculated for ankle, knee, and hip joints over the stance phase by combining anthropometric, kinematic, and ground reaction force data in a link-segment model [1].

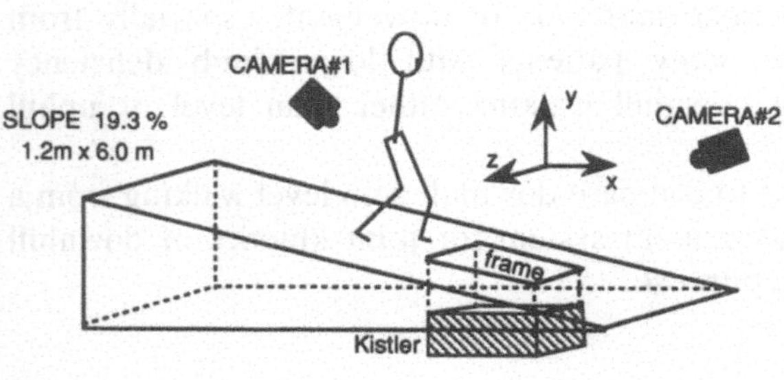

FIG. 1. Diagrammatic view of the experimental setup for downhill walking

Results and Discussion

Several values of kinematics and kinetics are compared between downhill and level walking and summarized in Table 1. The general shape and temporal occurrence of peaks in the ground reaction force, joint moment, and mechanical power curves at each joint for downhill and level walking were very similar; however, the magnitude of several selected values were remarkably different. Peak vertical ground reaction forces during early stance phase were found to be higher for downhill walking while the tendency was opposite during the late stance phase.

Since the body is being continuously lowered during downhill walking, the center of gravity of the body does not have to be lifted as vigorously as for level walking. This difference in mechanical work requirement is reflected in about 50% less muscle power generation at the ankle during push-off (1.60 W/kg for downhill and 3.10 W/kg for level).

Kinetic variables of the knee joint for downhill and level walking showed a different tendency from the ankle joint kinetics. Figure 2 shows a comparison

TABLE 1. Summary of comparison of maximum values of kinetic variables for downhill and level walking.

	Kinetic variable	Level	Downhill
GFR	Vertical—early stance	11.7 N/kg	16.1 N/kg
	Vertical—late stance	11.2 N/kg	7.9 N/kg
Ankle	Plantar flexion moment—late stance	1.14 Nm/kg	0.65 Nm/kg
	Power generation—late stance	3.10 W/kg	1.60 W/kg
Knee	Extension moment—early stance	1.16 Nm/kg	2.60 Nm/kg
	Power absorption—early stance	1.27 W/kg	7.50 W/kg
Hip	Extension moment—late stance	1.00 Nm/kg	1.30 Nm/kg
	Power generation—late stance	1.26 W/kg	1.80 W/kg

GFR, ground reaction forces.

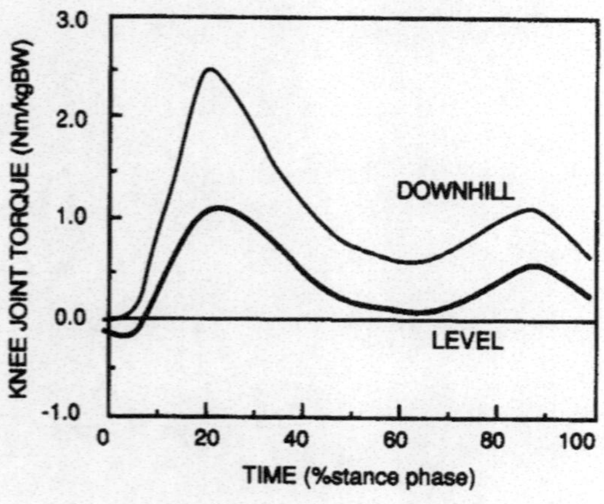

FIG. 2. Comparison of the changes of knee joint torque between downhill and level walking

of changes of joint torque at the knee joint during the stance phase between downhill and level walking. The curves represent the mean changes for downhill and level walking of 12 subjects normalized by the stance phase. Peak extension torque at the knee joint during downhill walking (2.60 N·m/kg) was 2.2 times larger compared to the value for level walking (1.16 N·m/kg).

The most remarkable difference between level and downhill walking occurs in the mechanical power requirement at the knee joint. The power absorption during the early stance phase was, on average, 5.9 times larger for downhill walking than for level walking (7.50 W/kg for downhill and 1.27 W/kg for level). This finding showed that much greater eccentric work was done on the knee extensor muscles during downhill walking than during level walking. This could be one of the answers for the question, "Why do lower limb-deficient people have difficulty in downhill walking?".

Acknowledgment. The authors would like to thank Mr. Rodney Robinson, Mr. David Oldland, Mr. Tony Roby, Mr. Alan Pearce, and Mr. Eric Harrison of the Department of Human Movement at the University of Western Australia for their devoted technical assistance.

Reference

1. Winter DA (1990) Biomechanics and motor control of human movement. Wiley and Sons, New York, pp 75–102

—Part IV—

Health and Physical Fitness

A Study of the Development Pattern of Physically Handicapped Students in Seoul

HYAE JA JEON and JONG SEOK KIM

Introduction

The best way to accommodate and integrate physically handicapped students is an important issue in an educational system that aims to provide equal opportunities for physical and intellectual development to all students during their school years. Since the recognition of problems related to this issue must be based upon a precise analysis of the current physical status of physically handicapped students, this study was conducted to assess the status of primary, middle, and high school students in Seoul who are physically handicapped.

Methods

Subjects

The status and physique of physically handicapped students who are in primary and secondary schools in Seoul were studied from October 1 to November 30, 1991. The educational statistics annuals and the average physical characteristics by the Seoul Education Office in 1990 were used for comparison.

Definitions of Physical Measurements

1. The definitions of height, weight, chest girth, and sitting height are subject to the students' physical examination guides developed by the Korean Ministry of Education.
2. Relative body weight: (weight/height) × 100
3. Relative chest girth: (chest girth/height) × 100
4. Relative sitting height: (sitting height/height) × 100
5. Rohrer index: $(\text{weight}/\text{height}^3) \times 10^5$
6. Kaup index: $(\text{weight}/\text{height}^2) \times 10^3$
7. Vervaeck index: (weight + chest circumference/height) × 100
8. Pelidisi index: $(\sqrt[3]{10 \times \text{weight}}/\text{sitting height}) \times 10^3$

Comparison with Physical Characteristics of Healthy Students

To determine the differences in physical growth, the characteristics of the handicapped were compared with healthy students (standard values). The standard physical characteristics were taken from the statistical annuals of the Seoul Education Office, which examined of a total of 6984 students including 3526 boys and 3458 girls 6–7 years of age (Table 1).

Results and Discussion

Values of Physical Measurement

Height

As shown in Fig. 1, the height of healthy boys increases linearly from 6 to 15 years of age and slows down thereafter, with an average of 171.06 cm at the age of 17. The height of physically handicapped students levels off between 9 and 10 years of age and becomes 165.9 ± 8.6 cm at the age of 17. In the case of girls, the average height increases linearly between 6 and 13 years of age, when it slows down and finally levels off at 158.77 cm at the age of 16. As with boys, the height of physically handicapped girl students also slows down between the age of 9–10 and it reaches 154.3 ± 65 cm at the age of 17. Girls' growth is more vigorous at the age of 9–11 than that of boys and, as referred to above, physically handicapped students' growth will be relatively slower between the age of 9–10. Although the reason is not clear, girls were 0.2–0.4 cm taller than boys at the age of 10–12 in the present study.

TABLE 1. Standard physical characteristics of students in Seoul[a].

	Height (cm)		Weight (kg)		Chest girth (cm)		Sitting height (cm)	
Age	M	F	M	F	M	F	M	F
6	119.37	118.31	22.41	22.52	58.51	56.80	66.38	65.66
7	124.79	124.01	25.20	24.52	60.73	59.45	68.88	68.30
8	130.02	129.60	28.28	27.50	63.09	61.66	71.04	70.68
9	135.14	134.37	31.32	30.75	65.19	63.83	73.55	73.02
10	140.38	141.35	35.64	35.58	68.74	67.26	75.70	76.36
11	145.66	147.28	39.99	39.44	71.77	70.24	78.17	79.03
12	152.85	152.48	45.30	44.48	74.48	74.75	81.48	82.63
13	159.54	156.16	50.13	48.76	77.54	77.52	84.82	84.67
14	165.81	157.37	55.60	51.17	81.20	79.23	88.40	85.61
15	169.55	158.95	60.05	53.14	84.84	80.36	91.04	86.47
16	170.88	158.61	61.14	53.73	86.26	81.12	91.89	86.27
17	171.23	158.70	64.18	55.49	88.09	82.10	92.38	86.46

[a] From the Seoul Education Statistical Annual, 1991.

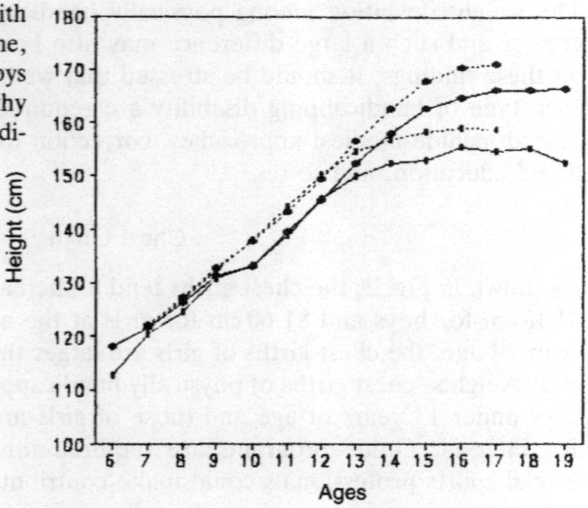

FIG. 1. Changes in height with age. Healthy boys (dashed line, closed circles); Handicapped boys (solid line, closed circles); Healthy girls (dashed line, bars); Handicapped girls (solid line, bars)

Body Weight

As shown in Fig. 2, the weight of boys increases linearly until the age of 15; that of girls increases until the age of 14, and both slow down thereafter. In the case of physically handicapped students, boys' weight essentially levels off at 13 years of age and reaches 57.5 ± 11.6 kg at the age of 16. Weight gain of girls starts to level off at 12 years of age. In other studies, the opposite pattern of growth between boys and girls was observed at the age of 8–10 years; however, the weight of healthy boys is heavier than that of girls at all ages. Even among physically handicapped students, the boys are consistently heavier than girls.

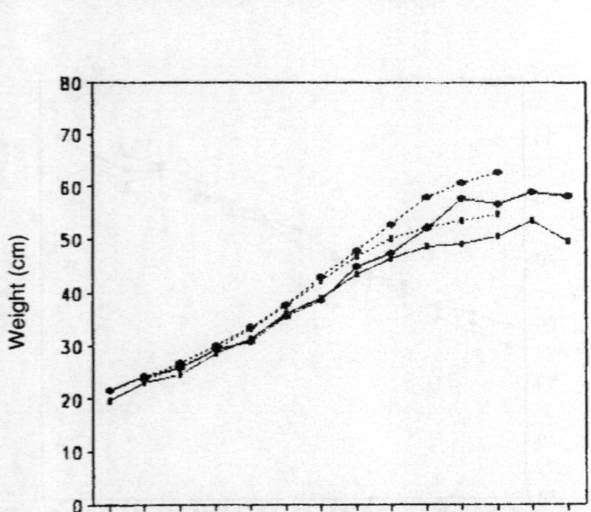

FIG. 2. Changes in weight with age

The weight deviation among physically handicapped students is considerably greater and such a large difference may also be found in body heights. Based on these findings, it should be stressed that well-designed services suitable for each type of handicapping disability are required for desirable growth. These should include medical approaches, correction for undersirable posture, nutritional education, and so on.

Chest Girth

As shown in Fig. 3, the chest girths tend to increase linearly with age and reach 87.18 cm for boys and 81.60 cm for girls at the age of 17. Between 11 and 14 years of age, the chest girths of girls are larger than those of boys. Contrary to body weights, chest girths of physically handicapped boys are larger the healthy boys under 13 years of age and those of girls are larger than in the observed age interval. Guide programs are required for balanced body growth, and special sports professionals could make contributions in various ways. Interest and participation in special sports in the daily life of the handicapped must be encouraged.

Sitting Height

As shown in Fig. 4, the sitting height of boys is 92.14 cm at the age of 17, and that of girls is 83.66 cm at the age of 13 with a more linear increase. The rate of increase slows down thereafter and reaches 86.36 cm at the age of 17. The growing pattern is similar to that of height. The growth of sitting height among physically handicapped boys slows down at the age of 9–10 years and reaches 87.9 ± 5.09 cm at 16 years of age; that of girls also slows down at 9–10 years and reaches 83.8 ± 5.1 cm at the age of 16.

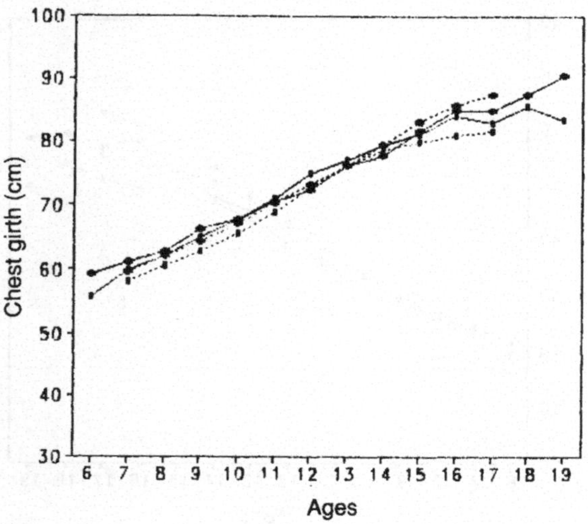

FIG. 3. Changes in chest girth with age

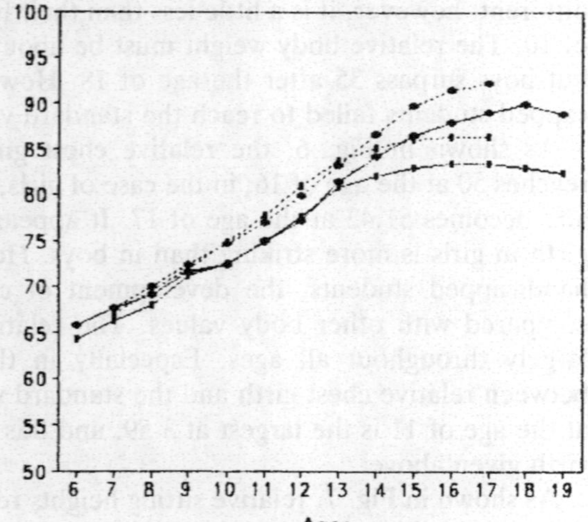

FIG. 4. Changes in sitting height with age

Index of Physical Growth

Relative Index

As shown in Fig. 5, the relative body weights of boys increase linearly to 36.53 at the age of 17, and of girls to 34.43 at the same age. That is to say, body weight is about one-fifth of height at 6 years of age and gradually increases to about one-third of height, and by such growth it seems that fruitful development is being made. Physically handicapped students are not significantly

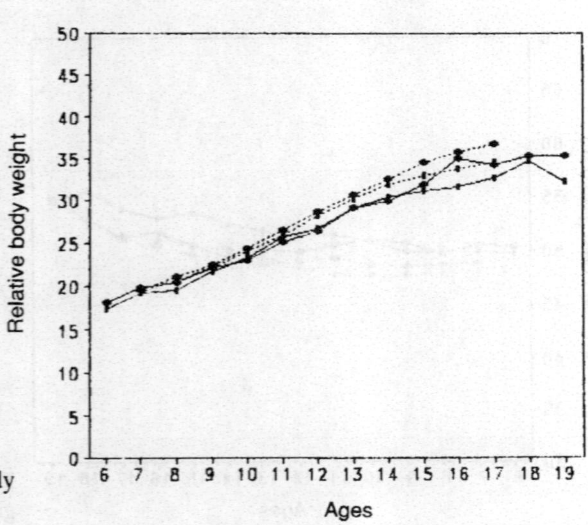

FIG. 5. Changes in relative body weight with age

different; however, it is a little less than their healthy counterparts after the age of 10. The relative body weight must be about 35 upon completion of growth, but boys surpass 35 after the age of 18. However, girls and physically handicapped students failed to reach the standard value.

As shown in Fig. 6, the relative chest girth remains at 48.19 or so and reaches 50 at the age of 16; in the case of girls, it increases from 13 years of age and becomes 51.43 at the age of 17. It appears that the development of chest girth in girls is more striking than in boys. However, in the case of physically handicapped students, the development of chest girth is closer to standard compared with other body values. The relative chest girth will also indicate largely throughout all ages. Especially in the case of girls, the difference between relative chest girth and the standard value at the age of 8 is 2.07; that at the age of 11 is the largest at 3.59, and this might reflect the results of chest girth given above.

As shown in Fig. 7, relative sitting heights reflect differences in the growth of the upper and lower parts of the body. According to the standard values, males are below 55.4 at the age of 7 and 53.23 at the age of 13, and this value does not increase thereafter. This indicates that the ratio occupied by sitting height becomes gradually smaller than body height, suggesting that the legs grow more rapidly than the upper part of the body during the ages studied. In case of females, it decreased from 55.28 at the age of 7 to 53.84 at the age of 11, and it falls behind that of males.

Nutritional Index

Rohrer's index (Fig. 8), the specific gravity of the human body, is usually assumed to be 1. In the case of boys, the standard value decreases from 1.31 at 7 years of age; however, that of girls gradually decreases after the age of 7 and

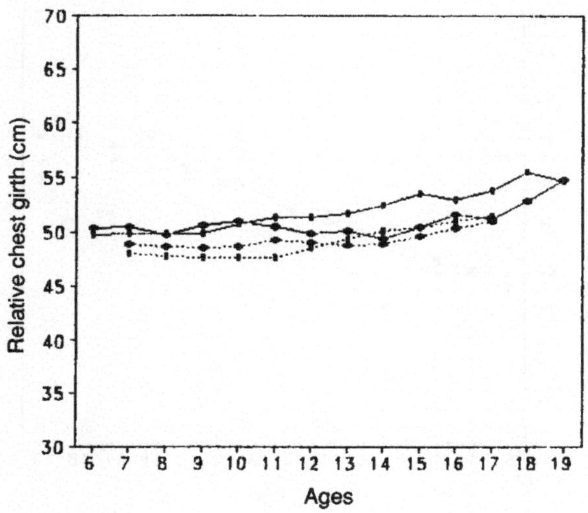

FIG. 6. Changes in relative chest girth with age

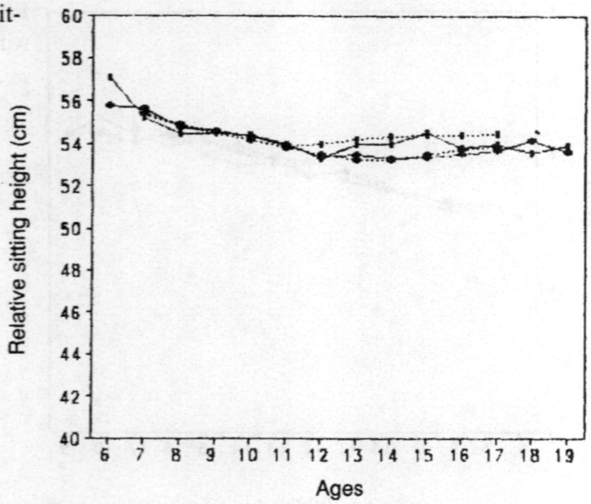

FIG. 7. Changes in relative sitting height with age

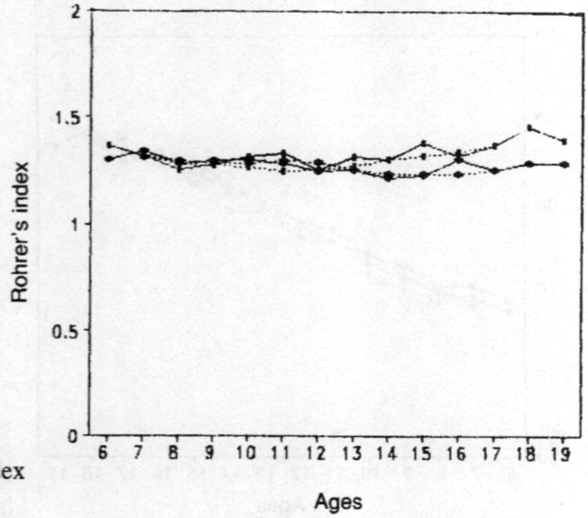

FIG. 8. Changes in Rohrer's index with age

reaches a minimum value of 1.25 at the age of 11–12. Thereafter, it increases considerably and, before the age of 13, that of boys is higher than girls.

Kaup's index (Fig. 9) is one of the nutritional indexes. If it is 2.0 or more, the growing condition is sufficient, and if it is less than 2.0 the growing condition is unsatisfactory. Among healthy students, the standard index value gradually increases with age and becomes 2.0 or more after the age of 14. In the case of physically handicapped students, however, it is somewhat lower than standard and reaches to 2.0 as late as 15–16 years of age.

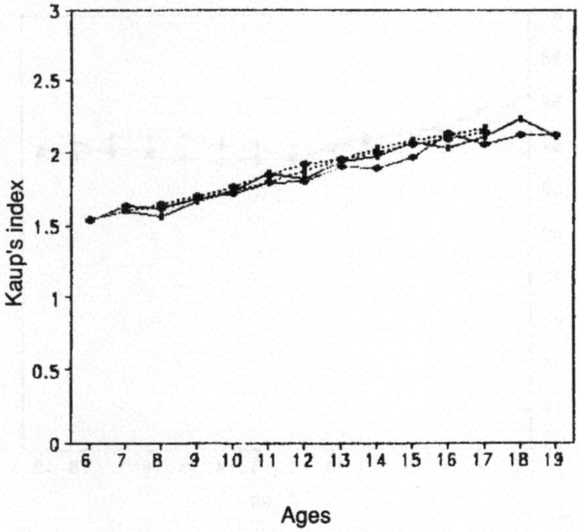

FIG. 9. Changes in Kaup's index with age

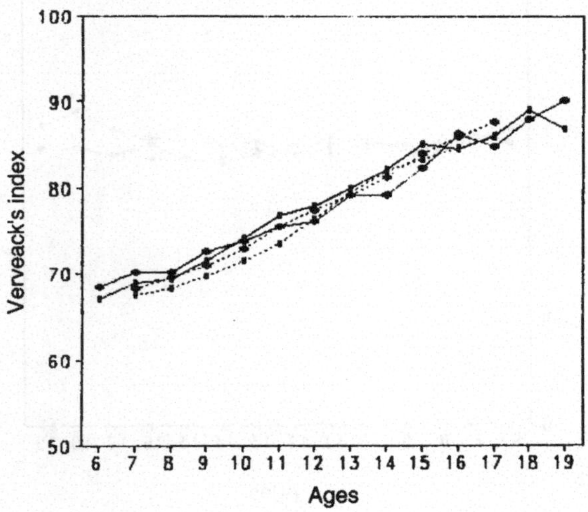

FIG. 10. Changes in Verveack's index with age

Verveack's index (Fig. 10) is regarded as normal when it is 90 or more. The standard value for boys is 68.34 at the age of 7 and for girls is 67.39 at the same age and will be 85–87 at the age of 17. Although the value does not reach 90, the nutritional condition seems to be good as the trend continues to increase. In the case of physically handicapped students, boys drop below the standard value by Verveack's value after 10 years, however, girls become higher than the standard value at the age of 1–3 years.

The Pelidisi index (Fig. 11) is about 100 for Western people. The standard value is lower than that in this study and is concentrated in the range 92–94.

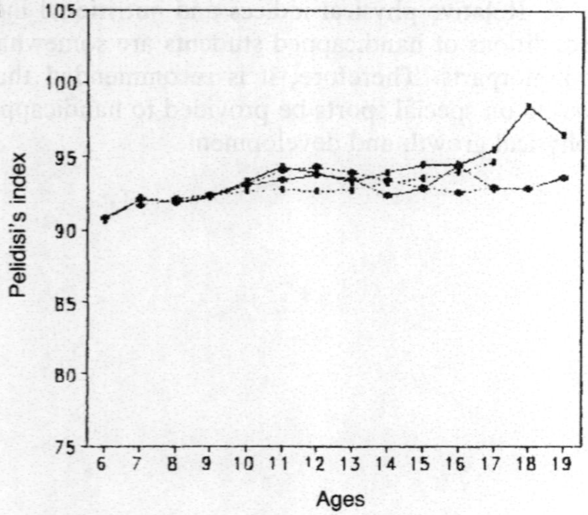

FIG. 11. Changes in Pelidisi's index with age

For boys, it is convex-shaped with age, with a peak at 12, whereas for girls, it keeps increasing.

Conclusions

This study was carried out to develop rehabilitation services through special sports and school health activies by analysis of the status and growing conditions of the physically handicapped student in regular public schools.

Physically handicapped students in regular schools were surveyed from October 1 to November 30, 1991.

The major findings are as follows:

1. The mean height of physically handicapped boy students was 165.9 ± 8.6 cm at the age of 17 years whereas of girls it was 155.0 ± 8.0 cm at the age of 16. This indicates that the relative growth rate slowed down after the age of 9–10.

2. The body weight of handicapped boys reached 57.5 ± 11.6 kg at the age of 16. That of handicapped girls reached 50.4 ± 8.8 kg at the age of 17, and their growth rates mainly slowed down around the age of 12–13. The standard deviation of height and body weight among the students is larger than among healthy students.

3. The chest girth of handicapped boys is 84.8 ± 6.4 cm at the age of 17; that of handicapped girls is 82.7 ± 5.5 cm. The development of height or weight of the handicapped is generally somewhat limited; only the chest girth shows greater development than the standard physique.

4. The sitting height of handicapped boys is 87.9 ± 5.0 cm at the age of 16 and of handicapped girls 83.3 ± 5.1 cm at the same age, and their growth rates both slowed down between the ages of 9 and 10.

5. Relative physical indices and nutritional indices also suggest that growth conditions of handicapped students are somewhat different from their healthy counterparts. Therefore, it is recommended that health education programs based on special sports be provided to handicapped students to promote better physical growth and development.

Effects of Aerobic Threshold Training on Aerobic Work Capacity in Hemiplegics

KAZUMI TSUKAGOSHI, MASARU IIDA, HIROSHI TAKAGI, NATU ODAJIMA, HARUMI OOKUBO, TOMOKO KIZAWA, and KYOKO TSUNEMI

Abstract. Twenty-six male hemiplegic patients participated in a 3-day/week, 16-week training program. Subjects were assigned to 3 groups of different training regimes. One group was assigned to walking, badminton, and table tennis playing at below the anaerobic threshold ($<$AT, $n = 10$). Another group was assigned to treadmill walking at the AT for 10 min in addition to playing badminton and table tennis (=AT, $n = 7$). The last was a control group which received no training (C, $n = 9$). Subjects were assessed for AT and $\dot{V}o_{2peak}$ before and after training, using a 30-s incremental protocol on a treadmill. After 16 weeks of training, significant improvement was observed in the AT ($P < 0.01$) and $\dot{V}o_{2peak}$ ($P < 0.05$) among the =AT after training compared with before training. The only significant change observed among the $<$AT was the increase in $\dot{V}o_{2peak}$ ($P < 0.05$). No significant change was seen in the C group. These results suggest that AT training in hemiplegic patients is effective in improving aerobic work capacity.

Introduction

It has been pointed out that many hemiplegics suffer from lower general endurance caused by long bed rest and reduced physical activities. Moreover, a drop in general endurance often affects their ability to look after themselves and take part in social activities. Therefore, it is important to increase their general endurance to promote smooth rehabilitation and enable them to resume an active social life.

The key to training for better general endurance is the setting of exercise intensity. In general, exercise intensity is expressed in relative terms against the maximum value of oxygen uptake (%$\dot{V}o_{2max}$) or heart rate (%HR_{max}). However, in the case of hemiplegics, it would be difficult to use the physiological index at the maximum exercise load as the standard. This is because many hemiplegics suffer from complications such as hypertension in addition to motor paralysis. Also, the degree of walking disorder from motor paralysis and the fall in endurance differ greatly from person to person. Therefore, the anaerobic threshold (AT), which can be measured at submaximal exercise levels, was used in this study as the exercise intensity standard to study the effect of training on hemiplegics.

Materials and Methods

Subjects

Twenty-six male hemiplegics who are or were institutionalized at the center participated in the study. They were divided into three groups based on training intensity: the first group who trained at the AT (=AT), and the second group who trained below the AT (<AT), and the third group who did not train (C). Descriptive characteristics of the subjects are presented in Table 1.

Measurement

An incremental load test using the treadmill was conducted before and after the 16-week training. The AT was measured from changes in the respiratory gas exchange during exercise, and the oxygen intake ($\dot{V}O_{2peak}$) was measured when the subjects stopped exercise. The protocol was as follows: after 4 min of warm-up at 5 m/min, the speed was increased every 30 s by 5 m/min until the maximum speed was achieved. While maintaining the speed, the incline was then increased every 30 s at a rate of 2%. The subjects used the paralytic side to hold on to the treadmill rail to prevent falling. Increase in the load was stopped when the subject complained of difficulty in walking, fatigue in the leg, or difficulty in breathing.

The gas analyzer (AE-280, Minato Medical Science, Tokyo, Japan) was used to measure the concentration and amount of the expired gas. The heart rate

TABLE 1. Physical characteristics and aerobic capacity of subjects.

	Age (years)	Height (cm)	Weight (kg)	Period from onset[a] (months)	AT (ml/min/kg)
<AT (n = 10)	47.9 ± 3.6[b]	166.2 ± 6.5	65.9 ± 6.7	19.3 ± 10.9	17.8 ± 3.4
=AT (n = 7)	44.8 ± 4.2	170.5 ± 5.6	67.9 ± 6.7	16.7 ± 8.2	16.2 ± 3.6
C (n = 9)	52.2 ± 3.6	162.5 ± 6.0	64.4 ± 8.0	55.6 ± 20.0	18.2 ± 2.8

Diagnosis
Cerebral hemorrhage (n = 19) Cerebral infraction (n = 7)

Br. Stage (L/E) III (n = 18) IV (n = 6) V (n = 2)

Involved side Right (n = 19) Left (n = 7)

AT, anaerobic threshold; C, control; Br, Brunnstrom.
[a] From onset of hemiplegia.
[b] Values are mean ± SD.

was measured with a telemeter electrocardiograph (DS-1044, Fukuda, Tokyo, Japan) using the chest bipolar leads method.

The AT was determined comprehensively by the rising point of $\dot{V}E/\dot{V}O_2$ without changes in $\dot{V}E/\dot{V}CO_2$, the soaring point of $\dot{V}CO_2$ and $\dot{V}E$, and the V-Slope method.

Training

The 70-min training was conducted three times a week for 16 weeks. Both the =AT and <AT groups participated in gait training, dribbling the ball, pulling the tire, badminton, table tennis, and other games. The treadmill walking at the AT for 10 min or longer was added to the =AT group. The heart rate of subjects during training was examined by hand and using a heart rate counter (Heart Rate Master, Canon, Tokyo, Japan).

Statistical Analysis

Statistical analysis was performed using *t*-tests for paired comparisons to evaluate differences between retraining values. A probability level of 0.05 was accepted as significant.

Results

Table 2 shows changes in variables of each group before and after training. Figure 1 shows changes of each group in AT. Significant improvement was identified in the time to complete the exercise, AT-$\dot{V}O_2$, $\dot{V}O_{2peak}$, and $\dot{V}E_{peak}$ among the =AT after training compared with before training. The only significant change identified among the <AT was the increase in $\dot{V}O_{2peak}$. No significant change was seen in the C group.

Discussion

No significant difference was identified among subjects in each group in terms of height, weight or AT-$\dot{V}O_2$ to weight prior to training. In other words, the aerobic work capacity level of subjects in each group was roughly the same. The initial AT-$\dot{V}O_2$ of each group was 1107–1184 ml/min. Davis et al. [1] measured and reported the pretraining AT of able males aged 43.0 ± 2.4 at 1361 ml/min. Although hemiplegics are reported to have lower aerobic work capacity [2], their AT was relatively close to that of able persons in this study. The use of the treadmill instead of a cycling ergometer for the loading device may account for the similar findings. Also, the relatively low degree of paralysis of subjects in the present study may have been a factor.

As a result of the 16-week training, significant improvement was identified among the =AT group, which combined ordinary training with 10 min of

TABLE 2. Comparison of pre- and post-training aerobic work capacity.

	=AT (n = 7)		<AT (n = 10)		C (n = 9)	
	pre	post	pre	post	pre	post
Weight	67.9	68.9	65.9	65.5	64.4	65.1*
(kg)	±6.7	±8.0	±6.7	±7.2	±8.0	±7.7
Exercise Time	7.7	9.0**	7.9	8.2	8.5	8.7
(min)	±1.0	±1.0	±1.1	±1.4	±1.6	±1.6
AT-$\dot{V}O_2$	1107	1268**	1166	1120	1181	1149
(ml/min)	±311	±273	±213	±230	±263	±264
AT-HR	109	108	114	111	116	111
(bpm)	±11	±15	±13	±17	±10	±12
$\dot{V}O_{2peak}$	1608	1821*	1504	1580*	1631	1632
(ml/min)	±552	±516	±263	±278	±385	±387
HR_{peak}	132	133	135	136	138	137
(bpm)	±15	±19	±17	±22	±11	±18
$\dot{V}E_{peak}$	58	64*	49	50	58	53
(l/min)	±11	±20	±9	±10	±18	±15

AT, anaerobic threshold; C, control; $\dot{V}O_2$, oxygen uptake; HR, heart rate; VE, minute ventilation.
* $P < 0.05$; ** $P < 0.01$.

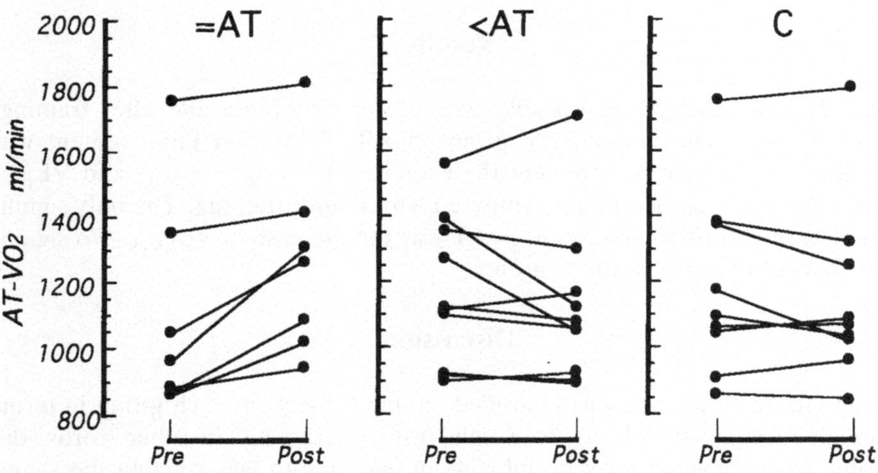

FIG. 1. Changes of oxygen uptake at anaerobic threshold (AT-$\dot{V}O_2$) in each group before (*pre*) and after (*post*) training

treadmill walking at AT, in the time to complete the exercise, AT-$\dot{V}O_2$, $\dot{V}O_{2peak}$ and $\dot{V}E_{peak}$. In the <AT group, a significant increase was observed only in the $\dot{V}O_{2peak}$. No significant change was seen in the C group, as expected. Many past reports on training based on AT or lactate threshold (LT) and their effects have identified an increase in AT and $\dot{V}O_{2max}$ [2–5] in training at or above AT

or LT. However, only a small number of reports have identified improvement in training at or below AT [3, 6]. This indicated that the exercise intensity of above AT is effective in improving aerobic work capacity. On the other hand, Gibbons et al. [3] reported an increase in AT and $\dot{V}o_{2max}$ among female college students who went through a 20-min training four times a week, at or below AT. This shows that, depending on the initial aerobic work capacity, exercise of even low intensity can be effective. This may account for the improvement in aerobic work capacity among subjects in the =AT and <AT groups in this study. In conclusion, the exercise stimuli in the AT intensity range must be continued for at least 10 min to improve the aerobic work capacity, particularly the AT of hemiplegics. The research also suggested the possibility of the use of AT in determining exercise intensity.

References

1. Davis JA, Frank MH, Wipp BJ, Wasserman K (1979) Anaerobic threshold alteration caused by endurance training in middle-aged men. J Appl Physiol 46(6):1039–1046
2. Tsukagoshi K, Iida M, Takagi H, Odajima N, Ookubo H, Kizawa T, Maruyama K, Yamanobe K (1993) Evaluation of general endurance in the hemiplegic patients, utilizing anaerobic threshold. Sogo Rehabiriteshon 21:585–591
3. Gibbons ES, Jessup GT, Wells TD, Werthmann D (1983) Effects of various training intensity levels on anaerobic threshold and aerobic capacity in females. J Sports Med 23:315–318
4. Henritze J, Arthur W, Robert LS, Kevin B (1985) Effects of training at and above the lactate threshold on the lactate threshold and maximal oxygen uptake. Eur J Appl Physiol 54:84–88
5. Ready AE, Quinney HA (1982) Alterations in anaerobic threshold as the result of endurance training and detraining. Med Sci Sports Exer 14(4):292–296
6. Sady S, Katch V, Freedson P, Weltman A (1981) Changes in metabolic acidosis: Evidence for an intensity threshold. J Sports Med 2:23–26

Endurance Training with an Adapted Device in the Visually Impaired

Hisakazu Saishoji and Hideo Nakata

Abstract. We designed a form of training in which the visually impaired walks while guiding himself or herself by following a rope affixed to a wall. The training is named "rope-guided walking" (RG-walking). The purpose of the present study was to examine the effects of endurance training using an adapted device on visually impaired subjects. The physiological exercise intensity of the 20-min RG-walking was 78.8 ± 6.7% peak$\dot{V}o_2$ and 72.5 ± 5.0% peak$\dot{V}o_2$ by the visually impaired subjects, and 69.3 ± 7.6% peak$\dot{V}o_2$ and 74.7 ± 4.05% peak$\dot{V}o_2$ by the sighted subjects. The visually impaired subjects peak$\dot{V}o_2$ increased by 12.4% from 30.6 ± 10.7 ml/kg/min to 34.4 ± 10.4 ml/kg/min by the fourth week of training. In addition, the four sighted subjects who participated in the training also showed an increase of 5.0% from 37.8 ± 4.7 ml/kg/min to 39.7 ± 3.3 ml/kg/min. By the eight weeks of training, the walking speed of the visually impaired subjects increased by 20.8% from 92.1 ± 15.3 m/min to 113.3 ± 14.6 m/min. As for the four sighted subjects, the walking speed increased by 28.2% from 107 ± 6.1 m/min to 137.4 ± 8.7 m/min. There were almost no changes with the control group. Consequently, RG-walking training is considered an exercise program that is effective in increasing the physical endurance of visually impaired persons.

Introduction

Because blind persons obtain only limited information from their surroundings, which limits their ability to exercise, it is assumed that their physical work capacity decreases. It has been reported that the physical performance of the blind is low [1]. If the exercise load is increased to make up for this lack of physical conditioning, an environment must be created in which blind people can exercise using their functioning senses.

According to Siegel et al. [2] and Sindou et al. [3], experimental research on the physical endurance of visually impaired subjects showed that exercise on a bicycle ergometer was effective in increasing the maximal oxygen uptake. Shapiro et al. [4] reported a statistically significant decrease in intraocular pressure during the ergometry performance on a bicycle ergometer. These findings suggest that adequate exercise may increase the physical strength and the effectiveness of rehabilitation treatment in the visually impaired. However, though bicycle ergometers have an advantage in that one can control the intensity of workload in his or her own pace, the movement of pedaling is rarely performed by visually impaired in their daily life. In addition, a relatively expensive piece of equipment is required.

Walking is an effective alternative to exercise on bicycle ergometers because it is a movement that visually impaired do every day. In this type of training, the visually impaired walks while guiding himself or herself by following a rope affixed to a wall. The training is thus named "rope-guided walking" (RG-walking).

The purpose of the present study was to examine the effects of endurance training using the adapted device on visually impaired subjects.

Methods

Subjects

The physical characteristics of the subjects are shown in Table 1. There were ten persons, including four visually impaired subjects (three men and one woman) between 18 and 67 years old living in a welfare center, and six sighted women, between 25 and 36 years old, working in a hospital affiliated with the center.

The sighted subjects were divided into two groups after a physical strength test (3-min distance walk, side step, grip strength, back strength, and standing long jump). Four were selected to participate in the training and the remaining two did not participate, for comparative purposes.

RG-Walking Device

Figure 1 shows the device used in RG-walking. It consists of a cotton rope 6 mm in diameter and 30 m in length and a polyvinylchloride (PVC) pipe 2.5 cm

TABLE 1. Physical characteristics of the subjects.

Group	Subj.	Age (years)	Gender	Degree of vision	Height (cm)	Weight (kg)	% Fat (%)	Peak $\dot{V}O_2$ (ml/kg/min)	Complication
Training	1. HS	18	M	M.M	165	45.0	10.0	44.5	—
Visually	2. EM	67	M	0.02	151	48.0	13.2	26.0	DM
impaired	3. HO	46	M	M.M	157	46.0	10.0	35.8	DM
	4. HK	47	F	M.M	153	76.0	51.2	15.9	FL HU
Sighted	1. ET	30	F	—	157	56.0	23.9	37.9	—
	2. HU	30	F	—	155	52.0	26.1	37.0	—
	3. TK	27	F	—	152	48.0	25.6	44.6	—
	4. UM	36	F	—	150	53.5	24.5	31.5	—
Control	1. MO	29	F	—	162	54.0	21.7	48.3	—
(sighted)	2. YK	25	F	—	157	47.0	24.5	37.4	—

MM, motus manus; DM, diabetes mellitus; FL, fatty liver; HU, hyperuricemia.

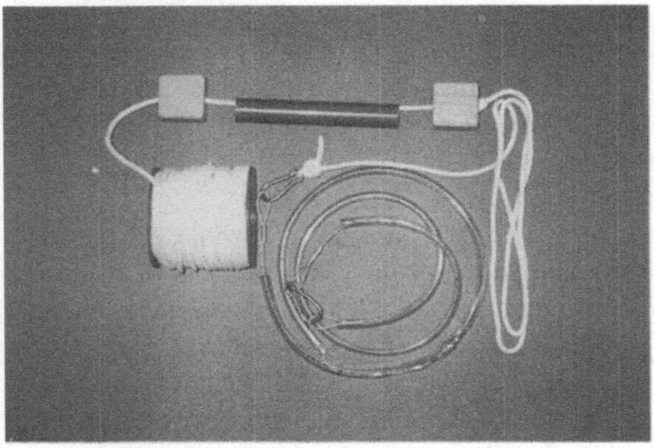

FIG. 1. Device used in rope-guided walking

in diameter and 17.0 cm in length. Each end of the rope, which is threaded through the pipe, is fixed onto a wall. Subjects slide the pipe along the rope as they walk. Subjects then walk back and forth along the length of the rope. So that visually impaired subjects can perceive the turning point, a wooden "stop-plate" is attached at the 0-m point (starting point) and at the 25-m point (returning point). The experimenter gives signals orally when a subject comes within 2–3 m of a stop-plate.

Experimental Design

Experiment 1

The oxygen uptake of the eight subjects selected above was measured during a 20-min RG-walking before training and then at the 4th week of training. The subjects' expired gas was measured once every 30 s with a respiratory mass spectrometer using a wireless transmission system. The data obtained were converted to 1-min values.

Experiment 2

The eight subjects did 20-min of RG-walking three times a week for 8 weeks. During the following 4 weeks, no training was done. As indexes of training effect, submaximal exercise by Modified Bruce protocol and the average walking speed during the 20-min RG-walking training were used.

Results

Experiment 1: Physiological Exercise Intensity

The physiological exercise intensity of the 20-min RG-walking, before and after training, as shown in Fig. 2, was 78.8 ± 6.7% peak$\dot{V}O_2$ and 72.5 ± 5.0%

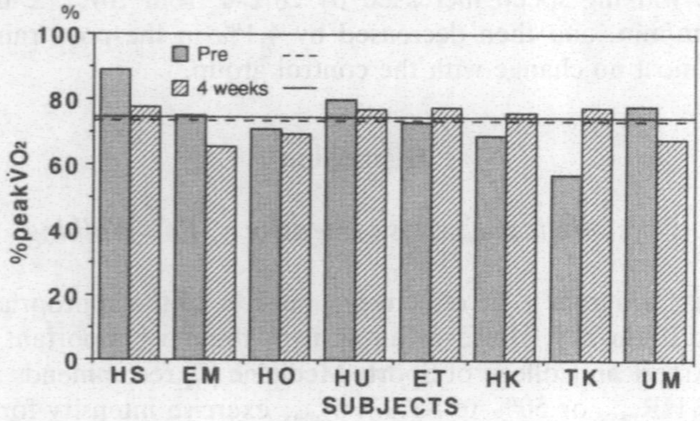

FIG. 2. %peak$\dot{V}O_2$ in each subject before and after training

peak$\dot{V}O_2$ by the visually impaired subjects, and 69.3 ± 7.6% peak$\dot{V}O_2$ and 74.7 ± 4.0% peak$\dot{V}O_2$ by the sighted subjects, respectively.

Experiment 2: Effects of Training

The results of experiment 2 are shown in Fig. 3. The visually impaired subjects' peak oxygen uptake increased by 12.4% from 30.6 ± 10.7 ml/kg/min to 34.4 ± 10.4 ml/kg/min by the 4th week of training. The four sighted subjects who participated in the training also showed an increase of 5.0% from 37.8 ± 4.7 ml/kg/min to 39.7 ± 3.3 ml/kg/min. The control group showed almost no change.

By the 8th week of training, the walking speed of the visually impaired subjects increased by 20.8% from 92.1 ± 15.3 m/min to 111.3 ± 14.6 m/min, but then it fell by 4.1% after the 4 post-training weeks. As for the four sighted

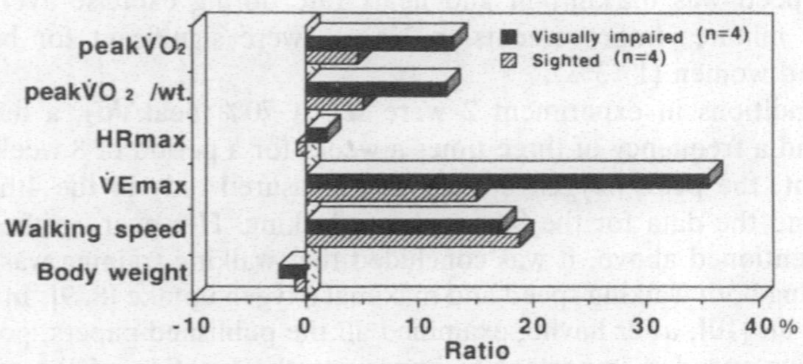

FIG. 3. Ratio of measured variables before and after training in visually impaired and sighted subjects

subjects, the walking speed increased by 28.2% from 107.1 ± 6.1 m/min to 137.4 ± 8.7 m/min, and then decreased by 4.1% in the post-training period. There was almost no change with the control group.

Discussion

Physiological Exercise Intensity of RG-Walking

For an exercise program to be effective, it must be of the appropriate intensity, duration, and frequency. However, intensity is the most important of the three [5, 6]. The American College of Sports Medicine [7] recommends a training of 60% to 90% HR_{max} or 50% to 85% $\dot{V}o_{2max}$ exercise intensity for 15–60 min, three to five times a week, as necessary to increase aerobic work capacity.

Exercise intensity of the 20-min RG-walking conducted in this study, as shown in Fig. 2, had an average value for all subjects of 74.0 ± 8.6% peak$\dot{V}o_2$ and 73.6 ± 4.7% peak$\dot{V}o_2$ at the pre-training and at the 4th week of training, respectively. It is thus proved that a 20-min RG-walking is in conformity with the necessary conditions mentioned above to improve aerobic work capacity.

Effects of Training

In Experiment 2, we examined how 20-min RG-walking of 70% peak$\dot{V}o_2$, performed as frequently as three times a week for 8 weeks, could influence the peak oxygen uptake and average walking speed during the test.

The peak oxygen uptake of the four visually impaired subjects and that of the four sighted subjects increased by 12.4% and 4.6%, respectively, by the 4th week of training. The increase in the average walking speed of the visually impaired subject and the sighted participants was 20.8% and 28.3%, respectively.

Jette et al. [8] studied sedentary 35- to 53-year-old men and women who walked 3 times per week for 12 weeks at speeds eliciting 60% $\dot{V}o_{2max}$. Mean walking speed was 6.2 km/min and heart rate during exercise averaged 132 beats per minute. Improvements in $\dot{V}o_{2max}$ were significant for both mem (9.7%) and women (17.3%).

The conditions in experiment 2 were set at 70% peak$\dot{V}o_2$, a duration of 20 min, and a frequency of three times a week, for a period of 8 weeks. In this experiment, the peak oxygen uptake was measured only in the 4th week of training and the data for the 8th week are lacking. However, in the previous studies mentioned above, it was concluded that walking training was effective in increasing both walking speed and maximal oxygen uptake [8, 9]. In addition, Porcari et al. [10], after having examined all the published papers, pointed out that walking speed is important in improving the function of the respiratory and cardiovascular systems.

Consequently, it can well be assumed that the peak oxygen uptake continued to increase until the 8th week as well as the average walking speed. RG-walking training is thus considered an exercise program that is effective in increasing the physical endurance of visually impaired persons.

References

1. Cumming GR, Goulding D, Baggley G (1971) Working capacity of deaf, and visually and mentally handicapped children. Arch Dis Childhood 46:490–494
2. Siegel W, Blomqvist G, Mitchell JH (1970) Effect of a quantitated physical training program on middle-aged sedentary men. Circulation, XL I:19–29
3. Sindou M, Kumagai S, Tanaka H (1987) Physical work capacity and effect of endurance training in visually handicaped boys and young male adults. Eur J Appl Physiol 56:501–507
4. Shapiro A, Wolf E, Feber I, Merin S (1983) The effect of physical activity on the intraocular pressure of glaucomatous patients. Eur J Appl Physiol 52:136–138
5. Shephard RJ (1968) Intensity, duration and frequency of exercise as determinants of the response to a training regime. Internationale Zeitschrift fuer Angewandte Physiologie Einschliesslich Arbeitsphysiologie 26:272–278
6. Sidney KH, Shephard RJ (1977) Maximum and submaximum exercise tests in men and women in the seventh, eighth, and ninth decades of life. J Appl Physiol 43:280–287
7. American College of Sports Medicine (1978) Quantity and quality of exercise for developing and maintaining fitness in healthy adults. Physician Sports Med 6:39–41
8. Jette M, Sidney K, Campbell J (1988) Effects of a twelve-week walking programme on maximal and submaximal work output indices in sedentary middle-aged men and women. J Sports Med Phys Fitness 28(1):59–66
9. Pollock ML, Miller HS, Janeway R, Linnerud AC, Robertson B, Valentino R (1971) Effects of walking on body composition and cardiovascular function of middle-aged men. J Appl Physiol 30:126–130
10. Porcari JP, Ebbeling CB, Ward A, Freedson PS, Rippe JM (1989) Walking for exercise testing and training. Sports Med 8(4):189–200

Aerobic Work Capacity of Quadriplegics and Exercise Intensity During the Twin-Basketball Game

YUKIHARU IKEDA, HISAKAZU SAISHOJI, TAKUMA MATSUMOTO, KENJI AKIHO, YUMIKO KUNIMI, MASAHIRO HOSHI, HARUNA ARAYA, and MASATO MIZUGUCHI

Abstract. The purpose of this cross-sectional study was to investigate the trainability of quadriplegics in terms of aerobic work capacity, and to investigate physiological exercise intensity during twin-basketball games. Ventilatory profile, alveolar gas exchange, and heart rate (HR) during the maximum effort arm-cranking exercise test was measured for ten male quadriplegic twin-basketball players (trained group) and ten male untrained quadriplegics (untrained group). HR was measured for seven subjects in the trained group during the twin-basketball game. The peak oxygen uptake ($\dot{V}O_{2peak}$) and peak HR (HR_{peak}) during the exercise test were significantly higher in the trained group (14.2 ± 1.9 ml/kg/min; 121.7 ± 18.2 bpm) than in the untrained group (10.3 ± 1.5 ml/kg/min; 101.5 ± 8.7 bpm). However, there was no significant difference between the two groups with respect to minute ventilation ($\dot{V}E$) and ventilatory equivalents for O_2 ($\dot{V}E/\dot{V}O_2$) at $\dot{V}O_{2peak}$ moment. The average HR during twin-basketball games was 112.5 ± 5.7 bpm, and the exercise intensity was 86.6 ± 7.9 $\%HR_{peak}$, and 75.1 ± 11.7 $\%\dot{V}O_{2peak}$. Thus, the trainability of quadriplegics in terms of aerobic work capacity was indicated. It is therefore concluded that twin-basketball is a sports activity that can effectively increase aerobic work capacity in quadriplegics.

Introduction

It is known that the aerobic work capacity of cervical cord-injured quadriplegics is low because they have few remaining functional muscles, low respiratory system function, and autonomic nervous system dysfunction.

This cross-sectional study investigated the trainability of quadriplegics in terms of aerobic work capacity. The aerobic work capacity of those who play wheelchair basketball (twin-basketball) regularly is compared with that of those who do not exercise regularly. The heart rate of quadriplegics during twin-basketball games was measured, and the exercise intensity was determined.

Methods

The subjects comprised ten male quadriplegics who regularly played twin-basketball (trained group), and ten male quadriplegics who did not exercise regularly (untrained group) (Table 1). All the subjects were quadriplegics with complete paralysis. The trained group comprised members whose levels of spinal cord functions (Zancolli's classification) [1] were C6B1 (one), C6B2 (three), C6B3 (two), C7A (three), and C7B (one). In the untrained group, there were C6B1 (two), C6B2 (four), C6B3 (two), and C8B (two). The trained group played twin-basketball three times a week, 2 h at a time. The subjects used a specially mounted electric-braked bicycle ergometer (Ergometer 829E, Monark, Sweden), so that they could use their arms to turn the ergometer for the incremental exercise test. The subjects remained in their wheelchairs, and the ergometer was placed on an adjustable-height table, which was set so that the crankshaft was at the same level as the subjects' shoulder joints. The ergometers' foot pedals were replaced with hand grips. Subjects' hands were fixed to the grips using bandages. The pedal rate was kept at 60 rpm for a 3-min warm-up period (0 W). Then the ramp load method was used to apply workload until the subjects became exhausted. The rate of increase of workload was 3 W/min for subjects who were C6B2 and below, and 4 W/min for those who were C6B3 and above.

Ventilatory profile and alveolar gas exchange during exercise was measured breath-by-breath with a respiratory mass spectrometer (Aeromonitor AE-280, Minato Medical Science, Tokyo, Japan).

The heart rate (HR) was measured with a telemeter electrocardiogram (Lifescope 6, Nihon Koden, Tokyo, Japan). The HR and oxygen uptake ($\dot{V}O_2$) per-minute values during the exercise test were recorded every 30 s. The highest values of HR and $\dot{V}O_2$ were determined as HR_{peak} and $\dot{V}O_{2peak}$. The HR-$\dot{V}O_2$ formula was obtained from the $\dot{V}O_2$ and HR measured at 1-min intervals.

TABLE 1. Physical characteristics and duration of twin-basketball experience.

Group[a] (n)		Age (years)	Weight (kg)	Level of function[b]	Duration from injury (months)	Twin-basketball experience (years)
Trained						
(10)	Mean	24.5	52.6	C6B1~C7B	76.4	4.0
	SD	2.9	9.6		38.8	3.3
Untrained						
(10)	Mean	25.0	56.3	C6B1~C8B	51.5	—
	SD	4.7	8.3		43.5	—

[a] All subjects are with complete paralysis. Mean ages, weights, and durations from injury were not significantly different between groups.

[b] After [1].

The wheelchair propulsion test was performed along a 25-m straight course set up in a corridor to determine how far subjects could propel themselves in 3 min. The subjects were instructed to propel themselves back and forth on the course as fast as they could.

HR for seven of ten subjects in the trained group, while playing twin-basketball, was measured with a portable heart rate memory device (Memory Mac, Vine, Tokyo, Japan) at 10-s intervals.

Results

The results of this maximum effort arm-cranking exercise test and the 3-min wheelchair propulsion test are shown in Table 2. Respiratory exchange ratio (R) of all subjects was over 1.0. The peak oxygen uptake ($\dot{V}o_{2peak}$), HR_{peak}, and the distances recorded for the 3-min wheelchair propulsion test were significantly higher among the trained group members than untrained group members. However, there was not a significant difference between the two groups with respect to minute ventilation ($\dot{V}E$) and ventilatory equivalents for O_2 ($\dot{V}E/\dot{V}o_2$) at $\dot{V}o_{2peak}$ moment.

There was a significant correlation ($P < 0.01$) between the 3-min wheelchair propulsion test results and $\dot{V}o_{2peak}$ values (Fig. 1).

The average heart rate during twin-basketball games was 112.5 ± 5.7 bpm, and the exercise intensity was 86.6 ± 7.9 %HR_{peak}, and 75.1 ± 11.7 %$\dot{V}o_{2peak}$.

Discussion

The $\dot{V}o_{2peak}$ and HR_{peak} of quadriplegics participating in these tests were similar to those found in other similar studies (Table 3). The results of the 3-min wheelchair propulsion test originally used by Hashitani et al. [2] to measure

TABLE 2. Comparison of physiological responses to maximum effort arm cranking test and 3-min wheelchair propelling distance.

Group (n)		$\dot{V}o_{2peak}$ (l/min)	$\dot{V}o_{2peak}$ (ml/kg/min)	HR_{peak} (beats/min)	$\dot{V}E^a$ (l/min)	$\dot{V}E/\dot{V}o_2{}^b$ (ml/ml)	R^c	3-minute distanct (m)
Trained								
(10)	Mean	0.800*	14.2**	121.7**	36.6	46.3	1.11	327.0**
	SD	0.215	1.9	18.2	12.4	7.5	0.08	51.7
Untrained								
(10)	Mean	0.602	10.3	101.5	30.6	60.9	1.09	215.3
	SD	0.105	1.5	8.7	10.5	25.6	0.69	65.2

* $P < 0.05$; ** $P < 0.01$ *vs* untrained.

[a] Minute ventilation at $\dot{V}o_{2peak}$ moment.

[b] Ventilatory equivalent for O_2 at $\dot{V}o_{2peak}$ moment.

[c] Highest values of respiratory exchange ratio during exercise test.

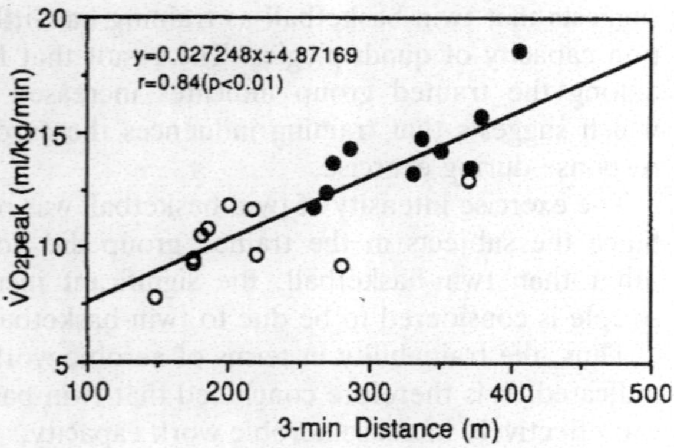

FIG. 1. Relationship between peak O_2 uptake and 3-min wheelchair propelling distance. *Solid circles*, trained (n = 10); *open circles*, untrained (n = 10)

TABLE 3. Comparison of $\dot{V}o_{2peak}$, HR_{peak} with quadriplegics in previous studies.

Authors	(year)	Subjects (n)	Mode of exercise	$\dot{V}o_{2peak}$ [a] (l/min)	$\dot{V}o_{2peak}$ [a] (ml/kg/min)	HR_{peak} [a] (beats/min)
Rhodes et al. [3]	(1981)	10	W/C Ergometer	0.91 ± 0.70	13.2 ± 1.7	97 ± 13.8
Lakomy et al. [4]	(1987)	2	Treadmill	1.15 ± 0.07	—	119 ± 8.5
Loan et al. [5]	(1987)	13	Arm cranking	0.80 ± 0.20	12.0 ± 3.3	109 ± 17.0
Figoni et al. [6]	(1988)	11	Arm cranking	0.66 ± 0.07	—	—
This study	Trained	10	Arm cranking	0.80 ± 0.22	14.2 ± 1.9	122 ± 18.2
	Untrained	10	Arm cranking	0.60 ± 0.11	10.3 ± 1.5	102 ± 8.7

W/C, wheelchair.
[a] Values are means ± standard deviations.

the endurance of patients with spinal cord injuries showed a significant correlation with $\dot{V}o_{2peak}$. Furthermore, because all the subjects' respiratory exchange ratio, which is one of the objective indices of maximum effort, was over 1.0, the method used in this study to apply workload was considered to be appropriate to measure quadriplegics' aerobic work capacity.

Generally, oxygen consumption of the active muscles, pulmonary ventilation capacity, and circulation function to active muscles are considered to be some of the factors that increase $\dot{V}o_{2peak}$. As for the increased oxygen consumption of active muscles, training effects can be expected to be the same in quadriplegics as in able-bodied persons. On the other hand, the fact that no significant difference was observed in $\dot{V}E$, and $\dot{V}E/\dot{V}o_2$, as an index of ventilation efficiency, at the $\dot{V}o_{2peak}$ moment between the trained and untrained groups, suggests that twin-basketball as training has little effect on pulmonary ventilation capacity of quadriplegics. The result that HR_{peak} was significantly higher among the trained group indicates increased circulation in active muscles, which suggests that training influences the cardiac autonomic nervous system response during exercise.

The exercise intensity of twin-basketball was relatively high for quadriplegics. Since the subjects in the trained group did not engage regularly in exercise other than twin-basketball, the significant increase of $\dot{V}O_{2peak}$ among these people is considered to be due to twin-basketball training.

Thus, the trainability in terms of aerobic work capacity of quadriplegics was indicated. It is therefore concluded that twin-basketball is a sports activity that can effectively increase aerobic work capacity.

References

1. Zancolli E (1975) Surgery for the quadriplegic hand with active, strong wrist extension preserved. Clin Orthop 112:101–113
2. Hashitani T, Hayashi T, Ando T (1989) Simple endurance measurement of the spinal cord injured. J Jpn Med Soc Paraplegia 2(1):70–71
3. Rhodes EC, McKenzie DC, Coutts KD, Rogers AR (1981) A field test for the prediction of aerobic capacity in male paraplegics and quadriplegics. Can J Appl Sports Sci 6(4):182–186
4. Lakomy HKA, Campbell I, Williams C (1987) Treadmill performance and selected physiological characteristics of wheelchair athletes. Brit J Sports Med 21(3):130–133
5. Loan MV, McCluer S, Loftin JM, Boileau RA (1987) Comparison of physiological responses to maximal arm exercise among able-bodied, paraplegics and quadriplegics. Paraplegia 25:397–405
6. Figoni SF, Boileau RA, Massey BH, Larsen JR (1988) Physiological responses of quadriplegic and able-bodied men during exercise at the same $\dot{V}O_2$. Adapt Phys Activity Quart 5:130–139

Assessment of Cardiovascular Regulation to Lower Body Negative Pressure in Bedridden Disabled Patients

Kumi Akataki, Kunihiko Itoh, Katsumi Mita, Nobuharu Suzuki, and Makoto Watakabe

Introduction

Disabled patients who are bedridden over a long period of time may be considered to be exposed to a continued weightlessness, similar to subjects in space flight. Cyanosis, edema, and cerebral anemia appear frequently in these patients simply because of passive orthostatic posture. These symptoms imply a deterioration in cardiovascular function which has occurred during the years of enforced bed rest in these patients. The purpose of the present study was to identify the cardiovascular response to lower body negative pressure (LBNP) in severely disabled patients during prolonged recumbency.

Methodology

Fifteen disabled subjects (20.3 ± 7.7 years, 21.2 ± 6.6 kg) and ten healthy volunteers (21.2 ± 2.4 years, 69.0 ± 9.4 kg) were included in this study. The disabled subjects were bedridden during the entire day for a period of longer than 5 years. LBNP was applied by enclosing the subject's lower body up to the iliac crest in an airtight box made of acryl. Air was partially removed from the box by a vacuum cleaner, and the pressure in the box was monitored by an aneroid manometer. After 5 min of supine rest for a control period, each subject underwent an LBNP test of −20 mmHg for 5 min. During supine rest and LBNP maneuver, heart rate (HR), stroke volume (SV), and mean blood pressure (MBP) were measured to investigate the hemodynamic response. Cardiac output (CO) was determined as the product of SV and HR. Plasma norepinephrine (NE) was used as a hormonal parameter associated with peripheral vasoconstriction. NE was determined in a blood sample from an antecubital vein at the end of the resting period and immediately after the LBNP test.

Results

In normal subjects, MBP showed a significant correlation between the resting control and LBNP test (Fig. 1). The solid line represents a linear regression

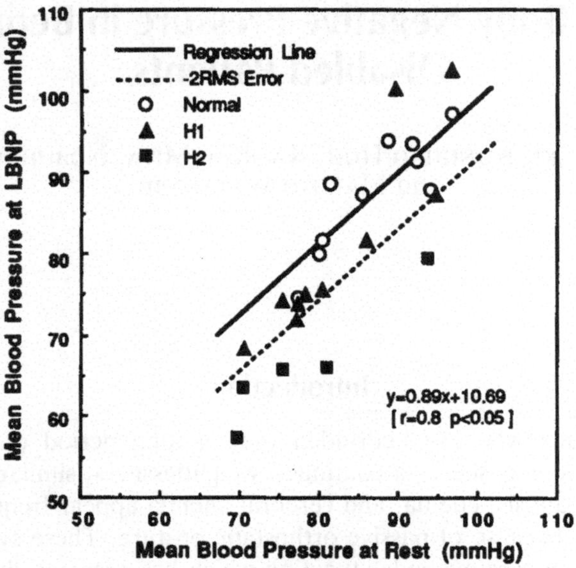

FIG. 1. Relationship of mean blood pressure (MBP) at rest and lower body negative pressure (LBNP) test. *RMS*: root mean square

and the broken line indicates a value twice the root mean square error (RMS error). Any response greater than the −2RMS error line is considered to represent the range of normal regulation. Based on this regression analysis in normal subjects, disabled patients were divided into two subgroups, H1 and H2. The H1 group consisted of the members whose blood pressure response was consistent with the normal group, and patients in the H2 group demonstrated a greater reduction in blood pressure, located below the −2RMS error line.

Resting Control

MBP at rest in the normal group was somewhat higher than in the disabled groups, however, no statistically significant difference among the three groups was observed (Fig. 2). SV and CO in both disabled groups were significantly less than in the normal group. This trend was also evident in the SV index and cardiac index (i.e., SV and CO normalized to body surface area). HR of 82 ± 8 beats/min in the H1 group and 105 ± 15 beats/min in the H2 group were both significantly higher than in the normal group, 71 ± 8 beats/min. The H2 group showed significantly higher plasma NE concentrations than the normal group. Although the resting NE concentration was higher in the H1 group, it was not significantly so. Generally, the difference of resting cardiovascular parameters between the normal group and each disabled group was greater in the H2 group than in the H1 group.

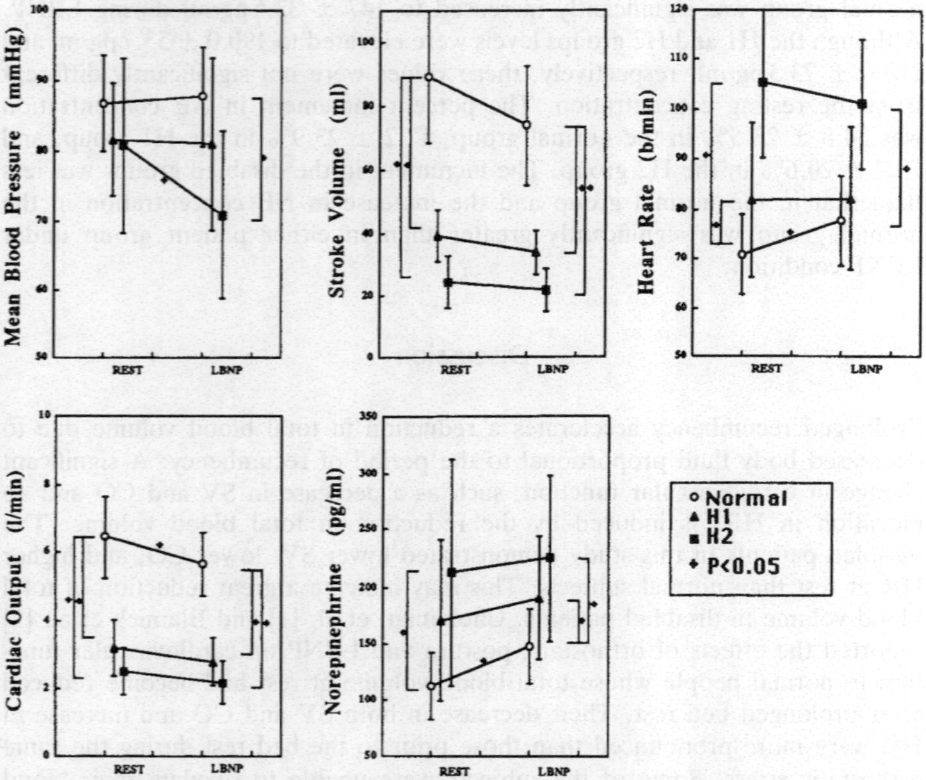

FIG. 2. Effect of −20 mmHg LBNP on MBP, stroke volume (*SV*), heart rate (*HR*), cardiac output (*CO*), and norepinephrine (*NE*) concentration

Lower Body Negative Pressure

The H1 and normal groups maintained a similar level of mean blood pressure during LBNP to that at rest (Fig. 2). MBP in the H2 group, however, decreased significantly by 9.9 ± 3.0 mmHg compared with the resting control. SV during the LBNP test was 73.8 ± 18.8 ml in the normal group, 33.6 ± 5.5 ml in the H1 group, and 21.5 ± 6.9 ml in the H2 group. Thus, disabled patients displayed a significantly smaller SV than normal subjects. A LBNP depression in SV of 15.5 ml was observed in the normal group. The decrease observed in the two disabled groups, however, was less than that in the normal group. The H1 and H2 groups demonstrated a decrease in SV of only 5.6 ml and 2.6 ml, respectively. CO responded to LBNP exposure similarly to SV as did SV index. HR in the normal group increased significantly during the LBNP test. The H1 group showed no distinct change in HR, and the H2 group demonstrated a slight but not statistically significant reduction. The NE concentration in the normal group was significantly increased to 147 ± 33.5 pg/ml during LBNP. Although the H1 and H2 groups levels were elevated to 190.0 ± 53.7 pg/ml and 225.0 ± 73.3 pg/ml, respectively, these values were not significantly different from the resting concentration. The percent increment in NE concentration was 34.8 ± 23.5% in the normal group, 17.2 ± 23.9% in the H1 group, and 10.7 ± 20.6% in the H2 group. The increment in the disabled groups was less than that in the normal group and the increase in NE concentration in the normal group was significantly greater than in either patient group under LBNP condition.

Discussion

Prolonged recumbency accelerates a reduction in total blood volume due to decreased body fluid proportional to the period of recumbency. A significant change in cardiovascular function, such as a decrease in SV and CO and an elevation in HR, is induced by the reduction in total blood volume. The disabled patients in this study demonstrated lower SV, lower CO, and higher HR at rest than normal subjects. This may indicate a great reduction of total blood volume in disabled patients. Chobanian et al. [1] and Blamick et al. [2] reported the effects of orthostatic posture and LBNP on cardiovascular function in normal people whose total blood volume at rest had become reduced after prolonged bed rest. Their decrease in both SV and CO and increase in HR were more pronounced than those prior to the bed rest during the same orthostatic stress. Some of the subjects were unable to regulate their blood pressure at the level of resting control. The authors concluded that their deterioration in cardiovascular function was caused mainly by reduced total blood volume due to prolonged recumbency. Disabled patients in the present investigation, however, showed a smaller decrease in SV and CO compared with normal subjects. Furthermore, they demonstrated either a smaller increase or a decrease in HR. These findings support those of Sather et al. [3]. Thus, a subject with low tolerance for LBNP exposure measured by onset of syncope demonstrated a smaller resting CO than an LBNP-tolerant subject. However, a range of presyncopal-limited LBNP exposures caused a similar reduction in CO in both low and high LBNP-tolerant subjects. This suggests that there is a limit to the reduction in CO due to increased orthostatic stress which is able to be tolerated without syncopal symptoms. In other words, high LBNP-tolerant people are endowed with a greater cardiac reserve in response to an increasing gravitational force. The disabled patients in this study already had an extremely small SV and CO at rest. Exposure to even a moderate LBNP of −20 mmHg produced a smaller CO than the limit reported by Sather et al. Conversely, the large decrease in SV and CO accompanying LBNP exposure was observed in normal subjects, however, these values during the LBNP test were still large compared with the limit value suggested by Sather et al. It may be noted also that the initial small SV and CO exhibited by disabled patients decreased their reserve for orthostatic stress and resulted in a smaller decreased response compared with normal subjects.

Chobanian et al. [1] and Blamick et al. [2] described a greater increase in HR during exposure to orthostatic stress after several weeks of bed rest compared with that before bed rest. The elevation in HR appears to be an exaggerated compensation for the decreased SV associated with prolonged recumbency. In contrast, Convertino et al. [4] demonstrated a smaller increase in HR after 30 days of bed rest than prior to recumbency in response to a LBNP challenge. They concluded that prolonged weightlessness significantly blunted the responsiveness and buffer capacity of the vagal barocardiac reflexes. The impaired baroreflex function appears to contribute to deterioration in cardiac regulation to orthostatic stress in addition to the accompanying decrease in blood volume. Our results in disabled patients are better understood in light of the above reports.

Peripheral vasoconstriction, which plays an important role in cardiovascular regulation, is also significantly affected by prolonged bed rest [4]. Peripheral vasoconstriction is activated by NE, a neurotransmitter released directly from sympathetic nerve endings in heart and vascular muscle. NE is released not only from the sympathetic nerve endings but also by sympathetic innervation of the adrenal medulla which responds to sympathetic excitement by releasing a large quantity of epinephrine and a small quantity of NE into the blood. These circulatory hormones bring about a generalized vasoconstriction. The measured plasma NE concentration thus reflects the total NE released from sympathetic nerve endings and the adrenal medulla. Wallin et al. [5] and Fiorica et al. [6] found a positive linear relationship between muscle sympathetic nerve activity and plasma NE concentration during progressive increase of orthostatic stress. The present study therefore used plasma NE concentration as a marker for the degree of vasoconstrictor activity during orthostatic stress.

Disabled patients demonstrated a smaller increase in plasma NE concentration to LBNP exposure compared with the normal subjects. These results suggest an attendant insufficient compensatory constriction of peripheral blood vessels in response to LBNP stress. Plasma NE concentration at rest was significantly higher in disabled patients than the normal control, suggesting a chronic sympathetic involvement which debilitates the effectiveness of the acute response to LBNP. This trend is consistent with Iwase et al. [7] who observed declining sympathetic nerve activity of aged people which they considered to be associated with orthostatic intolerance due to aging. The same reasoning may be applied to the ability of disabled patients in this study to respond effectively to LBNP stress. Thus we conclude that the cardiovascular deconditioning of disabled patients was caused not only by a decrease in total blood volume but also by impairment of baroreflex activity in the central and peripheral circulatory systems due to extremely prolonged recumbency.

Since it might be assumed that all the cardiovascular control mechanisms worked primarily to maintain blood pressure, disabled patients were classified into the H1 and H2 groups according to the degree of their change in blood pressure during exposure to LBNP. All the measured cardiovascular responses, as well as blood pressure in the H2 group, were inferior to the H1 group. This difference between the groups may be directly linked to their relative exposure to gravitational force during daily living. Most members in the H1 group were always supported in a sitting position either occasionally or regularly in their daily living while the H2 group received no orthostatic stimuli from a posture change. It is not easy to provide a disabled person with a regular orthostatic stimulus for any protracted period due to the severity of their illness and degree of their deformity and contracture. It has been established that regular LBNP exposure prevents body water loss induced by prolonged bed rest [8] and provides a potent stimulus to the baroreflex system [9]. LBNP is available to provide hydrostatic stress in a recumbent position and is thus a useful therapy for disabled patients who are unable to change posture independently and maintain an orthostatic position.

References

1. Chobanian AV, et al. (1974) The metabolic and hemodynamic effects of prolonged bed rest in normal subjecs. Circulation (XLIX):551–559
2. Blamick CA, et al. (1988) Leg vascular responsiveness during acute orthostasis following simulated weightlessness. Aviat Space Environ Med 59:40–43
3. Sather TM, et al. (1986) Cardiovascular dynamics associated with tolerance to lower body negative pressure. Aviat Space Environ Med 57:413–419
4. Convertino VA, et al. (1990) Head-down bed rest impairs vagal baroreflex responses and provokes orthostatic hypotension. J Appl Physiol 68:1458–1464
5. Wallin BG, et al. (1981) Plasma noradrenaline correlates to sympathetic muscle nerve activity in normotensive man. Acta Physiol Scand 111:69–73
6. Fiorica V, et al. (1985) Plasma norepinephrine, blood pressure and heart rate response to graded change in body position. Aviat Space Environ Med 56:1166–1171
7. Iwase S, et al. (1989) Effects of aging on muscle sympathetic nerve activity. Progr Biometeorol 7:73–78
8. Guezennec CY, et al. (1987) Fluid shifts and endocrine responses during lower body negative pressure and dynamic arm exercise. Aviat Space Environ Med 58:1066–1070
9. Victor RG, et al. (1987) Effects of lower body negative pressure on sympathetic discharge to leg muscles in humans. J Appl Physiol 63:2558–2562

Cardiorespiratory Adaptations of Heart Transplant Patients During a Constant Work Load Exercise at the Ventilatory Threshold

Alain Varray, Valérie Barthe, Jacques Mercier, Pierre Wintrebert, Bernard Albat, André Thévenet, and Christian Préfaut

Introduction

Cardiac transplantation has become a well-accepted and successful treatment for persons with end-stage heart disease. This is due to improvements in surgical techniques and overall management (donor and organ management), but also to the rapid progress in the treatment of rejection and medical complications after transplantation. The current survival rates reported on the basis of 1200 heart transplants are 81% for 1 year and 72% for 5 years [1]. Moreover, the patients also have an enhanced quality of life due to an increased functional capacity.

Several studies have been carried out to determine the specific problems that may be encountered in exercising transplant patients. The results have shown that these patients have a reduced maximal oxygen uptake [2–5] and increased lactic metabolism in response to exercise [6], leading to early exercise cessation. Others studies have shown that exercise training can improve their maximal oxygen uptake [6, 7]. The definition of a well-adapted training regimen, however, must include individually adapted training intensities. The validity of the ventilatory threshold has been confirmed for respiratory disease patients [8] and represents a highly suitable way for heart transplant patients (HTP) to ensure aerobic training [4]. The ventilatory threshold is closely related to the lactate threshold even in HTP [9] and it represents a particularly useful indicator for this population, given the early onset of anaerobiosis [6].

Generally, this technique requires close monitoring during the training sessions to control the adequacy of the real intensity used. The most common parameter used is the heart rate (HR). Unfortunately, the use of this parameter in HTP is questionable because of the surgical denervation. Indeed, during exercise the cardiac response is delayed [10]. During exercise training, the target HR would thus be lower than HR at ventilatory threshold. As the exercise adaptations have always been studied during incremental exercise, we have no indications concerning the cardiorespiratory adaptations of HTP during constant work load exercise. Without this prior knowledge, implementation of training at the ventilatory threshold could lead to inappropriate training intensities with important repercussions for the safety and efficacy of the training programs.

The purpose of this study was to analyze the cardiorespiratory adaptations during a constant work load exercise performed at the ventilatory threshold in heart transplant patients, and to specify the correction to be applied to the ventilatory threshold heart rate in order to ensure an adequate training intensity control.

Materials and Methods

Subjects

The study was carried out on seven orthotopic heart transplant patients who gave informed consent. The patients were New York Heart Association class IV at the time of transplant surgery, secondary to primitive cardiomyopathy ($n = 3$), or ischemic cardiomyopathy ($n = 4$). They were at 5.4 ± 1.4 months post-transplant (range 4–8) at the time of evaluation. All patients were receiving triple-drug immunosuppressive therapy (cyclosporin, azathioprine, and oral corticoids). They were 57.2 ± 1.9 years old (range 51–63) with the following anthropometric characteristics: body weight = 72.3 ± 2.8 kg, height = 172.7 ± 1.9 cm. None of these patients had yet been integrated into an exercise training program.

Measurements

The exercise testing was performed on a cycle ergometer (Ergometrics 900, Ergoline, Germany). Conventional 12-lead electrocardiographic recordings were obtained (Quinton 3000, Seattle, Wash., USA) while the subject breathed into a mouthpiece (dead space = 100 ml) connected to a CPX breath-by-breath respiratory analyzer (Medical Graphics, St. Paul, Minn., USA). Systolic and diastolic blood pressure levels were measured by a sphygmomanometer (Quinton 410). Cardiac output was estimated by the indirect CO_2 equilibrium rebreathing technique described by Collier [11] and Jones [12].

Protocol

Each patient performed two exercise tests at a 1-week interval. The first was an incremental exercise test (IT), and the second consisted of a 20-min constant work load exercise (CT) at the ventilatory threshold power output. For both the tests, the metabolic system was calibrated before testing for volume with a 3-l syringe. The gas analyzers were calibrated with a precision-analyzed gas mixture containing 12% oxygen, 5% carbon dioxide, and the balance of nitrogen. The oxygen uptake ($\dot{V}o_2$), CO_2 output ($\dot{V}co_2$), respiratory ratio (R), ventilation ($\dot{V}_E$), tidal volume ($\dot{V}_T$), and breathing frequency (f_b) were measured breath-by-breath and averaged over 30-s intervals. Blood pressure was recorded every 4 min.

Incremental Exercise Test

After a 1-min warm-up, the patients performed a 10-watt incremental exercise test. This test allowed us to determine the ventilatory threshold (VTh) according to the recommendations of Beaver et al. [13] and the symptom-limited oxygen uptake ($\dot{V}O_2$sl). Testing was terminated voluntarily by the subject or by the observation of established test-termination criteria [14].

Constant Work Load Exercise Test

The load used for this test was the load at which VTh had been measured during the incremental test. Its duration was 20 min, and cardiac output ($\dot{Q}$c) and stroke volume (SV) were measured in addition to the other variables. The $\dot{Q}$c and SV were assessed at rest, every 5 min during the exercise test, and at the 5th min of recovery.

Statistical Analysis

The data are expressed as the mean ± SEM (standard error of the mean). The cardiorespiratory variables were studied by a two-way ANOVA (time × subject). Mean comparisons were made by using the Tukey test [15]. The plateau values (during CT) were defined by the mean of the values recorded at the 16th, 18th, and 20th min, if their comparisons showed no statistical difference with a β error level at 0.01. These plateau values were compared to those recorded at VTh during IT with a paired Student's *t*-test. A stepwise regression analysis was used to predict the plateau HR (during CT) from the values of the VTh heart rate during IT, the anthropometric characteristics, and the post-transplant delay. The predictive character of the equation was then evaluated with the Bland and Altman procedure [16].

Results and Discussion

The two tests were very well tolerated by all the patients.

Incremental Test

The mean $\dot{V}O_2$ at the VTh was 821.3 ± 38 ml/min and the power exhibited was 42.8 ± 4.8 watts. The VTh heart rate was 104.8 ± 4.2 beat/min.

Constant Work Load Exercise at VTh

During the constant work load exercise at VTh, the HTP were able to reach a steady state for all the respiratory variables (Fig. 1) and the cardiovascular parameters after the 5th min, except for HR (Fig. 2). Indeed, HR increased during exercise more slowly but reached a plateau after the 6th min (Fig. 2). At 5 min of recovery, these values were not different from the pre-exercise values, except for HR, which was always significantly higher ($P < 0.001$).

The plateau values during the constant work load exercise were higher than those recorded at VTh during the incremental exercise test: 10.5% for HR ($P < 0.01$), 23% for $\dot{V}O_2$ ($P < 0.01$), 34% for $\dot{V}CO_2$, ($P < 0.001$), and 43% for $\dot{V}E$ ($P < 0.001$). The stepwise regression analysis showed that the HR plateau (HR_p) can be easily predicted from two independent variables: the HR at VTh (HRVTh in beat/min during IT exercise) and the time after transplantation (time in months). The predictive equation is the following:

$$HR_p = (1.38{*}HRVTh) - (3.18{*}time) - 11.81$$
$$r = 0.95$$
$$Syx = 6.03$$

The agreement between the real values of HR_p and those derived from the equation is presented in Fig. 3.

These results show that the HTP are able to perform constant work load exercise at their own VTh, and under these conditions, can reach a metabolic steady state within 5–6 min. The delay in cardiac adaptation during exercise and recovery is due to the cardiac denervation subsequent to transplantation [10]. It is striking to note that the delay in HR increase is compensated by a very sharp increase in SV, so that cardiac output reaches a steady state quite quickly, indicating very good adaptation to this kind of exercise. In the absence of vagal tone, the exaggerated HR values during recovery are compatible with the high level of blood catecholamines measured in normal subjects [17]. Indeed, the epinephrine levels are constant for 20 min of exercise and this may explain the HR plateau during steady state exercise [10, 18]. It is thus possible to obtain a steady state, even for HR, in HTP exercising at the VTh intensity. This point is of prime importance because it directly concerns the control of individualization of training. Nevertheless, in our study, the HR plateau values were always higher than those recorded at VTh during the IT exercise. A very safe solution to compensate this discrepancy was the discovery of a highly predictive equation which took into account the HR at VTh and the time elapsed between transplantation and exercise.

The practical utility of this equation is that the HR value to control during training sessions can be determined without a second exercise test. In addition, the interpretation of this equation is logical. Indeed, the equation gives an higher value for the HR at VTh but this is partially compensated by the time interval after transplantation. This is compatible with the studies Mercier et al. [19] and Labovitz et al. [20], who pointed out that the delay in heart rate

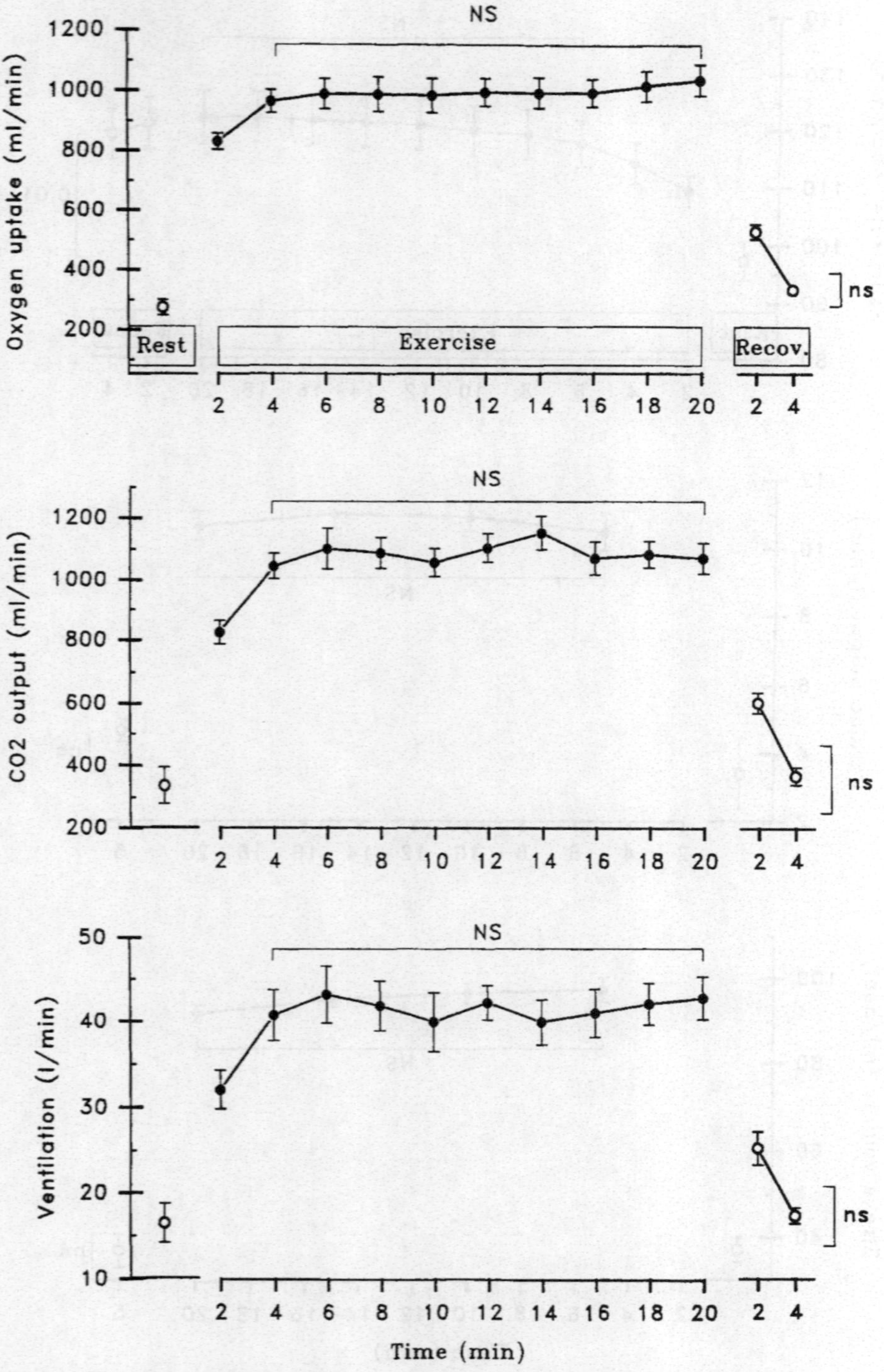

FIG. 1. Respiratory variables measured during the 20-min constant work load exercise. *Brackets* at the right of each figure represent the comparison between the resting value and the last value recorded during recovery

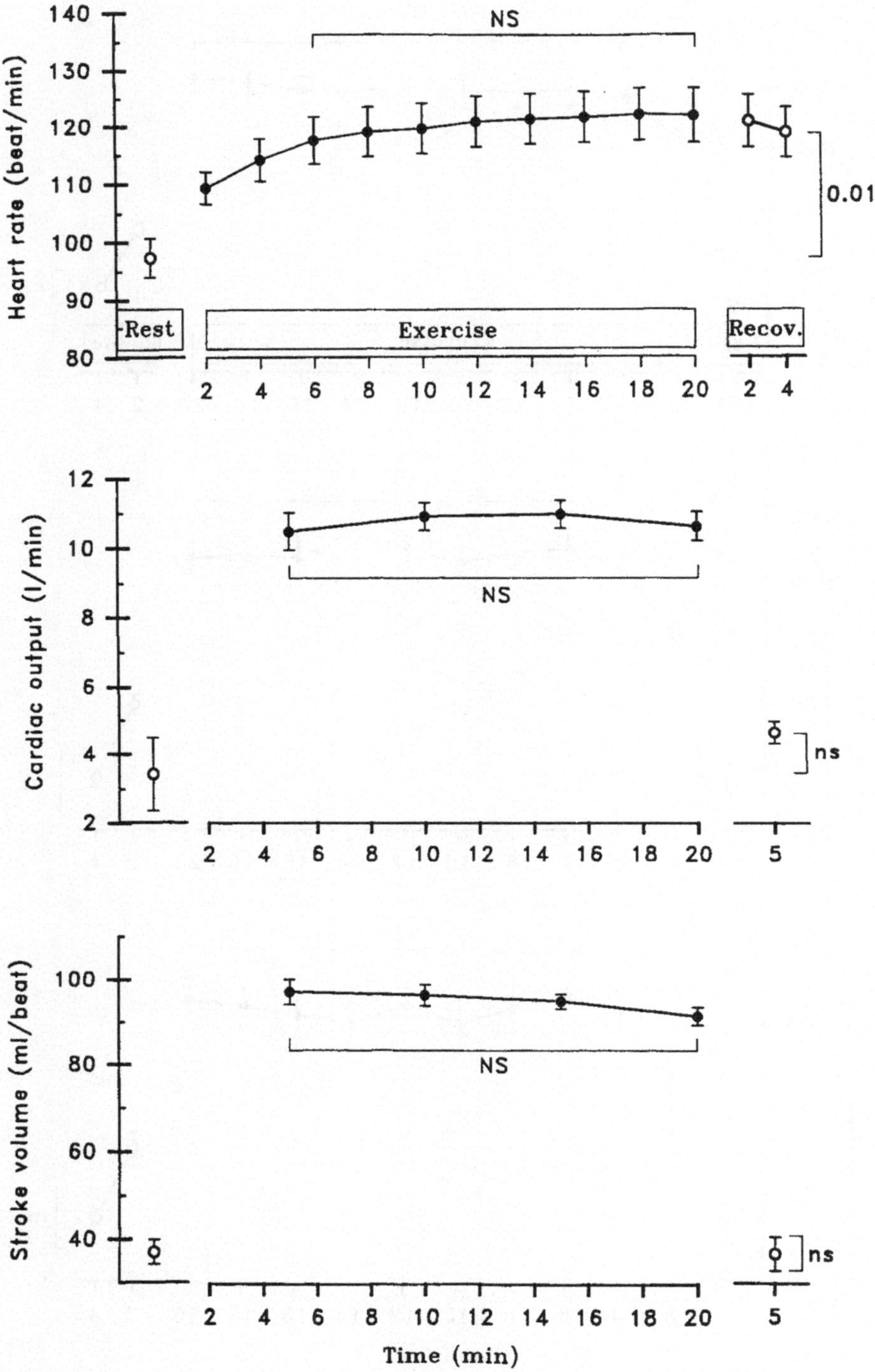

FIG. 2. Cardiovascular variables measured during the 20-min constant work load exercise. *Brackets* at the right of each figure represent the comparison between the resting value and the last value recorded during recovery. *NS*, not significant

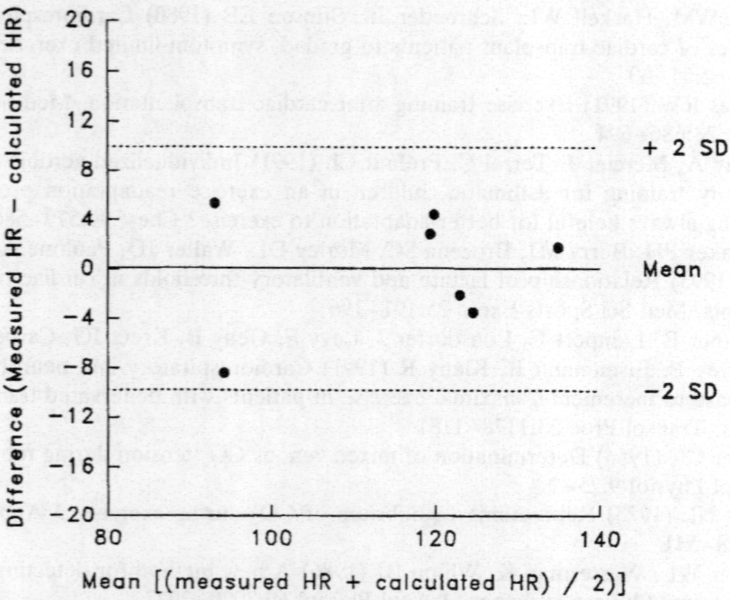

FIG. 3. Graphical presentation of the agreement between the measured plateau heart rate values and those derived from the predictive equation. *SD*, standard deviation

response decreases proportionally with the time after transplantation, probably due to increased myocardium sensitivity to circulating catecholamines [21, 22] or perhaps by partial reinnervation [23].

In conclusion, a steady state exercise at the ventilatory threshold is possible and very well tolerated in heart transplant patients. In addition, the heart rate to be reached during the training sessions can be accurately predicted from the heart rate at ventilatory threshold and the time elapsed since transplantation.

References

1. Kriett JM, Kaye MP (1990) The registry of the international society for heart transplantation: seventh official report—1990. J Heart Transplant 9:323–330
2. Cerretelli P, Grassi B, Colombini A, Caru B, Marconi C (1988) Gas exchange and metabolic transients in heart transplant recipients. Resp Physiol 74:355–371
3. Degre SG, Niset JM, Desmet JM, Ibrahim T, Stoupel E, et al. (1987) Cardiorespiratory response to early exercise testing after orthotopic cardiac transplantation. Am J Cardiol 60:926–928
4. Kavanagh T, Yakoub MH, Mertens DJ, Kennedy J, Campbell RB, Sawyer P (1988) Cardiorespiratory response to exercise training after orthotopic cardiac transplantation. Circulation 77:162–177
5. Mercier J, Ville N, Wintrebert P, Caillaud C, Varray A, Albat B, Thévenet A, Préfaut Ch (to be published) Influence of post-surgery time on transplanted heart rate in orthotopic cardiac transplant patients during exercise. Med Sci Sports Exerc

6. Savin WM, Haskell WL, Schroeder JS, Stinson EB (1980) Cardiorespiratory responses of cardiac transplant patients to graded, symptom-limited exercise. Circulation 62:55–60
7. Squires RW (1991) Exercise training after cardiac transplantation. Med Sci Sports Exerc 23:686–694
8. Varray A, Mercier J, Terral C, Préfaut Ch (1991) Individualized aerobic and high intensity training for asthmatic children in an exercise readaptation program: is training always helpful for better adaptation to exercise? Chest 99:579–586
9. Brubaker PH, Berry MJ, Brozena SC, Morley DL, Walter JD, Paolone AM, Bove AA (1993) Relationship of lactate and ventilatory thresholds in cardiac transplant patients. Med Sci Sports Exerc 25:191–196
10. Mettauer B, Lampert E, Lonsdorfer J, Levy F, Geny B, Kretz JG, Carpentier A, Haberey P, Eisenmann B, Kieny R (1991) Cardiorespiratory and neurohormonal response to incremental maximal exercise in patients with denervated transplanted hearts. Transpl Proc 23:1178–1181
11. Collier CR (1956) Determination of mixed venous CO_2 tension during rebreathing. J Appl Physiol 9:25–29
12. Jones NL (1973) Rebreathing equilibrium of CO_2 during exercise. J Appl Physiol 35:538–541
13. Beaver WL, Wasserman K, Whipp BJ (1986) A new method for detecting anaerobic threshold by gas exchange. J Appl Physiol 60:2020–2027
14. American College of Medicine (1986) Guidelines for exercise testing and prescription, 4th edn. Lea and Febiger, Philadelphia
15. Wilkinson L (1990) Systat: The system for statistics. Systat Evanston
16. Bland JM, Altman DG (1986) Statistical method for assessing agreement between two methods of clinical measurement. Lancet 8:307–310
17. Kjaer M, Christensen NJ, Sonne B, Richter EA, Galbo H (1985) Effect of exercise on epinephrine turnover in trained and untrained male subjects. J Appl Physiol 59:1061–1067
18. Quigg RJ, Rocco MB, Gauthier DF, Creager MA, Hartley LH, Colucci WS (1989) Mechanism of the attenuated peak heart rate responsiveness after orthotopic cardiac transplantation. J Am Coll Cardiol 14:338–344
19. Mercier J, Wintrebert P, Caillaud C, Varray A, Albat B, Thévenet A, Préfaut Ch (1994) Adaptations cardiorespiratoires à l'exercice du transplanté cardiaque: influence du délai post-transplantation. Science & Sports 9:1–8
20. Labovitz AJ, Drimmer AM, McBride LR, Pennington DG, Wilman VL, Miller LW (1989) Exercise capacity during the first year after cardiac transplantation. Am J Cardiol 64:642–645
21. Lurie KG, Bristow MR, Reitz BA (1983) Increased β adrenergic receptor density in an experimental model of cardiac transplantation. J Thorac Cardiovasc Surg 86:195–201
22. Yusuf S, Theodoropoulos S, Mathias CJ, Dhalla N, Wittes J, Mitchell A, Yacoub M (1987) Increased sensitivity of the denervated transplanted human heart to isoprenaline both before and after beta-adrenergic blockage. Circulation 75:696–704
23. Wilson RF, Christensen BV, Olivari MT, Simon A, White CW, Laxon DD (1991) Evidence for structural sympathetic reinnervation after orthotopic cardiac transplantation in humans. Circulation 83:1210–1220

Cardiorespiratory Function of Educable Mentally Retarded Boys

UI-SOO KIM and KWANG-HO KIM

Abstract. The purpose of this study was to see if educable mentally retarded (EMR) boys differ from intellectually normal boys in cardiorespiratory function. Nineteen EMR boys were matched with nineteen normal boys of comparable age. Both groups took the Balke/Ware treadmill test in which the protocol involved maintaining a constant speed of 3.4 mph while increasing the grade, from horizontal at the first minute, one degree each subsequent minute until the subject became exhausted. In analyzing the group test scores, it was found that the cardiorespiratory function of the EMR group was 20%–30% lower (HR $P < 0.01$, oxygen uptake ($\dot{V}O_2$) $P < 0.01$, $\dot{V}O_2$/kg $P < 0.01$, $\dot{V}O_2$/kg lean body mass (LBM) $P < 0.01$, $\dot{V}_E$ body temperature, pressure, saturation (BTPS) $P < 0.01$) than the normal group, but there were no significant differences in O_2 pulse and $\dot{V}_{E_{max}}$.

Introduction

Modern society has been continually preoccupied with different ways in which to improve the quality of life for all of mankind, and the handicapped also have a right to pursue happiness without discrimination and prejudice. A disability means that a person has a limitation that precludes certain activities. The number of people with inherited disabilities are about 4 in every 1000. According to a national sampling result in 1985 in Korea, there were almost one million handicapped people.

Demographically, the most common type of handicap is speech impediments, followed by hearing disabilities, mental retardation, and blindness. Because of the indifference of society, of the government, and of customs in Korea, special education is far behind the advanced countries.

While there are approximately 50 000 mentally handicapped youth, residential educational, and welfare facilities are in great demand, as with other handicapped groups. It is recommended that the mentally handicapped at schools with an intergrated curriculum be given careful consideration.

It is true that the handicapped not only have limited physical capacity compared with able-bodied students, but they also tend to avoid physical activity and become overweight. Therfore, physical education plays are important role for them. For effective physical education, after understanding their basic traits, teachers have to provide a properly intergrated educational program for the handicapped.

Cardiorespiratory function maximum oxygen uptake are useful parameters to evaluate each individual's physical strength. Cardiorespiratory function is a useful index to evaluate personal health such as cardiac endurance and aerobic ability [1]. Also, maximal oxygen uptake has not only been used as an index of physical activity, but provides valuable information about oxygen transportation and maximal aerobic ability [2]. Sharkey [3] insisted that maximal oxygen uptake ($\dot{V}O_2$) reflects uptake, transportation, and utilization of oxygen, and it is the best way to assess the physical strength.

Cardiorespiratory function plays a significant role for the mentally retarded as well [4–8]. Physical activity at a suitable level is essential for everyone, especially for the handicapped, while many retarded people require a physical strength of high level to compensate for decreased coordination and physical defects [9, 10]. They also require more opportunity for physical activity to improve physical strength than do normal people [11]. In Korea, this has been accomplished by studying maximal oxygen uptake in normal elementary school students, adolescents, youth, and in middle-aged people. However, there is little research on basic physical strength of the mentally retarded people.

The purpose of this study was to show whether educable mentally retarded (EMR) boys differ from normal boys in cardiorespiratory function, thus providing the basic data to develop a physical education curriculum for boys with mental retardation.

Methods

Subjects

Table 1 shows the characteristics of the subjects. Nineteen EMR boys were matched with 19 normal boys of comparable age.

Procedures

Figure 1 shows the detailed experimental procedures in a block diagram.

A period of orientation and adaptation was very important for mentally retarded subjects. Subjects were requested to arrive at the laboratory by 10 O'clock in the morning. The researcher explained the important information concerning the experiment for 20–30 min.

After a 10-min warm-up and treadmill adaptive period, the subjects were allowed to take a rest for 10 min.

At maximal exercise, each subject ran on the treadmill with a modified Balke/Ware protocol (Table 2). It was maintaining a constant speed of 3.4 mph

TABLE 1. Characteristics of subjects.

Group	IQ	Age (years)	Height (cm)	Weight (kg)	% body fat[a,b] (%)
EMR	61 ± 5.5	15.7 ± 1.2	162.4 ± 9.5	57.4 ± 13.0	25.3 ± 7.7
Normal	110 ± 8.2	15.4 ± 0.7	166.9 ± 6.2	54.7 ± 9.2	19.4 ± 5.9

EMR, educable mentally retarded.
[a] After [12]. Body density = $1.098 - 0.060\ l_{og\ \times(chest)}$.
[b] After [13]. % fat = (4.95/Body density) − 4.50 × 100.

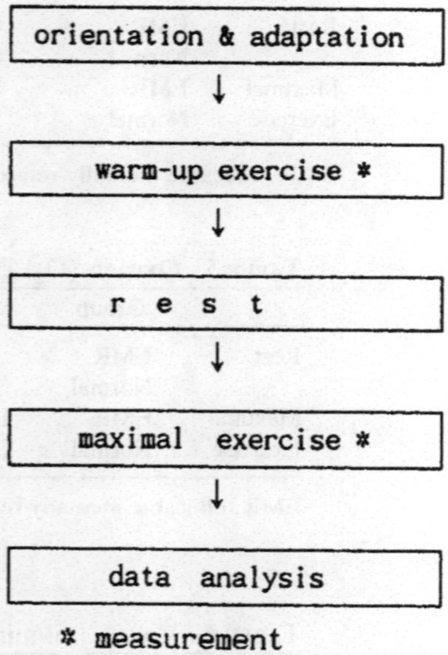

FIG. 1. Experimental procedures

TABLE 2. The modified Balke/Ware protocol (uphill walking).

	1	2	3	4	5	6
Time (min)	1	1	1	1	1	1
Speed (mph)	3.4	3.4	3.4	3.4	3.4	3.4
Degree (%)	0	1	2	3	4	5

while increasing the grade from a horizontal degree at the 1st min in 1-degree increments each subsequent minute until the subject became exhausted.

Heart rate, O_2 pulse, $\dot{V}o_{2max}$, $\dot{V}o_{2max}$/kg, and ventilation ($\dot{V}E$) were measured and analyzed during the maximal exercise as well as the rest period by a Sensor Medics Auto gas analyzer.

TABLE 3. Maximum heart rate (beat/min).

	Group	Mean	SD	*t*-test	df	*P*
Rest	EMR	83.16	9.92	0.26	36	0.793
	Normal	82.32	10.16			
Maximal	EMR	163.94	18.39	−5.62	35	0.000
Exercise	Normal	190.21	8.52			

EMR, educable mentally retarded; df, degree of freedom.

TABLE 4. Maximum oxygen uptake $\dot{V}o_{2max}$ l/min.

	Group	Mean (l/min)	SD	*t*-test	df	*P*
Rest	EMR	0.28	0.1	0.56	36	0.580
	Normal	0.26	0.1			
Maximal	EMR	2.06	0.53	−3.87	35	0.000
Exercise	Normal	2.63	0.36			

EMR, educable mentally retarded; df, degree of freedom.

TABLE 5. Oxygen (O_2) Pulse (ml/beat/min).

	Group	Mean	SD	*t*-test	df	*P*
Rest	EMR	3.29	1.05	0.65	36	0.520
	Normal	3.08	0.95			
Maximal	EMR	12.81	3.41	−1.47	35	0.151
Exercise	Normal	14.19	2.19			

EMR, educable mentally retarded; df, degree of freedom.

TABLE 6. $\dot{V}o_{2max}$ (ml/min/kg).

	Group	Mean	SD	*t*-test	df	*P*
Rest	EMR	4.75	1.55	−0.36	36	0.724
	Normal	4.96	1.89			
Maximal	EMR	36.05	6.36	−5.85	35	0.000
Exercise	Normal	48.86	6.93			

EMR, educable mentally retarded; df, degree of freedom.

TABLE 7. $\dot{V}o_{2max}$ (ml/LBM/min).

	Group	Mean	SD	*t*-test	df	*P*
Rest	EMR	6.55	2.29	0.54	36	0.589
	Normal	6.14	2.40			
Maximal	EMR	49.72	8.10	−3.84	35	0.000
Exercise	Normal	59.87	7.98			

EMR, educable mentally retarded; LMB, lean body mass; df, degree of freedom.

TABLE 8. $\dot{V}_E$ (l/min).

	Group	Mean	SD	t-test	df	P
Rest	EMR	9.92	3.39	−0.31	36	0.757
	Normal	10.37	4.90			
Maximal	EMR	57.88	14.31	−3.34	35	0.002
	Normal	74.55	15.98			

EMR, educable mentally retarded; df, degree of freedom.

TABLE 9. Ventilation VE($\dot{V}_{E_{max}}/\dot{V}_{O_{2max}}$).

	Group	Mean	SD	t-test	df	P
Rest	EMR	36.91	10.47	−0.83	36	0.413
	Normal	39.96	12.19			
Maximal	EMR	28.44	3.53	0.13	35	0.898
Exercise	Normal	28.28	4.19			

EMR, educable mentally retarded; df, degree of freedom.

Statistical Analysis

The statistical technique applied for data analysis was student's two-tailed t-test. The level of significance was set at 0.05.

Discussion

Previous studies have shown that the cardiorespiratory function of mentally retarded boys is 20%−40% less than normal boys [14]. We started this study under the assumption that the basic physical strength differs between the two groups, and this study focused on its cause and alternatives.

The low HR_{max} influenced cardiorespiratory function. McArdle and Magle [15] showed that mentally retarded boys, as evidenced by treadmill and bicycle ergometer experiments, is 20%−40% less than normal boys in HR_{max}. The main reason seemed to be due to fatigue of local muscles, low motivation, and the lack of muscular practice. Also, mentally retarded boys have lower HR_{max} due to the inherited disability, thus limiting maximal oxygen uptake.

In this study as well, at interview with subjects right after the experiment, all subjects with a low level of cardiorespiratory function said that the reason the exercise was ceased was not because they were out of breath, but due to lack of power to support their legs.

Additionally, we think it would be useful to evaluate mentally retarded boys before and after training to confirm its effectiveness.

According to our results, while maximal oxygen uptake per weight for the EMR group was 36.05 ± 6.36 ml/kg/min, maximal oxygen uptake per weight for the normal group was 48.86 ± 6.96 ml/kg/min, thus confirming the earlier findings that normal boys have a 20%–30% higher cardiorespiratory function than mentally retarded boys. These findings are consistent with the study of Burkett and Ewing [16] which showed that the maximal oxygen uptake of mentally retarded boys was approximately 27–43.6 ml/kg/min, even higher than the values reported by Burkett and Ewing [16] 30–27.6 ml/kg/min and Millar [17] 27.6 ml/kg/min using a treadmill.

Furthermore, our results are comparable with those of Coleman et al. [18], Yoshizawa et al. [19] by PWC 170, and Maksud and Hamilton [20] by bicycle ergometer.

As shown in Table 1, the fact that mentally retarded boys are comparatively overweight and their increased percentage of body fat is reflected in their maximal oxygen uptake per weight values. Some of the important factors that educators must consider when preparing an exercise regimen include: physical education, diet education, and physical curriculum.

On the other hand, there was no significant difference between the two groups in max O_2 pulse or in $\dot{V}E_{max}$. Although contrary to the stereotype that mentally retarded boys have lower than normal physical strength, it is possible for mentally retarded boys improve physical strength if they participate in a regular exercise program [21].

If only experimental results are used to judge cardiorespiratory function clinically, there is a chance that error will be introduced. Because boys with mental retardation have less muscular strength than boys without a handicap. There might be chance hurt the subjects with mental retardation if $\dot{V}O_{2max}$ is be taken at more than 70% level of the expected HR_{max} and expected VO_{2max}.

It has been well known that the treadmill is the best way to evaluate cardiorespiratory function of mentally retarded boys because the mechanical speed and pace can be controlled.

Although the physical strength of mentally retarded boys is far behind that of normal boys due to inactivity and the lack of motivation, endurance, and muscular strength, educators must provide a useful strategy for them.

Conclusions

On the basis of the results analyzed in this study, the following conclusions were reached:

1. A significant difference was observed in HR_{max} between the EMR group and the normal group.
2. A significant difference was observed in $\dot{V}O_{2max}$ between the EMR group and the normal group.
3. A significant difference was not observed in O_2 pulse between the EMR group and the normal group.
4. A significant difference was observed in $\dot{V}O_{2max}$/kg between the EMR group and the normal group.

5. A significant difference was observed in $\dot{V}O_{2max}$/LBM between the EMR group and the normal group.
6. A significant difference was observed in $\dot{V}O_{2max}$ between the EMR group and the normal group.
7. A significant difference was not observed in $\dot{V}E_{max}$ (ventilatory equivalent) between the EMR group and the normal group.

References

1. Astrand PO (1952) Experimental studies of physical working capacity in ventilation to sex and age. Einar Munkagaard, Copenhagen
2. Hermansen L, Andersen KL (1965) Aerobic work capacity in young Norwegian men and women, J Appl Physiol 20(3):425–431
3. Sharkey BJ (1984) The physiology of fitness. Human kinetics, Champaign IL
4. Andrew GM, Reid JG, Beck S, McDonald W (1979) Training of the developmentally handicapped young adults. Can J Appl Sport Sci 4:289–293
5. Beasley CR (1982) Physical of a jogging program on cardiovasular fitness and work performance of mentally retarded adults. Am J Mental Defic 86:609–613
6. Nordgren B (1970) Physical capacity in a group of mentally retarded adults. Scand J Rehab Med 2:125–132
7. Nordgren B (1971) Physical capacity and training in a group of young adult mentally retarded persons. Acta Paediatr Scand 217(Suppl):119–121
8. Rarick GL, Dobbins DA, Broadhead GD (1976) The motor domain and its educationally handicapped children. Prentice-Hall, Englewood Cliffs, NJ
9. American Alliance for Health, Physical Education, Recreation and Dance (1972) Special fitness test manual for mildly mentally retarded persons. Reston, VA
10. Winnick JK (1980) Project UNIQUE. State Unversity of New York, College at Brockport; BEH-US Office of Education
11. Eichstaedt CB, Wang P (1980) A study of physical fitness levels of mentally handicapped children and adolescents in Illinois. Illinois State University
12. Parizikova J (1961) Total body fat and skinfold thickness in children. Physical Culture Institute, Prague
13. Siri WE (1961) Body composition from fluid spaces and density: Analysis of methods. In: Brozek J, Henschel A (eds) Techniques for measuring body composition. Nat Acad Sci Res Council, Washington, DC, pp 223–244
14. Fernhall S, Tymeson GT, Webster GE (1988) Cadiovascular fitness of mentally retarded individuals. APA Quart 5:12–28
15. McArdle WD, Magle YR (1970) Physical work capacity and maximal oxygen uptake in treadmill and bicycle exercise, Med Sci Sports 2:118–123.
16. Burkett LN, Ewing N (1984) Max Vo_2 uptake on five trainable, mentally retarded high school students. In: Kroll W (ed) Abstracts of research papers presented at the Anaheim, CA, Convention of the American Alliance of Health, Physical Education, Recreation and Dance. American Alliance for Health, Physical Education, and Dance, Reston, VA
17. Millar AL (1984) The effect of endurance training on Vo_{2max} of Down's syndrome adolescents and young adults, Doctoral dissertation, Arizona State University
18. Coleman AE, Ayoub MM, Friedrich DW (1976) Assessment of the physical work capacity of institutionalized mentally retarded. Am J Mental Defic 80:629–635

19. Yoshizawa S, Ishizaki T, Honda H (1975) Aerobic capacity of mentally retarded boys and girls in junior high schools, J Hum Ergol 4:15–26
20. Maksud MG, Hamilton LH (1974) Physiological responses of EMR children to strenuous exercise. Am J Mental Defic 79:32–38
21. Schurrer R, Weltman A, Brammerl H (1985) Effects of physical training on cardiovascular fitness and behavior patterns of mentally retarded adults. Am J Mental Defic 90:167–170

Adaptation in Students with Down Syndrome: An Experimental Study on the Trainability of Strength and Power

Otto J. Schantz

Abstract. Based on an ecological model of adaptation, the development of physical strength and power is evaluated as an educational objective for mentally retarded persons with Down syndrome (DS) using the approach of the theory of sports training. The purpose of this study was to compare different kinds of strength and power of students with DS and trainable mentally retarded (TMR) peers without DS, and to compare and evaluate the feasibility and effects of strength training in school in these 2 groups. 115 students (CA 12 to 18) participated in this experiment, which was designed to have a high ecological validity. The results show differences in strength and power between the 2 groups, depending on sex and the kind of skill. Similar progress was noted in both groups; however, differences in some tasks diminished significantly between the 2 samples. The implications for curriculum development are discussed.

Introduction

Different kinds of physical strength and power are important for motor skills in daily and professional life, but particularly for physical education and sports. Physical strength is a condition indispensable to movement and exercise. Consequently, the improvement of physical strength and power figures in nearly all curricula for mentally retarded persons. The main purpose of my study was to evaluate the capacity of adaptation in students with Down syndrome (DS), especially the effects of strength training under normal conditions in school.

Review of Related Literature

Numerous studies show the influence of etiology on motor performances of mentally retarded people (for a review of literature see [1–4]). In general, persons with DS show weaker performances than other handicapped people [5, 6]. Low muscle tone and low strength of children and adults with DS have been reported [7–9]. Sex differences seem to be similar in nonretarded and in retarded populations [10]. Experiments concerning the capacities of adaptation or the trainability of mentally retarded persons are rare, especially for trainable or profoundly mentally retarded people [11]. Most of these studies lack methodological rigor or external validity [12, 13]. Few experiments deal with the trainability of muscular strength of people with DS. Weber [14] studied the effects of two different training programs on the muscular strength of 15 DS boys and girls aged between 13 and 18 years. At the conclusion of a 6-week treatment, groups enrolled in a circuit strength exercise program showed significantly greater gains in muscular strength than experimental groups involved in circuit weight training. No research dealing with the trainability of DS subjects compared to retarded without DS has been done. Skrobak-Kaczynski and Vavik [15] confirms that the strength of mentally retarded persons with DS improves after training.

Hypotheses

1. The levels of maximal strength, power, and muscular endurance of mentally retarded students with DS are inferior to those of the nonretarded. Depending on the kind of strength and skill, the range of these differences is more or less distinct.
2. The strength levels of mentally retarded students with DS are inferior to those of retarded students with other etiologies.
3. The physical strength of mentally retarded students with DS can be improved under regular school conditions.
4. The improvement of mentally retarded students with DS is similar to that of their retarded peers.

Methods

Motor and biomechanical tests were used to measure these following categories of strength: (1) adapted 20-m-dash, (2) modified sit-ups, (3) modified standing broad jump, and (4) modified medicine ball throw.

All tests were modified and adapted to be comprehensible and feasible for trainable mentally retarded students. Especially, the specific motivation of retarded persons was taken into consideration. Maximal strength, explosive strength, and "starting power" were measured by biomechanical tests [16] with the aid of a special computer-controlled system developed by the author. A strength-time curve was recorded during a maximal and explosive voluntary contraction against an immovable resistance. To increase motivation, a column of polychromatic lights indicated the changes of strength. The following six parameters were measured:

(1–2) Maximal static strength of elbow and knee extension, defined by the peak of the recorded time-strength curve

(3–4) Explosive strength of elbow and knee extension, defined by maximal power
(5–6) "Starting power" of elbow and knee extension, defined as the force at 30 ms after beginning of contraction

The intraclass reliability coefficients of these tests varied between $R_{tt} = 0.87$ and $R_{tt} = 0.98$.

Subjects

The total sample consisted of 136 retarded male (61) and female (54) students attending special schools. Of these, 25 were persons with DS (11 males, 14 females). Both etiologic groups were divided into experimental and control groups. The average age was 16.1 ± 2.6 years. A sample of 329 high school peers served as the non-handicapped control group.

Etiologic factors taken into consideration were based on medical examinations. All retarded students were reared at home, but institutionalized in special schools 5 days a week. They were found to have an IQ below 75 on the HAWIK scale (Wechsler scale). None of them had major physical, visual, or hearing disorders.

Experimental Schedule

After pretesting the whole sample, the experimental groups were enrolled in a special strength training program over a period of 4 months. This program took place during regular physical education classes for 20 min per week.

Statistical Analysis

The statistical analysis was mainly based on different kinds of analysis of variance (factorial ANOVA, repeated measure ANOVA, multivariate techniques). Z-scores were computed to compare performances in diverse tests. Statistical significance was assumed at P values smaller than 0.05.

Results

Nonretarded students, both boys and girls, performed better in all test items than their retarded peers ($P < 0.01$). The range of these differences, however, depends significantly on the kind of skills and abilities tested ($P < 0.01$). Compared to nonretarded, retarded students with and without DS performed best in the medicine ball throw and in the biomechanical tests. In the 20-m dash, the standing broad jump, and the sit-ups, their results were comparatively weak. For these tests, the differences were more than 3 standard deviations (SD) between pupils with and without DS, and sometimes even more than 4 SD (Fig. 1a,b). Profiles showing the range of test results among the non-

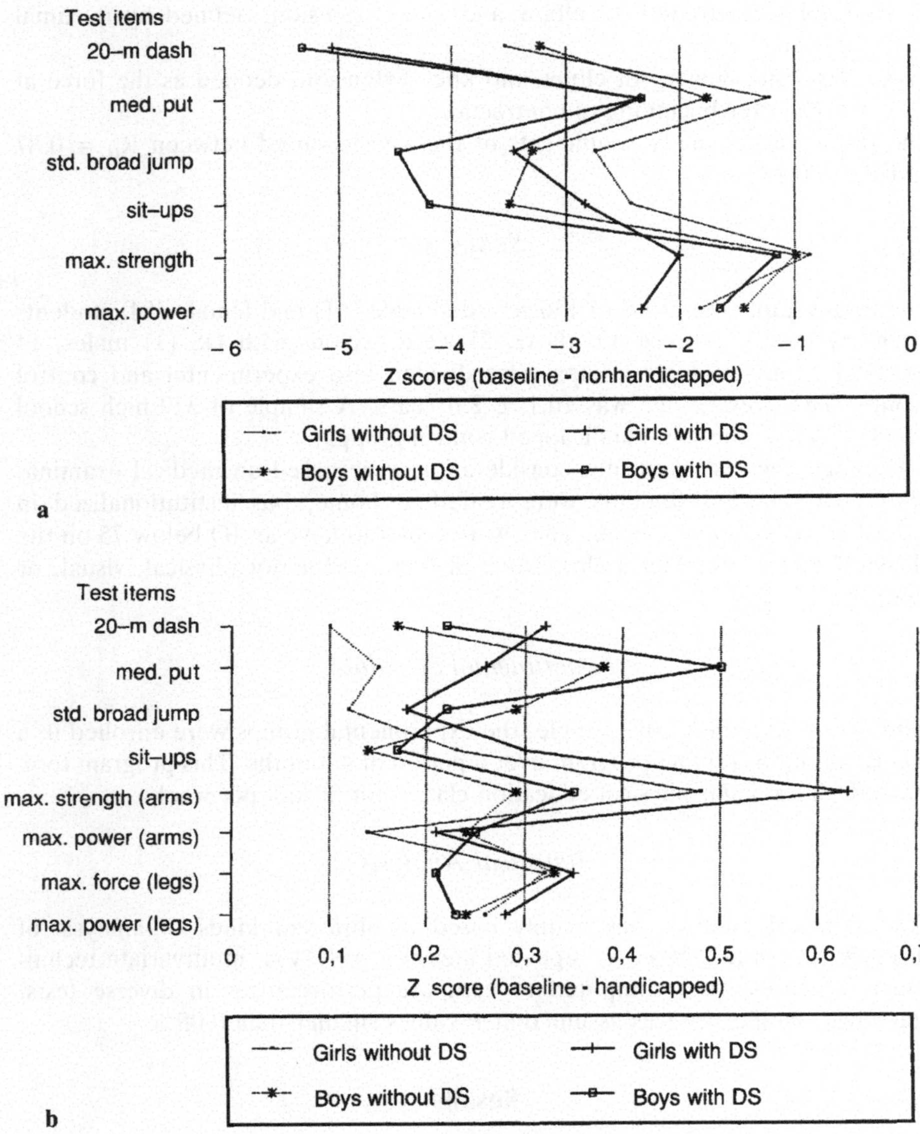

FIG. 1. Z-scores of **a** pretest results and **b** improvement after training (boys and girls). *med.*, medicine; *std.*, standing; *max.*, maximal

handicapped students are very similar (despite the different amounts) for both etiologic subgroups of retarded boys and girls.

Table 1 shows the pretest results of this study. All test results of boys with DS were inferior to those of their retarded peers, DS boys and girls needed about 0.4 longer than their retarded peers to run 20 m ($P \leqslant 0.045$). Average

TABLE 1. Pretest results.

Tests	Boys with DS (*n* = 11) M	SD	Boys w/o DS (*n* = 50) M	SD	Girls with DS (*n* = 14) M	SD	Girls w/o DS (*n* = 40) M	SD
20-m dash (s)	4.65	0.59	4.18	0.66	5.04	0.73	4.68	0.73
med. ball put (m)	2.91	0.89	3.61	1.45	2.42	0.78	2.64	0.76
st. broad jump. (m)	1.03	0.34	1.31	0.51	0.93	0.32	1.14	0.34
sit-ups (n)	7.45	2.11	8.50	2.64	6.79	2.12	7.45	2.34
F max arms (N)	333.7	132.8	364.4	166.6	193.5	73.7	267.6	88.6
F max legs (N)	602.4	379.9	619.4	334.7	357.9	133.2	475.9	225.3
ex. power a.(N/ms)	1.83	0.71	2.31	1.75	0.95	0.53	1.65	0.79
ex. power l.(N/ms)	2.16	1.10	2.89	1.92	1.61	0.65	2.27	1.29

DS, Down syndrome; w/o, without; med., medicine; st., standing; F, force; ex., explosive; a., arms; l, legs.

differences in the medicine ball put and standing broad jump are statistically significant (70 cm, 28 cm; $P \leqslant 0.045$) within the group of boys. Girls differed only 22 cm in the medicine ball put ($P = 0.19$); their average difference in the standing broad jump results (18 cm) is nearly significant at 0.065. DS boys and girls demonstrated about 90% of the muscular endurance level of their retarded peers. This inferiority, however, was not significant ($P > 0.05$).

Girls with DS performed significantly worse than the handicapped controls in biomechanical tests of maximal strength, explosive power, and starting power of arms and legs ($P < 0.024$). They showed only about 73% of the maximal muscular strength of upper and lower limbs (193 *vs* 267 N, 358 *vs* 476 N). Differences in explosive power were even more pronounced. Their average performances reached 60% for the explosive arm extension and 70% for the knee extension (0.95 *vs* 1.56 N/ms; 1.6 *vs* 2.27 N/s).

There was not much difference in maximal strength of elbow (337 *vs* 362 N) and leg extension (602 *vs* 619 N) between retarded boys with DS and other handicapped students ($t \leqslant 0.53$; $P > 0.05$), but their capacities to produce the different kinds of explosive strength were—except for the explosive knee extension ($t = 1.61$; $P = 0.06$)—much less developed in male DS subjects ($P \leqslant 0.05$). Their explosive power was about 25% less important than the one of the handicapped controls.

Retests resulted in clear-cut differences favoring retarded students (boys and girls) having taken part in our strength training program over retarded subjects of the control groups ($F \geqslant 4.23$; $P < 0.05$). If we just take into consideration the subgroup of students with DS, improvement is evident for all tests except for power legs and starting power of arms and legs ($P \leqslant 0.022$). Progress in muscular endurance of the trunk is only significant at the 0.07 level.

Girls improved their performances in all tests ($P \leqslant 0.038$) except explosive power of the arms and starting power of the upper and lower limbs ($P \geqslant 0.16$). Among DS boys only the improvement in running performance and of medicine ball put scores were statistically significant ($P \leqslant 0.03$).

No sex difference of trainability could be found; the progress of boys and girls was similar ($P \geqslant 0.20$). DS students and their retarded peers demonstrated almost identical amelioration of performances. There is no significant relation between etiology and trainability ($P \geqslant 0.288$) except for the running performance wherein DS girls showed greater gains than the retarded controls ($P = 0.14$). All experimental groups of retarded students improved their maximal strength and explosive power during the training period, whereas the strength levels of the control groups remained the same ($F \geqslant 4.52$; $P < 0.05$). Results for "starting power" are not presented because they are highly correlated with explosive power ($r > 0.89$); the results for both kinds of strength are very similar.

Within both etiologic groups, the retarded boys enrolled in our training program showed the best improvement in the medicine ball put, and girls developed best in maximal strength. The boys' range between test and retest was low for sit-ups. Girls showed relatively little progress in jumping performance and explosive power of the upper limbs, as was the case with girls without DS in running. These ranges of improvement for the different kinds of strength are only significant within the group of retarded girls without DS who improved their maximal strength more than their running performance ($P < 0.05$).

Discussion

The results relating to the strength level of mentally retarded persons correspond to the results of other researchers [10, 17]. The low level of explosive power of DS children is confirmed by the study of Oseland [18]. The lack of capacity to perform an explosive muscular contraction can be explained by the low muscular tonus, which, in general, is a characteristic of this population [9, 14, 19]. Obesity could also help to explain lower performances of DS subjects in running and jumping [20]. Morphological differences, measured by a body-mass index, were evident in our sample ($P < 0.001$).

Our study showed that ranges of test differences between retarded and nonretarded students with and without DS grew in accordance with the complexity of skills. Ranges of difference were relatively low for the biomechanical tests, but high for running and jumping. Kral [21] and Burwitz et al. [22] also found similar results. These variations seem to be caused by a lack of motor coordination capacities which is probably—at least partly—due to a lack of movement experience [23, 24].

Skrobak-Kaczynski and Vavik [15] and Katsimpalis [25] report improvements of maximal strength varying from 33% to 53%. These results agree with ours. The greatest gains we found amount to 42% for maximal strength of retarded girls. Studies about the special trainability of different kinds of strength are not known. The slight differences in trainability found in our study can be explained by an unequal accentuation of the training and the different training levels at the pretest. It is easier to make progress starting from a low level. This could partly explain the significant interaction between etiology and trainability concerning the running performances of girls.

The relatively limited progress in muscular endurance is perhaps due to a lack of motivation among the retarded students. Compared to nonretarded, they are less likely to accept unpleasant feelings of fatigue to attain an abstract objective. The sit-ups test administered to evaluate muscular endurance is exhausting and requires great will power. One reason why some control groups of retarded students showed re-test results of muscular endurance significantly inferior to the pretest may be that they remembered the discomfort of the pretest.

Conclusion

The experiment demonstrates that mentally retarded students with DS are able to improve all the different kinds of tested physical strength under normal conditions in school. The progress of students with and without DS is similar, except for running performance, wherein DS girls improved more easily than their retarded peers. A lack of motor experience due to overprotection might explain the lower starting level of performance and therefore the higher trainability. Future curricula for mentally retarded persons must take into account this potential of DS students which seems insufficiently developed. As the training program was feasible for handicapped and non-handicapped students and as both groups benefited from this program, it seems possible to organize similar programs for training sessions where retarded and nonretarded are enrolled in the same training groups.

References

1. Henderson SE (1985) Motor skill development. In: Lane D, Stratford B (eds) Current approaches to Down syndrome. Holt, Rinehart and Winston, London, pp 187–218
2. Henderson SE (1986) Some aspects of the development of motor control in Down's syndrome. In: Whiting, HTA, Wade MG (eds) Themes in motor development. Martinus Nijhoff, Boston, pp 69–92
3. Reid G (1985) Physical activity programming. in: Lane D, Stratford B (eds) Current approaches to Down syndrome. London, pp 219–241
4. Block MR (1991) Motor development in children with Down syndrome: A review of the literature. APAQ 8:179–209
5. Nordgren B (1970) Physical capabilities in a group of mentally retarded adults. Scand J Rehabil Med: pp 125–132
6. Henderson SE, Morris J, Ray S (1981) Performance of down's syndrome and other retarded children on the Cratty Gross-Motor-Test. Am J Mental Defic 85: pp 4:416–424
7. Davis WE, Kelso JAS (1982) Analysis of "invariant characteristics" in the motor control of Down syndrome and normal subjects. J Motor Behav 14:194–212

8. Davis WE, Sinning WE (1987) Muscle stiffness in Down syndrome and other mentally handicapped subjects. A research note. J Motor Behav 19:103–144
9. Morris AF, Vaughan, SE, Vaccaro P (1982) Measurement of neuromuscular tone and strength in Down syndrome children. J Mental Defic Res 26:41–46
10. Rarick GL (1981) Die motorische Leistungsfähigkeit geistig behinderter Kinder. In: Rieder H, Buttendorf T, Höss, H (eds) Förderung der Motorik geistig Behinderter. Berlin, pp 1–38
11. Bauer A, Pellens C, Van der Schoot P (1981) Dokumentation und Bericht zum Stand der Forschung im Bereich Motorik und Sport bei geistig Retardierten. In: Jochheim K-A, Van der Schoot P (eds) Behindertensport und Rehabilitation. Teil I: Psychisch Behinderte, Geistig Retardierte. Schorndorf, pp 55–466
12. Wessel JA, Vogel PG, Knowles CJ (1977) Studies related to moderately (trainable) persons. In: Aahper (ed) The best of challenge, vol 3, pp 104–108
13. Schantz O (1990) Konditionelle Adaptationsfähigkeit geistig behinderter Schüler. Eine empirische Untersuchung über die Ausprägung und Trainierbarkeit ausgewählter sportmethodischer und sportbiomechanischer Kraftparameter von Sonderschülern. Doc diss, Mainz
14. Weber RC (1985) Effects of strength development training programs for Down's Syndrome adolescents. Doc diss, University of Utah, Salt Lake City
15. Skrobak-Kaczynski J, Vavik T (1980) Fysisk arbeidskapasitet og dens trenbarhet hos personer med Down's syndrom (mongolisme). In: Den norske laegeforening 100:(19/21):1210–1213
16. Schmidtbleicher D, Baumann W (1987) Kraft. In: Beyer E (ed) Wörterbuch der Sportwissenschaft. Schorndorf, pp 347–348
17. Londeree BR, Johnson LE (1974) Motor fitness of TMR v. EMR and normal children. Med Sci Sports 6 (4):247–252
18. Oseland DJ (1980) Physical fitness comparison between Down's Syndrome students and moderately mentally impaired students. Master's thesis, Illinois State University, Springfield
19. Chiva M, Rutschmann Y (1979) L'étiologie de la débilité mentale. In: Zazzo R (ed) Les débilités mentales. Paris, pp 87–148
20. Cronk CE, Chumela WC, Roche AF (1985) Assessment of overweight children with Trisomie 21. Am J Mental Defic 89:433–436
21. Kral P (1972) Motor characteristics and development of retarded children: successful experience. Educ Training Ment Retard 7 (1):14–21
22. Burwitz L, Daggett A, Harrïson PW, Davies B (1978) Cognition and gross motor performance in ESN children. Am Correc Ther J 32(4):123–126
23. Schantz O (1985) Quelques aspects concernant 1'évaluation de la condition physique des handicapés mentaux. In: CTNERHI (ed) Corps, mouvement, déficience mentale, société. Paris, pp 197–200
24. Schantz O (1991) Adaptation in mentally retarded compared to non-retarded persons. 8th International ISAPA Symposium. Miami
25. Katsimpalis TP (1968) The effect of isometric exercise on the educable mentally retarded. Doc diss, Colorado State College, Greeley

Decreasing Motor Ability in Adults with Down Syndrome

TAKASHI NAKAYA, KATSUHIKO KUSANO, and KYONOSUKE YABE

Abstract. The rate of decline in motor abilities with aging in adults with Down syndrome (DS) was examined over a period of 10 years. There were 12 motor tests administered, including a run test, muscle strength test, flexibility test, agility test, and balance test. Except for the trunk flexion and extension test, the DS group showed lower motor ability when compared to the retarded without DS (R) group and much lower ability when compared to the nonretarded (NR) group. The DS group showed a more rapid decline in motor abilities, except for trunk flexion and extension, than both the R and NR groups. These results were discussed in terms of the clinical and pathological characteristics of Down syndrome.

Introduction

There is evidence that some aging processes in people with Down Syndrome (DS) begin earlier and progress more rapidly than in the general population. Early changes in skin, hair, and posture, early occurrence of Alzheimer's disease [1–4], and a shorter life expectancy [5, 6] suggest that the motor abilities of people with DS decrease more rapidly than those of nonretarded or retarded people without DS. However, there are very few reports discussing this phenomenon. This study was designed to examine longitudinally the rate of decline in motor ability in adults with DS over a period of 10 years. The changes in their motor ability were compared with those of the retarded without DS from the same institution to insure accuracy in comparison.

Subjects and Methods

The subjects of this test were 10 adults with DS (DS group) and 10 retarded adults without DS (R group) from the same institution for the mentally retarded. Twelve motor tests were administered: a 50-m run, a 1000-m run, a trunk flexion test, trunk extension test, a vertical jump, a standing broad jump, a running broad jump, a grip strength test, a back strength test, a handball throw, a balance test, and a zigzag run. The tests were administered once a year from 1982 to 1992. The subjects' ages in the first year ranged from 16 to 32. The means and standard deviations for the nonretarded group were adopted from Meshizuka's data [7].

Results

Table 1 presents the means and standard deviations of the 12 motor tests for the DS group, the retarded (R) group, and the nonretarded (NR) group. The

TABLE 1. Means and standard deviations of the 12 motor tests for the Down syndrome group, the retarded without Down syndrome group, and the nonretarded group.

	Age	15–24 mean (SD)	25–34 mean (SD)	35–44 mean (SD)
Trunk flexion	Down	17.0 (6.4)	13.7 (5.5)	14.3 (7.5)
(cm)	Retarded	3.1 (7.9)	4.1 (6.3)	2.4 (3.6)
	Nonretarded	15.7 (6.2)	12.0 (6.2)	9.6 (6.1)
Trunk extention	Down	59.8 (6.4)	55.5 (7.5)	38.6 (12.3)
(cm)	Retarded	41.6 (8.1)	41.4 (10.3)	44.3 (6.0)
	Nonretarded	56.2 (8.2)	52.5 (8.0)	43.6 (6.4)
Back strength	Down	67 (20.9)	73 (22.3)	43 (19.4)
(kg)	Retarded	86 (20.1)	94 (29.8)	93 (23.6)
	Nonretarded	148 (25.5)	151 (25.0)	141 (24.5)
Grip strength	Down	27.3 (4.4)	26.6 (5.3)	20.4 (4.2)
(kg)	Retarded	30.6 (6.6)	32.2 (7.0)	41.9 (4.8)
	Nonretarded	46.1 (7.1)	46.6 (6.8)	45.1 (6.5)
Foot balance	Down	58.2 (60.0)	24.4 (32.3)	11.9 (7.8)
(sec)	Retarded	137.0 (59.0)	98.6 (78.3)	158.0 (62.2)
	Nonretarded	—	—	—
50-m run	Down	9.8 (1.27)	10.5 (1.58)	12.1 (2.04)
(sec)	Retarded	8.4 (1.16)	9.1 (0.90)	8.8 (0.36)
	Nonretarded	7.4 (0.47)	7.7 (0.51)	8.1 (0.55)
Zigzag run	Down	17.7 (1.93)	18.1 (2.41)	19.0 (2.13)
(sec)	Retarded	14.3 (2.03)	15.5 (1.93)	16.5 (1.72)
	Nonretarded	—	—	—
Handball throw	Down	12.3 (3.2)	11.1 (2.6)	9.2 (2.6)
(m)	Retarded	14.4 (4.4)	13.2 (4.6)	13.8 (3.2)
	Nonretarded	28.5 (5.2)	25.8 (4.8)	22.5 (4.0)
Running broad jump	Down	236 (60)	204 (49)	167 (41)
(cm)	Retarded	305 (54)	277 (56)	267 (17)
	Nonretarded	446 (50)	425 (52)	403 (50)
Standing broad jump	Down	161 (26)	139 (30)	127 (20)
(cm)	Retarded	171 (21)	163 (33)	162 (12)
	Nonretarded	232 (27)	220 (26)	206 (26)
Vertical jump	Down	32.0 (8.7)	25.7 (6.5)	23.8 (6.2)
(cm)	Retarded	36.3 (7.2)	32.1 (6.9)	29.8 (4.6)
	Nonretarded	56.8 (7.8)	51.0 (7.9)	45.5 (7.5)
1000-m run	Down	364 (54)	404 (49)	435 (76)
(sec)	Retarded	275 (37)	278 (36)	264 (15)
	Nonretarded	—	—	—

DS group showed greater ability than both the NR and R groups on both the trunk flexion and the trunk extension tests. Except for the trunk flexion and extension tests, the DS group showed lower motor ability compared to the R group and much lower ability compared to the NR group.

Figure 1 shows the completion time of the 1000-m run for the DS group and the mean time for all three groups. Though there was some fluctuation in completion times, the mean time increased with age. The DS group showed a more rapid increase in completion time over the testing period than did the R group.

Figure 2 shows the results of the standing broad jump for the DS group and the mean results for all three groups. The DS group showed a more rapid decline in ability than the R group. The same tendency for more rapid decline in motor ability in the DS group was observed in all other tests except for the trunk flexion and trunk extension tests.

Figure 3 shows the results of the trunk flexion test. The DS group showed better performance in this test than both the NR and R groups, and the rate of decline was less than that of the NR group.

Discussion

The DS group showed the highest score in the trunk flexion test, and this is consistent with earlier reports that DS subjects have diminished muscle tone [8, 9]. This abnormality (hypotonia) permits greater flexibility of the joint. Therefore, high scores do not necessarily indicate higher ability in the DS

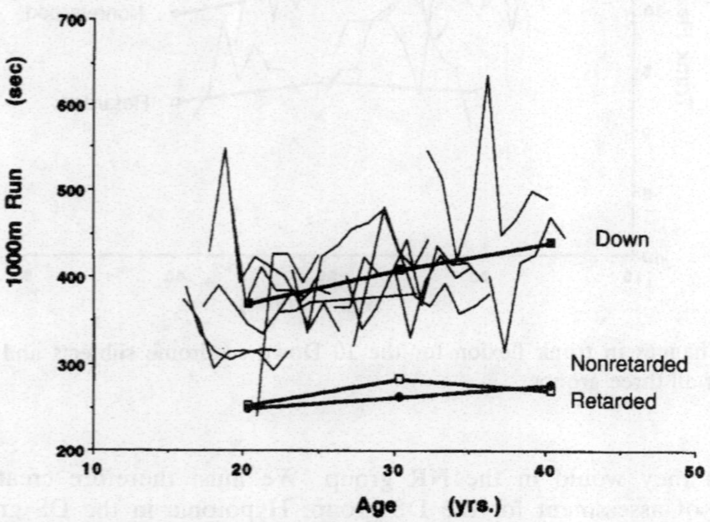

FIG. 1. Changes in 1000-m run for the 10 Down syndrome subjects and the mean record for all three groups

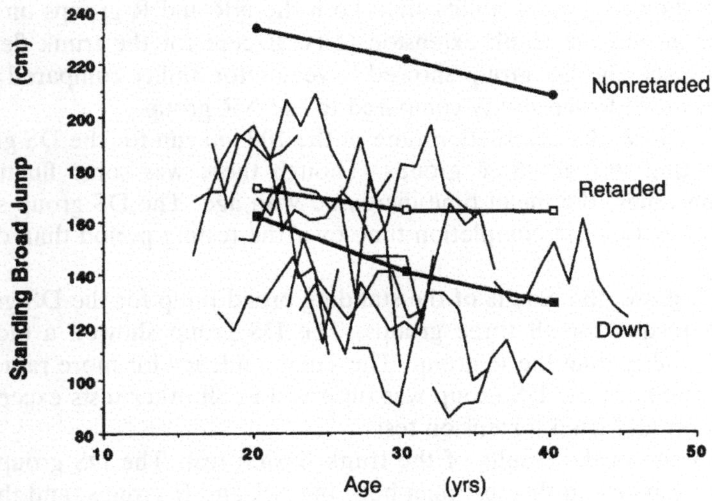

FIG. 2. Changes in standing broad jump for the 10 Down syndrome subjects and the mean record for all three groups

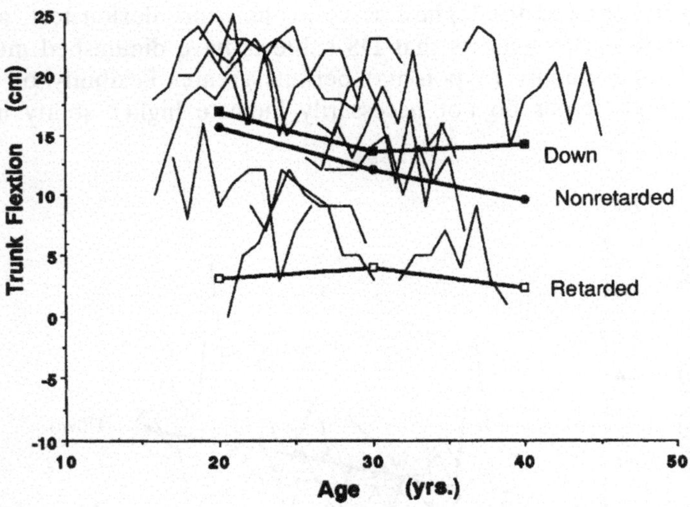

FIG. 3. Changes in trunk flexion for the 10 Down syndrome subjects and the mean record for all three groups

group as they would in the NR group. We must therefore create a new standard of assessment for the DS group. Hypotonia in the DS group may explain the lower muscle strength (grip strength and back strength) and muscle power (50-m run, running broad jump, vertical jump) seen in this group.

The rapid decline in motor ability with age in the DS subjects is attributed primarily to clinical and pathological problems associated with DS including hypogonadism, age-related increase in hypothyroidism, age-related increase in seizures, increased incidence of neoplasms, and degenerative vascular disease [1, 9–11]. Such changes can be expected to directly accelerate the decline of motor ability.

Lack of physical activity in daily life also contributes to lower motor ability and the rapid decrease in performance. Long periods of inactivity or apathy are often associated with Alzheimer's disease, a higher incidence of which occures in those with DS than in the general population [11]. We should therefore encourage DS patients to engage in more physical activity on a regular basis by developing an adapted physical exercise program.

References

1. Benda CE (1969) Down's syndrome-mongolism and management. Grune and Stratton, New York, pp 44
2. O'Hara PT (1972) Electron microscopic study of the brain in Down's syndrome. Brain 95:681–684
3. Oliver C, Holland AJ (1986) Down syndrome and Alzheimer's disease: A review. Psychol Med 16:307–322
4. Solitaire GB, Lamarche JB (1966) Alzheimer's disease and senile dementia as seen in mongoloids; neuropathological observations. Am J Ment Defic 11:79–84
5. Fryers T (1986) Survival in Down's syndrome. J Ment Defic Res 30:101–110
6. Masaki M, Higurashi M, Iijima K (1981) Mortality and survival for Down's syndrome in Japan. Am J Hum Genet 33:629–639
7. Mesizuka T, Himaru T, Nagata S (1970) Nihonjin no Tairyoku Hyojunchi (Physical fitness of Japanese people). Fumaido, Tokyo, pp 109–230
8. Cowrie V (1970) A study of the early development of mongoloids. Pergamon, Oxford, pp 1–27
9. O'Connor N, Berkerson G (1963) Eye movement in normals and defectives. Am J Ment Defic 68:85–90
10. Brown WT (1985) Genetics of aging. In: Janicki MP, Wisniewski HM (eds) Aging and developmental disabilities: Issues and approaches. Brookes, Baltimore, pp 185–194
11. Zigman WB, Schupf N, Zigman A, Silverman W (1993) Aging and Alzheimer's disease in people with mental retardation. Int Rev Res Ment Retard 19:41–70

—Part V—

Physical Activity for the Elderly

Dynamic Balance Training by Balance Board for the Elderly

Katsuo Fujiwara, Hitoshi Asai, Hiroshi Toyama, Kenji Kunita, Akiyoshi Miyaguchi, Tadahiko Yamashina, and Sotoyuki Usui

Abstract. Focusing attention on falls, a dynamic balance training program using a balance board was carried out by a group of elderly persons for 3 weeks. We investigated dynamic balance and physical fitness factors before and after training. The subjects included 54 young adults and 58 elderly persons. Of these, the number of subjects assigned to the training groups were 27 and 35, respectively. We measured balance when a horizontal board was quickly inclined; various physical fitness factors were expected to be closely related to balance ability. The following results were obtained: (1) The dynamic balance of elderly persons was remarkably inferior to that of young persons. (2) Balance board training had a considerable effect for elderly persons. (3) The only physical fitness factor which showed a significant change after training in all subject groups was the hip joint extension limit. In addition, training increased the muscle strength of plantar flexion in elderly men, and the percentage of body fat decreased in elderly women. (4) The physical fitness factors which showed a significant correlation to dynamic balance differed between men and women, and between the young and the elderly.

Introduction

How elderly persons are to live a healthy and safe life in an aging society is an important social problem awaiting a solution. Many elderly persons suffer accidents by falling, and they occasionally suffer a serious injury that requires a long recovery. It has been suggested that some accidents may be caused by a decrease in equilibrium function, and some researchers [1–4] have investigated the relationship between falls and balance. They have reported that the subjects who experience falls show a slightly lower stability than those who have not fallen. However, stability was measured while maintaining a quiet standing posture. Since the falls often occur in dymamic conditions, it seems reasonable to measure dynamic balance under conditions which approximate the falls as closely as possible. There are some reports that suggest equilibrium function is improved by changing daily activities and by balance training. On the other hand, the balance response to a disturbance stimulus and the adaptation of dynamic balance has hardly been investigated. Therefore it is desirable to systematically analyze whether dynamic balance training is effective, and to determine which items of physical fitness are associated with a training effect.

In this study, focusing attention on falls, the training of dynamic balance using a balance board was carried out by elderly persons for 3 weeks. We investigated the relationship between physical fitness factors and dynamic balance before and after training.

Methods

Subjects

Subjects included 54 young adults (31 men and 23 women) and 58 elderly persons (25 men and 33 women). Mean and standard deviation (SD) of their ages were 19.4 ± 1.31, 20.4 ± 2.14, 68.9 ± 4.61, and 68.3 ± 3.42 years, respectively. Differences in sex were not significant. The number of subjects assigned to the training groups were 14, 13, 14, and 21 of the above subjects, respectively. Subjects with hypertension and orthopedic conditions which might affect equilibrium were excluded.

Training of Dynamic Balance

Dynamic balance training was conducted for 3 weeks. The training device was a balance board which consisted of a 24.5 × 50 × 2.2 cm wooden board with a 2.2 × 24.5 × 2.2 cm wooden square pillar attached in the center. When the board was rocked from side to side, the maximum possible inclination was 5°. The subjects stood on the training device with their eyes open. To maintain the training device in a horizontal position, the center of foot pressure (CFP) had to be maintained in the base area of the square pillar (Fig. 1). Once inclinations commenced in an anteroposterior direction, the subjects were required to return the training device to the horizontal position as soon as possible. Standing foot positions coincided with the following three points being aligned with the square pillar: the middle of the longitudinal foot arch, the thenar eminence, and the distal end of the tibia. According to our previous study [5] those positions were at about 45%, 75%, and 25% from the heel, using the foot length (FL) as 100%. When the CFP was maintained within the base of the square pillar at each foot position, the subjects maintained a quiet standing, forward-leaning, and backward-leaning posture. If these forward or backward postures were unable to be maintained, an extreme forward- or backward-leaning posture was maintained. Training time at each position was 2 min for a total of 6 min a day.

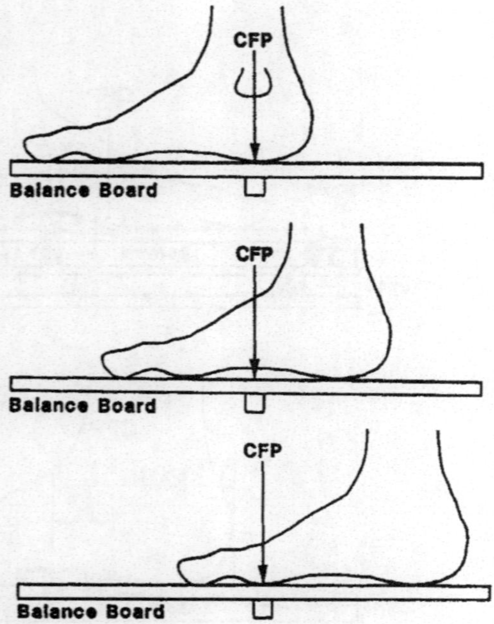

FIG. 1. Training method for dynamic balance using balance board. *CFP*, center of foot pressure

Measurements of Dynamic Balance and Physical Fitness

Dynamic Balance

Dynamic balance was evaluated by the reaction speed required by the subjects to return the leaning board to a horizontal position after an equilibrium disturbance. The disturbing stimulus was the rapid inclination of the floor while subjects stood on the leaning board. The subjects stood with the axis of the leaning board at a point 45% of the total foot length from the heel and maintained a forward- and backward-leaning posture with the CFP at 60% ± 1 cm and 30% ± 1 cm. Under these conditions, when a stopper under one end of the leaning board was removed using a solenoid, the leaning board tilted 5° by gravity. The subjects tried to return the leaning board to a horizontal position. This was the third trial. When the leaning board inclined at 5°, its end contacted the ground. The rapidity of equilibrium response was evaluated by the contact time with the ground (Fig. 2).

Forward and Backward Limits of Stability Base Area

The CFP was monitored while extreme forward- and backward-leaning postures were maintained on a force plate for 10 s. The monitoring was done by using equipment with a luminous diode on the pen part of a pen recorder, which was placed 1 m in front of the subjects. Forward and backward limits of stability

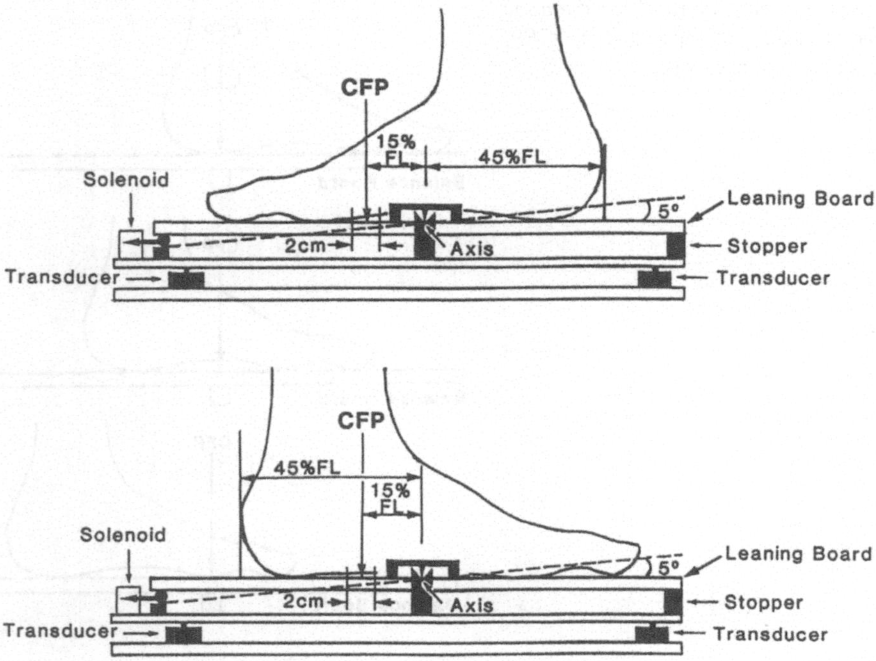

FIG. 2. Equipment to measure rapid postural reaction to floor tilt

base area were evaluated by the mean position of CFP in those leaning postures.

Joint Position Sense

The ability to sense trunk flexion (20°) and ankle plantar flexion (20°) was measured by the angular reproducible method. The former was measured with the trunk fixed by a bar and the lower limbs fixed beside a vertical bar while standing. The latter was measured in a supine position with the foot in a neutral position. The measurements were carried out five times with the eyes closed after an examiner verbally indicated the target position twice. These absolute errors from the target position were calculated.

Simple Body Reaction Time

Basic dynamic posture was maintained on a force plate and the subjects jumped vertically on a light signal [6]. Subjects had five experimental trials. Three periods were analyzed: (1) from the light signal to the start point of the jump (start time), (2) from the start point of the jump to the take-off point of the foot (movement time), and (3) from the light signal to the take-off point (reaction time).

Flexibility

Ranges of motion of ankle dorsal flexion, plantar flexion, and hip joint flexion and extension were measured by the TODAI goniometer method. Ankle range of motion was measured in a prone position and with the foot in a neutral position, while hip range of motion was measured with the front of the trunk fixed on a wall and with the right leg non-weight bearing and free to move.

Muscle Strength

Muscle strength of plantar flexion and dorsal flexion were measured with the hip, knee, and foot joints flexed at 90 degrees. The measurements on the right foot were carried out twice. The higher value of the two was used.

Physique

The items measured were height, weight, upper leg girth, lower leg girth, percent body fat, and lean body mass. The percent body fat was calculated by the formulas of Nagamine [4] and Brozek [7] using values of subcutaneous fat thickness.

The level of statistical significance was set at 5%.

Results

Dynamic Balance

The time from when the stopper under the leaning board started to move until the leaning board contacted the ground did not differ significantly among all subject groups. The mean and SD were 50 ± 10.51 ms in the anterior tilt and 44.0 ± 10.43 ms in the posterior tilt.

The contact time did not show a significant correlation between age groups. Mean and SD of the contact times before and after dynamic balance training are shown in Fig. 3. When the subjects could not maintain the standing posture at the target CFP position, they shifted to a maintainable extreme forward- or backward-leaning posture.

In both the young and elderly groups, the contact time before training was not significantly different by sex. The contact times for the elderly subjects were considerably longer than for the young subjects. The ratio of elderly subjects to young subjects was 1.51:1 for men and 1.6:1 for women before training and 1.6:1 for men and 1.65:1 for women after training. A comparison of tilt directions showed that the contact time in posterior tilt was significantly longer than in anterior tilt.

The contact time before training was not significantly different between the trained and the untrained groups. There was no change in the measurements taken before and after training in the untrained group. A significant decrease

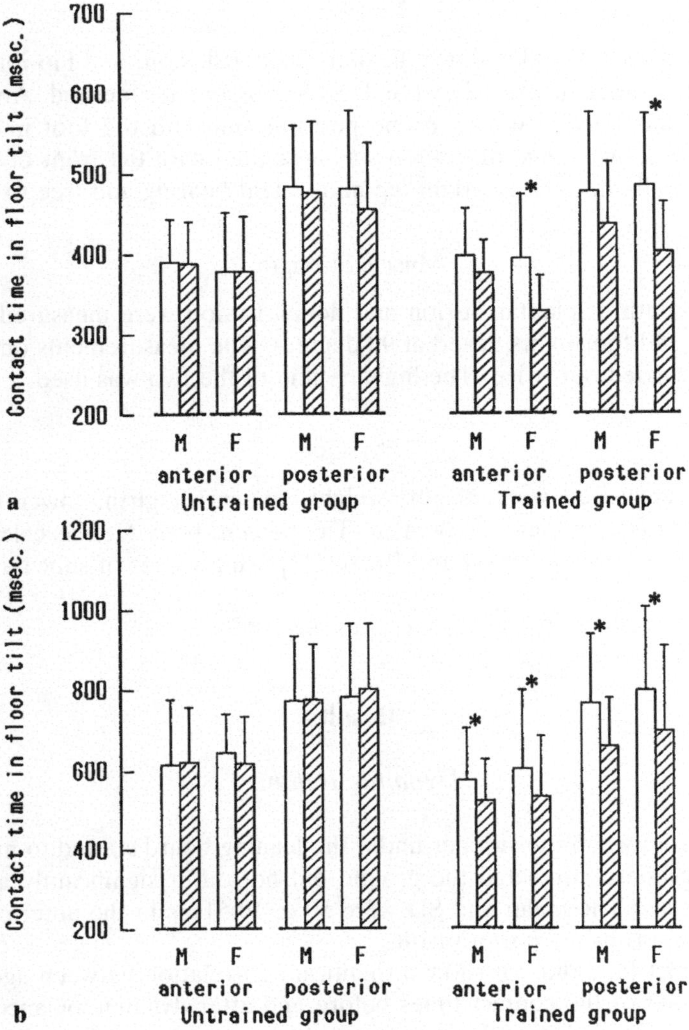

FIG. 3. Contact time in floor tilt in **a** young and **b** elderly subjects. *Open bars*, pretraining; *hatched bars*, posttraining; M, men; F, women

of the contact time by the training was recognized in posterior tilt for young women, and in anterior and posterior tilt for elderly men and women.

Forward and Backward Limits of Stability Base Area

Mean and SD of the CFP positions in the extreme forward- and backward-leaning postures are shown in Fig. 4. The forward CFP position showed no significant difference between young men and women and between the trained

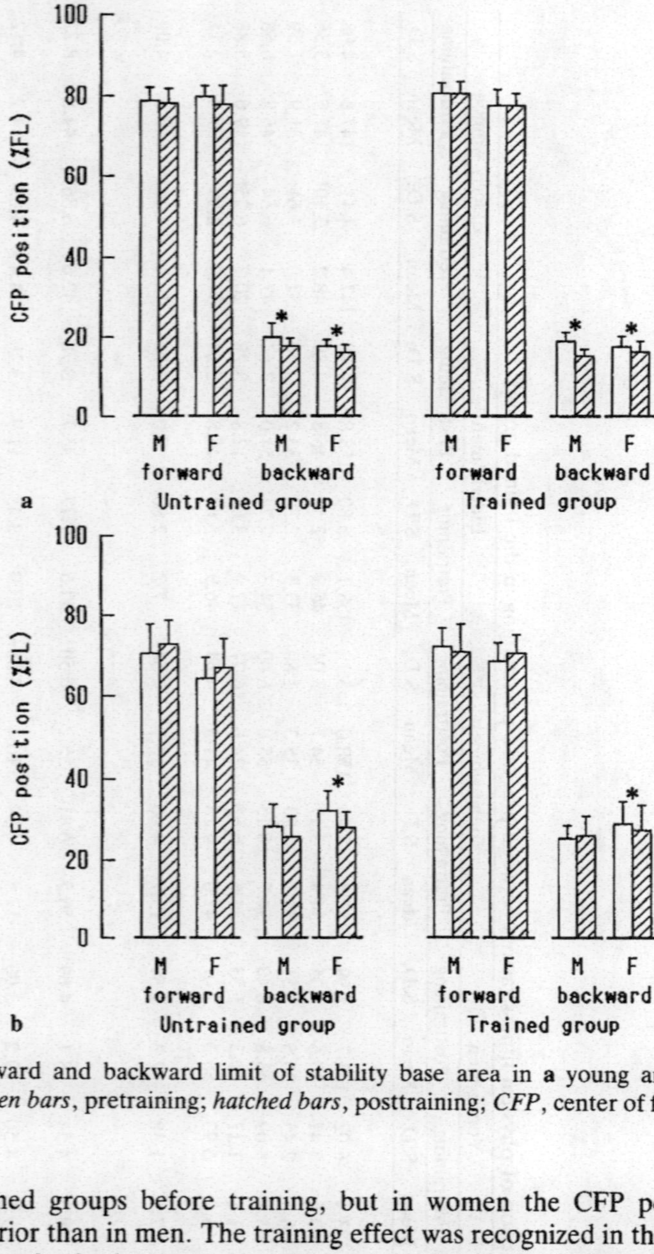

FIG. 4. Forward and backward limit of stability base area in **a** young and **b** elderly subjects. *Open bars*, pretraining; *hatched bars*, posttraining; *CFP*, center of foot pressure

and untrained groups before training, but in women the CFP position was more posterior than in men. The training effect was recognized in the backward CFP position for both sex groups. However, a significant backward change of that position was also recognized in the untrained group.

In elderly persons, the stability base area was significantly narrower as compared with young persons, and in women compared with men. Training in women caused a significant backward shift in the CFP position in the extreme backward-leaning posture.

TABLE 1. Comparison of physical fitness factors between pre- and posttraining in the trained groups.

	Young men				Young women				Elderly men				Elderly women			
	Pretraining		Posttraining		Pretraining		Posttraining		Pretraining		Posttraining		Pretraining		Posttraining	
Item	Mean	S.D.	Mean	S.D.	Mean	S.D.	Mean	S.D.	Mean	S.D.	Mean	S.D.	Mean	S.D.	Mean	S.D.
Physique (cm)																
Height	173.4	6.02	173.7	5.99	157.8	5.46	158.0	5.19	158.1	5.80	158.8	4.48	147.4	4.11	147.6	4.08
Upper leg girth	50.6	3.47	50.6	3.35	54.9	3.17	54.7	3.04	46.9	2.51	46.8	2.89	48.2	3.10*	47.5	3.36
Lower leg girth	36.3	2.45	36.5	2.51	35.1	1.83	35.3	1.80	33.3	2.32	33.2	2.30	32.0	1.61	31.9	1.59
Weight (kg)	63.1	8.09	63.8	8.40	54.7	6.13	55.0	6.00	54.3	7.74	54.0	7.64	47.1	6.54	46.8	6.58
Body fat (%)	11.1	1.17	11.3	1.33	24.6	6.63	24.6	6.77	12.9	3.07	12.8	3.28	20.7	6.25*	19.6	5.88
Lean body mass (kg)	56.0	6.93	56.3	7.07	41.0	4.28	41.3	4.64	46.9	5.62	46.8	5.24	37.0	2.99	37.2	3.11
Body fat mass (kg)	7.1	1.38	7.3	1.59	13.7	4.60	13.7	4.54	7.2	2.80	7.0	3.00	10.1	4.19*	9.5	4.09
Flexibility																
Plantar flex. (degree)	48.3	4.54	48.1	4.69[a]	56.5	6.91	55.2	6.50	30.6	7.77	33.7	8.78	42.6	6.86*	44.8	8.22
Dorsal flex. (degree)	19.1	4.50	19.2	3.00	17.5	4.34	16.4	3.55	10.9	3.43	11.9	3.10	14.4	4.03	14.2	4.12
Hip flex. (degree)	76.9	7.97*	80.4	9.19[a]	79.6	5.94	80.0	6.44	67.8	9.23*	75.3	8.65	69.9	10.82*	74.6	8.95[a]
Hip ext. (degree)	23.9	4.06*	27.9	3.06	30.3	4.21*	35.5	5.19	18.2	4.62*	25.1	4.33	21.0	8.01*	23.4	6.56

Muscle strength																
Plantar flex. (kg)	121.6	16.36	123.8	22.85[a]	96.8	16.41	98.8	13.92	83.0	16.95	87.5	18.79	58.9	11.66*	62.5	12.47
Dorsal flex. (kg)	28.7	5.77	27.5	4.43	23.0	3.92	22.3	2.73	20.3	4.22	19.9	3.74	13.6	2.59	13.0	2.47
Plantar flex./ Weight	1.94	0.241	1.95	0.284[a]	1.77	0.189	1.79	0.127	1.53	0.221	1.62	0.242	1.26	0.240*	1.35	0.247
Dorsal flex./ Weight	0.45	0.086	0.43	0.067	0.42	0.064	0.40	0.046	0.38	0.072	0.37	0.070	0.30	0.077	0.28	0.059
Body reaction time (ms)																
Start time	152.2	12.55	157.8	21.34	161.8	12.87	169.5	12.80[b]	236.4	44.03	223.8	47.39	269.2	69.92	244.0	47.35
Movement time	144.3	25.32	155.4	21.32	162.4	23.04	176.1	22.30	194.6	16.46	199.9	15.70	232.7	33.19	238.7	40.18
Reaction time	296.5	33.66	313.4	38.79	324.7	26.00	345.7	26.79	431.0	52.50	423.6	55.72	502.0	96.60	473.4	85.93
Sensibility (degree)																
Trunk flex.	2.2	1.16	2.4	1.61	2.8	0.95	2.3	1.59	3.6	1.98	3.6	2.65	4.6	2.53	3.4	2.39
Ankle plant. flex.	2.7	1.64	3.3	1.59	5.1	2.04*	3.0	1.04	5.5	6.02	3.3	2.22	3.8	2.93	3.3	2.13

Flex., flexion; ext., extension; plant., plantar.

* $P < 0.05$.

[a] significant increase in the untrained group.

[b] significant decrease in the untrained group.

Changes in Physical Fitness After Training

Mean and SD of each item for physical fitness are shown in Table 1 for both young and elderly groups. Improvements in the dynamic balance after training are marked with an asterisk. Items that changed after the training period in the untrained group are marked with a plus (a) or a minus (b).

In young persons, items that changed specifically in the training group were hip extension range for men and women and ankle plantar flexion for men. In elderly persons, hip extension and flexion range changed for men; and upper leg girth, percent body fat, body fat mass, plantar flexion range, hip flexion and extension range, plantar flexion strength, and plantar flexion strength per weight for women also changed significantly.

Correlation Between Dynamic Balance and Physical Fitness

Items for physical fitness that had a significant correlation with contact time in posterior and anterior tilt are shown below, classified according to age. For young men, the items were plantar flexion strength per weight, movement time, and reaction time in anterior tilt; and movement time, reaction time, and ankle plantar flexion sense in posterior tilt. For young women, the items were height and backward limit of stability base area in anterior tilt, and height and lean body mass in posterior tilt. For elderly men, the items were height, upper leg girth, lower leg girth, weight, lean body mass, plantar flexion strength, plantar flexion strength per weight, forward and backward limits of stability base area, trunk flexion, and ankle plantar flexion in anterior tilt; and plantar flexion strength per weight in posterior tilt. For elderly women, there were no correlations in anterior tilt; in posterior tilt, the item was trunk flexion.

Discussion

Postural Control in Dynamic Balance Test

It is apparent from the tilting time of the leaning board that the subjects cannot produce a postural reaction before the leaning board contacts the ground. In addition, even if some postural control is produced prior to the tilt, it was not sufficient to prevent the leaning board from contacting the ground. The time point when the stopper was removed could be anticipated because a preparatory periodic signal was given before the stopper was taken off. Therefore, it is conceivable that anticipatory postural control exists in this condition. Evidence for the preparatory postural control is that when the signal was given but the stopper was not removed, the CFP sometimes moved in the opposite direction in which the subjects anticipated the board would move.

Change in Dynamic Balance with Aging

It is conceivable from the values of contact time that the dynamic equilibrium for the elderly is inferior to that for young adults. Two models for the decline in equilibrium function with aging were introduced by Woollacott [8]. The first describes a linear physiological decline in balance. The second suggests that balance continues at a high level unless a serious injury or disease causes a rapid decline. Woollacott favored the latter model. Valid evidence which supports the second model is elderly without diseases affecting equilibrium function do not show remarkable differences compared with young persons. In our study, a pathological examination was not done. However, the fact that the distributions of the contact time in young and elderly adults scarcely crossed each other does not provide support for the latter model. In our previous studies [9, 10], the magnitude of body sway while maintaining a quiet standing posture showed no significant difference between average students and gymnasts at Tsukuba University, and the results did not change when the test was repeated. On the other hand, when the test was conducted with a sinusoidally vibrating standing plate, dynamic equilibrium showed a significant difference between those student groups and was improved by repeating the test. Those results were presumably produced by the difficulty of the task. The task of dynamic balance in this study was probably more difficult and the test more sensitive for equilibrium function.

Training Method of Dynamic Balance

It may be important to have a clear objective for postural control in the equilibrium training. In this study, that objective was to maintain the CFP within the base (width 2.2 cm) of a square pillar. The difficulty of dynamic balance changes with the width of the base. The width in this study was decided by referring to the range in an anteroposterior direction of the CFP fluctuation while maintaing a quiet standing posture for 1 min. The average of the range is about 2 cm in young persons and 3 cm in elderly persons [11]. These ranges are larger in a forward- and backward-leaning posture than in a quiet standing posture [2, 3, 5, 12]. Hence, the leaning board inevitably tilts while a standing posture is maintained, and it is conceivable that this training was effective for many adults and was especially difficult for elderly persons. The forward and backward limits of the stability base area may be additional factors that determine the difficulty of training. Considering these factors, the training of dynamic balance would certainly be more difficult for elderly persons, especially in the backward-leaning posture.

However, a training effect was not recognized only in young men. One reason for this result may be that the balance board base was wide, so the training may have been too easy for them. It is also conceivable that young men have many daily experiences similar to the training task on the balance board [13, 14].

The contact time in anterior tilt showed significant correlations to many factors of physical fitness for elderly males and nothing for elderly females. In contrast, in posterior tilt, plantar flexion strength per weight for elderly men and only trunk flexion for elderly women correlated significantly. These results suggest that, in daily life, experiences such as maintaing a backward-leaning posture under unstable conditions are unusual, especialy for elderly people. Elderly women may experience few situations that require maintenance of a forward-leaning posture under unstable conditions. We infer that in such cases, a suitable neural program for maintaining such a dynamic posture is not formed. In contrast, we infer that such a program is formed for elderly men and so the dynamic balance is affected by many physical fitness factors.

Some physical fitness factors were improved by the training such as range of hip extension for all subject groups. In addition, we observed improved plantar flexion for young women, hip flexion range and plantar flexion strength per weight for elderly men, and physical fitness factors associated with decreased body fat for elderly women. It may be impossible to determine to what degree these factors are associated with the improvement of dynamic balance, because as mentioned above, the relationship between dynamic balance and physical fitness is complex.

In conclusion, training by balance board is effective in improving dynamic balance and various physical fitness factors for elderly persons.

References

1. Fernie GR, Gryfe CI, Holliday PJ, Llewellyn A (1982) The relationship of postural sway in standing to the incidence of falls in geriatric subjects. Age Ageing 11:11–16
2. Hasselkus BR, Shambes GM (1975) Aging and postural sway in woman. J Gerontol 30(6):661–667
3. Lord SR, Clark RD, Webster IW (1991) Postural stability and associated physiological factors in a population of aged persons. J Gerontol 46(3):69–76
4. Nagamine S, Suzuki S (1964) Anthropometry and body compositon of Japanese young men and women. Human Biol 36:8–15
5. Fujiwara K, Ikegami H, Okada M, Koyama Y (1982) Contribution of age and muscle strength of lower limbs to steadiness and stability in standing posture. J Anthrop Soc Nippon 90(4):385–400
6. Ikai M, Asami T, Shibayama H (1961) Straingauge-vertical jump reaction time measurement equipment and its application. Olympia 7:18–28
7. Brozek J, Grande JT, Anderson A, Keys A (1963) Densitometric analysis of body composition: Review of some quantitative assumptions. Ann NY Acad Sci 110: 113–140
8. Woollacott MH (1989) Aging, posture control and movement preparation. In: Woollacott MH, Shumway-Cook A (eds) Development of posture and gait across the life span. University of South Carolina Press, Columbia, pp 155–175
9. Fujiwara K, Toyama H, Asai H, Miyaguchi A, Yamashina T, Demura S (1992) Evaluation of adaptability of equilibrium function in the old. Descente Sports Sci 13:262–271

10. Fujiwara K, Ikegami H (1984) The characteristics of postural response in upright stance to the floor vibration. Jpn J Phys Ed 29(3):251–261
11. Yagi K, Fujino A, Tokumasu K, Iho K, Yoneda S (1987) Study on stabilometry in normal upright standing: the change depending on age-grade. Equilibrium Res 46(4):343–349
12. Stelmach GE, Phillip J, Di Fabio RP, Teasdale N (1989) Age functional postural reflexes, and voluntary sway. J Gerontol 44(4B):100–106
13. Oida Y, Nagamatsu T, Arao H, Minegishi Y, Ebashi H (1991) A study on the development of the new method to evaluate the capacity of daily living in the elderly: the measurement of postural stability. Bull Phys Fit Res Inst 78:1–9
14. Sakamoto M, Watanabe H, Mobara S, Ibusuki T, Sakamoto S (1989) Influence of the amount of daily activity on movement of the center of gravity in standing posture. J Phys Ther Sci 1:21–24

Ten-Year Longitudinal Evaluation of Physical Fitness in the Elderly

MISAKA KIMURA, TAMON ARAI, and YASUKO OKAYAMA

Abstract. Of a local group of aged individuals who were followed up for 10 years, the results of physical fitness tests were reviewed in 11 men (aged 65–81 years, mean 69.5 years, at the initial examination) and 49 women (aged 65–79 years, mean 69.3 years, at the initial examination), in whom all the data from these 10 years were available, to longitudinally evaluate the physical fitness of the elderly. When the data from the 10 years in these subjects were compared with our previous cross-sectional data, (1) the changes in the muscle strength, muscle power, and equilibrium were nearly in agreement with those shown by the cross-sectional study, and the performance declined markedly after 75–80 years; (2) the changes in agility and flexibility showed different patterns from the cross-sectional results; and (3) comparison of the total fitness scores in these subjects with those of the cross-sectional study indicated that the former belonged to a relatively unfit group at the initial examination, but their fitness level deteriorated insignificantly during the 10 years. Although none of our subjects practiced any sport, they were interested in exercise such as gymnastics and walking and were participating in various social activities including our fitness evaluation program. Such an active lifestyle is considered to contribute to prevention of the age-associated decline of physical fitness.

Introduction

To remain fit and active is an essential factor in healthy longevity. On the assumption that retaining a sufficient cardiopulmonary reserve and exercise ability is important for healthy old age, we have quantified these elements of fitness in the elderly by safer methods [1, 2]. Using a battery of tests, we have obtained reference values of physical performance of the elderly from cross-sectional data of about 900 subjects [3] and reported that fitness can be maintained by regular light exercise in daily life [4]. In this study, fitness of the elderly was evaluated longitudinally in a local group of aged individuals whom we have followed up for more than 10 years.

Methods

Of the 333 individuals (118 men and 215 women) who participated in the health class held annually at the Kyoto Welfare Center for Aged Citizens for the first time betwen 1980 and 1983, 109 (28 men and 81 women) were still participating after 10 years. Eleven men (aged 65–81 years, mean 69.5 years, at the first participation) and 49 women (aged 65–79 years, mean 69.5 years, at the first participation) of these individuals regularly underwent a battery of physical performance tests (annually for the first 5 years, after 7 years, and after 10 years), and the data of all items evaluated during the 10-year period were available for analysis.

The battery of tests used in this study was a modified version of the physical performance tests for middle-aged individuals devised by the Ministry of Education, Culture and Science for aged individuals. It consisted of 6 items that require relatively mild exertion, i.e., grip strength (muscle strength), vertical jump (muscle power), balancing on one leg with eyes closed (equilibrium), stepping (agility), anterior trunk flexion in sitting with the legs extended (flexibility), and breath holding time (endurance). The performance in each item was scored according to a 5-grade scale, and the total score was calculated.

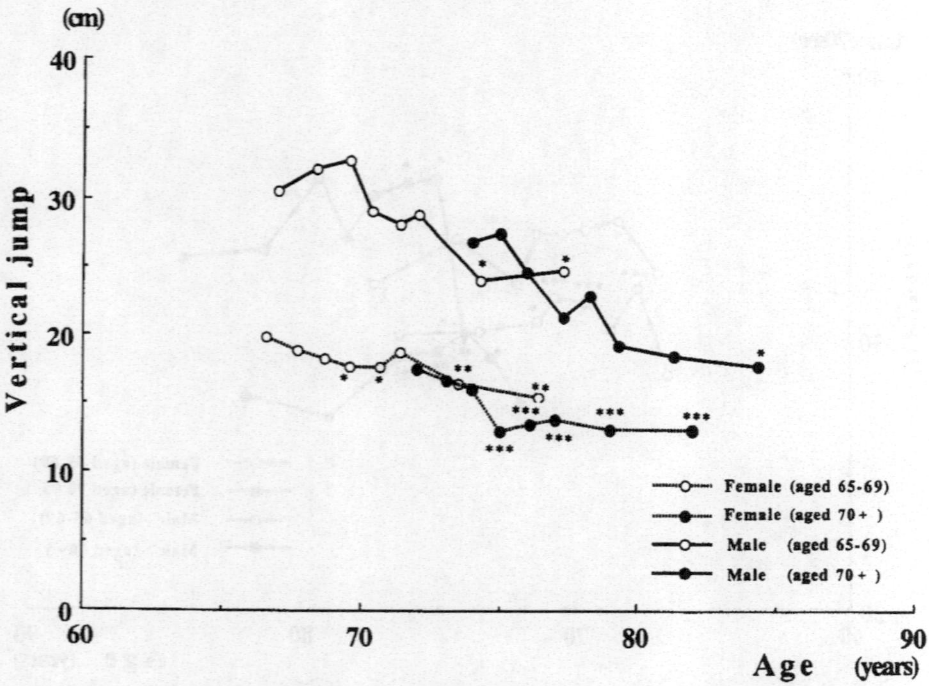

FIG. 1. Changes in vertical jump performance in two age groups (65–69, 70+years) during a 10-year period. $*P < 0.05$; $**P < 0.01$; $***P < 0.001$ by t-test in comparison with the values at the initial examination

The values on follow-up examination were evaluated separately between those aged 65–69 years (7 men and 25 women) and those aged 70 years and above (4 men and 24 women) at the first examination.

Results

Figure 1 shows the mean values of the performance of vertical jump in the two age groups (65–69 and 70+years) over the 10 years. The height of vertical jump clearly decreased with age despite some fluctuations. In both age groups, the decrease was significant after 7 and 10 years in men and after 3 or more years in women as compared with the values at the first examination. Similar age-related changes were also observed in grip strength and balancing on one leg with closed eyes, and the performances after more than 5 or 7 years were significantly reduced as compared with those at the initial examination. The results of balancing on one leg varied widely both for each individual and among individuals, and showed marked declines after about 70 years; they were 0–5 s in about 90% of the subjects after 75 years.

Figure 2 shows changes in stepping performance. The performance improved significantly for the first 2–3 years or 4–5 years and deteriorated gradually

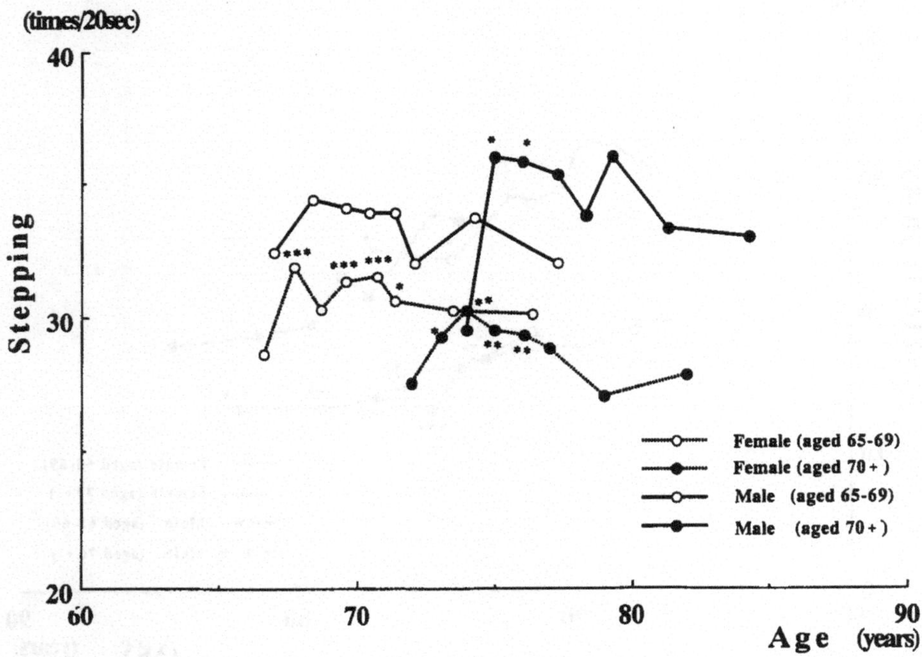

Fig. 2. Changes in stepping performance in two age groups (65–69, 70+years) during a 10-year period. $^{*}P < 0.05$, $^{**}P < 0.01$, $^{***}P < 0.001$ by *t*-test in comparison with the values at the initial examination

thereafter, but the performance after 7 and 10 years was comparable to or slightly better than that at the first examination in both sexes and both age groups. Anterior flexion and breath holding showed no age-associated changes in either sex or age group.

Figure 3 shows changes in the total score of physical performance with regression lines of the total score of physical performance against the age in individuals with (upper line) and without (lower line) a habit of regular exercise in the previous cross-sectional study. The total score tended to improve for the first 2–3 years but decreased progressively thereafter, and it was significantly reduced in women after 5 or more years as compared with the initial value. The mean values for both age groups of our subjects ranged between these two regression lines.

Discussion

Physical performance is known to change with age. We have reported earlier on the basis of cross-sectional data of about 900 subjects that changes in

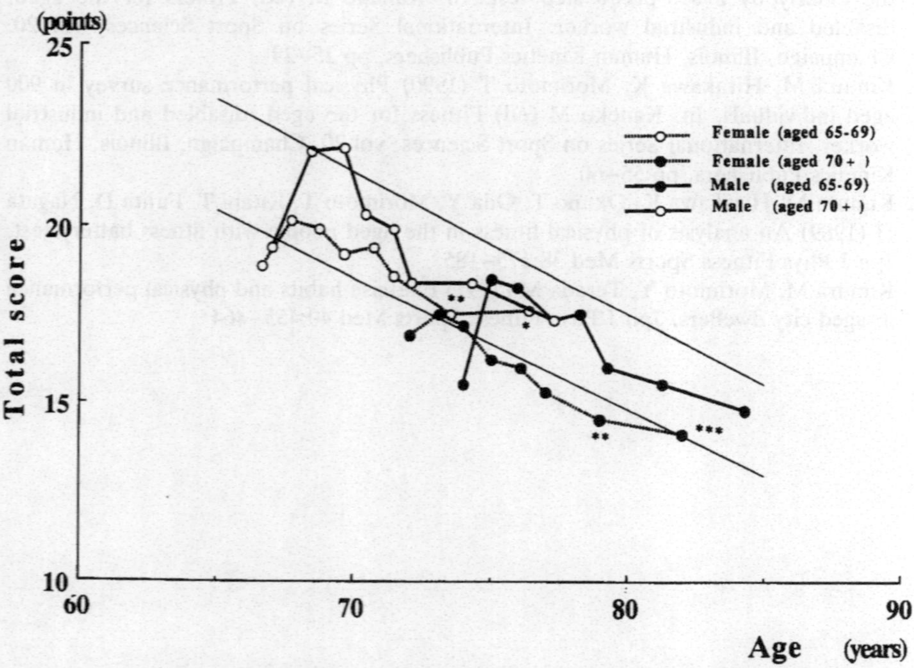

FIG. 3. Changes in the total score of fitness in two age groups (65–69, 70+years) during a 10-year period. $^{*}P < 0.05$, $^{**}P < 0.01$, $^{***}P < 0.001$ by *t*-test in comparison with the values at the initial examination. The two thin lines are regression lines of the total score of fitness against the age for individuals having (*above*) and not having (*below*) habits of regular exercise

physical abilities in old age are basically an extension of those in youth and middle age and that they change similarly in men and women despite differences among elements of fitness and age levels [2, 3]. In this study, the muscle strength, muscle power, and equilibrium decreased markedly at 75 years and above as was indicated by the earlier cross-sectional study [2, 3]. In these subjects, however, the pattern of changes in agility and flexibility were different from the cross-sectional study, and the decline in the total score was smaller. According to the reference values obtained by the earlier cross-sectional study, the total score of fitness of the subjects in the present study at the initial examination suggests that they belonged to a poor-performance group. From these observations, efforts to maintain a healthy life style with regular light exercise, such as that provided by the health class, is considered to have contributed to the delay in the decline of physical performance in these subjects.

References

1. Hirakawa K, Oda Y, Kimura M, Morimoto T (1990) Evaluation of work capacity in the elderly by a self-paced step test. In: Kaneko M (ed) Fitness for the aged, disabled and industrial worker. International Series on Sport Sciences, vol 20. Champaign, Illinois, Human Kinetics Publishers, pp 25–29
2. Kimura M, Hirakawa K, Morimoto T (1990) Physical performance survey in 900 aged individuals. In: Kaneko M (ed) Fitness for the aged, disabled and industrial worker. International Series on Sport Sciences, vol 20. Champaign, Illinois, Human Kinetics Publishers, pp 55–60
3. Kimura M, Hirakawa K, Okuno T, Oda Y, Morimoto T, Kitani T, Fujita D, Nagata H (1989) An analysis of physical fitness in the aged people with fitness battery test. Jpn J Phys Fitness Sports Med 38:175–185
4. Kimura M, Morimoto Y, Terada M (1991) Exercise habits and physical performance in aged city dwellers. Jpn J Phys Fitness Sports Med 40:455–464

The Credo Project: Adapted Physical Activity for Autonomous Active and Sedentary Elderly

Denis Drouin, Marc-André Delisle, René Larouche,
Roselyne Normand, and Clermont Simard

Abstract. Holistic research was conducted to measure the physical, psychological, and social health perception of autonomous elderly between the ages of 55 and 85 years. The theoretical framework comprised current research trends using subjective measures with elderly persons and Travis (1981)/Pender (1982) promotional health models. The hypothesis tested was that active elderly—those participating in regular physical activity programs (indoor physical exercise, outdoor activities, or both)—will have higher health perception scores than sedentary elderly. To test this hypothesis, five perception measures were used. Testing sessions were always supervised, the ratio being one supervisor per ten participants, and lasted 3 months. The sample included 1060 persons. The research design had 240 variables [samples (5), age groups (4), schooling (3), status (2), gender (2)]. The results confirmed our hypothesis since the active elderly obtained higher perception scores for physical, psychological, and social health. Data for variables such as age group, schooling, status, and gender also reveal trends in health perception.

Introduction

The quality of life of older persons cannot be ignored by society. When we use the term "quality of life" with the elderly, it refers to physical, psychological, and social needs, that is, to everyday living conditions. Today the aging process is receiving new attention from gerontological research. It is now more appropriate to refer to aging not only as a state but also as a process, during which one continues to develop in all human dimensions, that is, physiologically, psychologicaly, spiritually, and socially.

With respect to the physiological dimension, current research suggests that as much as 50% of age-related deterioration is the result of inactivity. Many studies of the elderly have investigated the difference between active and sedentary lifestyles. It appears that an active lifestyle leads to better quality of life and consequently to a more positive perception of health and wellness. Active elderly persons develop a positive mental state which contributes to greater self-sufficiency and life satisfaction.

This project was initiated to evaluate the impact of physical activities and an active lifestyle on the physical, psychological, and social health of autonomous elderly persons living in rural areas.

Problem

In this study, self-perception is associated with the evaluative dimension as described by Breytspraak and George [1]. Elderly persons were requested to self-evaluate their perception of physical, psychological, and social health.

Hypothesis

Elderly persons who participate in formal physical education programs will obtain significant higher perception scores for physical, psychological, and social health.

Methodology

Sample

To obtain a random sample of the autonomous elderly of a rural population, the models of Cochran [2] and Yamane [3] were utilized. The sample included five categories of participants: (1) those participating on a weekly basis in the physical fitness program, each session lasting about 90 min; (2) elderly persons participating in outdoor activities (walking, skiing, cycling, etc.) at least once a week; (3) those engaged in both programs; (4) those doing physical exercises on their own, without any formal administrative structure; and (5) sedentary elderly persons. The elderly participants represented four age groups: 55–64, 65–74, 75–84, and 85 years and older; the sample included women and men having different levels of education and social status.

Perception Measuring Scale

To evaluate physical, psychological, and social health, the Linn and Linn [4] scale was used. This specific self-evaluation scale includes 41 items which measure six different factors: (1) physical autonomy, (2) symptoms of aging, (3) self-esteem, (4) social satisfaction, (5) depression, and (6) personal control. The French version of the instrument was validated by Drouin et al. [5]. The questionnaire takes about 20 min to complete.

Data Collection

Every volunteer participant received letters of information and agreement. Testing sessions were supervised; the ratio was about one supervisor per ten participants. Every questionnaire was verified by the supervisor, and to be included in the analysis, 85% of the scale had to have been completed.

Analysis

Analysis of variance (ANOVA) for unbalanced cells was employed since the research design had 240 variables; five categories, four age groups two genders, three schooling levels, and two social status.

Results and Discussion

Table 1 presents sampling identification and distribution while Table 2 shows age group, gender, schooling level, and social status. Table 3 shows ANOVA for all variables, while Table 4 indicates the means from elderly samples.

TABLE 1. Sampling identification and distribution.

Elderly persons	*n*
1 Sedentary Did not participate in any form of physical exercise	113
2 Physically active Participated by himself in some physical exercise at least once a week for the last 3 months (walking, skating, skiing)	312
3 Physical conditionning Participated in the weekly program	163
4 Outdoor activity Participated in the weekly program	113
5 Physical conditionning and outdoor activities Participated in both programs	365

TABLE 2. Age group, genders, schooling level and social status.

	n
Age (years)	
55–64	278
65–74	485
75–84	268
85+	40
Gender	
Men	315
Women	745
Schooling level	
Elementary (grades 1–7)	315
Secondary (grades 8–12)	321
Post-secondary	97
Social status	
Married	692
Others (single, divorced, etc.)	384

TABLE 3. ANOVA for sampling, age group, gender, schooling level and social status.

	n	MS	M	F	*P*
Sample	1059	761.49		7.37	0.0001*
Age group		239.53		2.32	0.073
Gender		124.73			
Men	291		139.01	1.23	0.26
Women	704		138.09		
Schooling level		188.77		1.87	0.15
Post-secondary	94		139.83		
Secondary	302		138.66		
Elementary	610		138.05		
Social status		439.33		4.43	0.03*
Married	640		139.4		
Others	367		136.58		

* Significant.

TABLE 4. Sample mean perception scores for physical, psychological, and social health.

	n	Mean	*P*
Physical conditioning and outdoor programs	362	140.35	
Outdoor programs	113	139.27	
Physically active	310	138.56	
Physical conditioning	161	137.06	0.05*
Sedentary	113	131.71	0.05**

* Significant from physical conditioning and outdoor program.
** Significant from four other samples.

ANOVA results point out significant health perception scores for the variables "sampling" and "social status."

Our main hypothesis was confirmed since the data show significant perception (p = 0.0001) scores between active and sedentary elderly persons; this result confirms current literature trends. The second significant perception (p = 0.03) score is observed between married elderly couples and those having other social status.

For other variables, age group, genders, and schooling level there were no significant health perception scores.

When specific factors of the Linn and Linn [4] questionnaire are analyzed, data indicate that men's perception scores are different for physical autonomy and symptoms of aging; women obtained higher perception scores for social satisfaction. With regard to physical autonomy, it refers to the degree of independence for visiting friends, doing errands, and completing daily routine work; symptoms of aging concern physical pain, lack of energy, and nervousness. The concept of social satisfaction refers to the frequency of meeting with parents and friends, the practice of physical activities, and leisure.

When variable schooling level is considered, the results indicate that significantly higher perception scores for self-esteem and personal control were calculated for post-secondary education. In the Linn and Linn [4] scale, self-esteem refers to personal qualities, positive attitude, and self-achievement while personal control deals with success and self-responsibility.

In reference to social status, married elderly couples obtained significant perception scores for physical autonomy and depression; the latter refers to loneliness and anxiety about health.

Samples

Many studies reported a positive relationship between life/social satisfaction, health, and physical exercise [6–9]. Other studies maintain that physically active elderly people seem to have positive attitude toward work, are in better health, and seem to cope well with stress and tension [10–12]. Rosenberg [13] suggested that physically active elderly people increase their perception in life satisfaction, life quality, and happiness. Our results are in agreement with these studies since our sample of autonomous active rural elderly obtained much better perception scores for physical, psychological, and social health.

Age Groups

According to Morganti et al. [14] wellness—which refers to life satisfaction, self-esteem, and personal control—sometimes increases [15, 16], decreases [17, 18], or does not change with age [19, 20]. Our data indicate that there is no difference in physical, psychological, and social health among the different age groups (55–64, 65–74, 75–84; and 85 years and older) and are in agreement with Edwards and Klenmack [19] and Hunter et al. [20].

Gender

No significant differences in perception scores were observed between elderly men and women (n = 745). Morganti et al. [21] showed that scores for life satisfaction are generally higher for women of different age groups (14–16; 25–34; 45–54; 60–69; 79–79, and 80 and older). Our analysis indicates that men obtained higher perception scores for factors of physical autonomy and symptoms of aging, while women got better scores for social satisfaction.

Education

Some studies endorse the concept that a higher level of education contributes to better perception of well-being [22, 23]. Our results showed that perception scores for factors of self-esteem and personal control were significantly higher for elderly people having completed post-secondary education. As already mentionned by Larson [24], the health status of older people is the dimension that is most strongly related to subjective well-being.

In considering our results, it is appropriate to mention that physical, psychological, and social health perception of elderly people was affected by lifestyle (active life versus sedentary life) and social status. On the other hand, variables such as gender and schooling level affected factors of autonomy, symptoms of aging, social satisfaction, self-esteem, and personal control. Our data indicate that age did not have any effect on health perception scores.

Acknowledgements. This study was supported by grants from the Ministry of Health and Social Services, Quebec, Canada; the Ministry of Recreation, Hunting, and Fishing, Quebec, Canada; and the Arthur-Caux Social Service Center, Laurier Station, Lotbinière, Quebec, Canada.

References

1. Breytspraak LM, George LK (1979) Measurement of self-concept and self-esteem in older people: state of the art. Exp Aging Res 5:137–148
2. Cochran WG (1977) Sampling technique. John Wiley and Sons, New York
3. Yamane T (1967) Elementary sampling theory. Prentice-Hall, Englewood Cliffs, New Jersey
4. Linn WM, Linn BS (1984) Self-evaluation of life function scale: A short comprehensive self-report of health for elderly adults. J Gerontol 39(5):603–613
5. Drouin D, Rice K, Simard C (1989) Self-evaluation of life function scale for autonomous elderly adults: A cross-cultural validation (abstract). 7th International Symposium on Adapted Physical Activity. West Berlin
6. Kelly JR, Steinkamp MW, Kelly JR (1987) Later-life satisfaction: does leisure contribute? Leisure Sci 9:189–200
7. Reddick LC (1985) Life satisfaction determinants of older males and females. Leisure Sci 7:47–63
8. McGuire FA (1984) A factor analytic study of leisure contraints in advanced adulthood. Leisure Sci 6:313–326
9. Mancini JA, Quinn WH (1981) Dimensions of health and their importance for morale in old age: A multivariate examination. J Comm Health 7:118–128
10. Heinzelman F, Bagley RW (1970) Response to physical activity programs and their effects on health behavior. Public Health Depot 85:905–911
11. Schaie KW, Geiwitz J (1982) Adult development and aging. Boston, Little Brown
12. Hogan PI, Santomier JP (1984) Effect of mastering swimming skills on older adults self-efficacy. Res Quart Exercise Sport 55:294–296
13. Rosenberg E (1986) Sport voluntary association involvement and happiness among middle-aged and elderly Americans. In: McPherson BC (ed) Sport and aging, Human kinetics, Champaign, Ill., pp 45–52
14. Morganti JB, Nehrke MF, Hulicka IM (1980) Resident and staff perceptions of latitude of choice in elderly institutionalized men. Exp Aging Res 6:367–384
15. Hess A, Bradshaw HL (1974) Positiveness of self-concept and ideal self as a function of age. J Gen Psychol 117:56–67

16. Staats S (1974) An experimental psychology class, internal versus external locus of control for three age groups. Int J Aging Hum Dev 5:7–10
17. Bloom KL (1961) Age and the self-concept. Am J Psych 118:534–548
18. Bradley RH, Webb R (1976) Age-related differences in locus of control orientation in three behavioral domains. Hum Dev 19:49–55
19. Edwards JN, Klenmack DL (1973) Correlates of cycle satisfaction. J Gerontol 28:497–502
20. Hunter KL, Linn MW, Harris R (1981–1982) Characteristics of high and low self-esteem in the elderly. Int J Aging Hum Dev 14:117–126
21. Morganti JB, Nehrke MF, Hulicka IM, Cataldo JF (1988) Life span differences in life satisfaction, self-concept, and locus of control. Int J Aging Hum Dev 26:45–56
22. Campbell A (1976) Subjective measures of well-being. Am Psychol 31:117–124
23. Speake DL, Cowart ME, Pellet K (1989) Health perceptions and lifestyles of the elderly. Res Nursing Health 12:93–100
24. Larson R (1978) Thirty years of research on the subjective well-being of older Americans. J Gerontol 33:109–125

Osteoporosis Risk Prevalence Among Intellectually Disabled Women

BERNADETTE FOSTER and JEFF WALKLEY

Abstract. This paper describes a major community health problem affecting up to half of the elderly female population of industrialized countries. Although it is known that there are a number of significant risk factors that increase the probability of developing osteoporosis, there exists some controversy between the exact causal relationships. Current research is focusing on the benefits of achieving the optimum peak bone mass in young adulthood, decades before the clinical symptoms of osteoporosis become manifest. Diet and physical activity have been reported to aid this process.

Introduction

Intellectually disabled women are susceptible to many of the significant risk factors associated with the development of osteoporosis. However, few studies have investigated the incidence of the disease in this population. If these women do display a higher incidence of osteoporosis than in the general population, early intervention strategies to increase their bone density are required.

Risk Factors for Osteoporosis

Osteoporosis has been identified as the most common metabolic disorder of the skeletal system [1]. It is characterized by a reduction in bone mass that affects the strength and biomechanical integrity of the skeleton which subsequently leads to an increased risk of bone fracture. Fracture sites most commonly associated with osteoporosis are at the proximal femur and verlebrae, but as bone can be lost throughout the entire skeleton, fractures also result at other sites.

The development of osteoporosis is largely determined by changes in the metabolism and structure of the skeleton. In their lifetime, women will lose approximately 35% of cortical (compact) bone and 50% of trabecular (cancellous) bone. In contrast, men lose approximately two-thirds of these amounts.

The significance of the problem has been underlined by recent evidence from a range of international researchers which shows that the ocurrence of both osteoporosis and vertebral and hip fractures is increasing [2]. Results of similar studies in Australia predict an 83% increase in bed occupancy rates due to proximal femoral fractures between 1986 and 2011 [3].

The major underlying cause of age-related fracture is increased bone fragility due to bone loss [1]. An independent risk factor for fractures is also the increased susceptibility of the elderly to suffer falls, due to poor coordination, failing eyesight, slowed reflexes, neurological diseases, and the use of sedatives and other drugs.

Miller [4] performed a retrospective analysis of the outcomes of 360 people with fractures of the hip. His research showed that after one year, 27% of the patients had died, and 22% remained nonambulatory. This loss of mobility usually resulted in decreased independence and a greater probability of becoming institutionalized.

Incidence of Osteoporosis in Australia

The Australian Bureau of Statistics reported that between the years 1986 and 2011, the Australian population over the age of 65 years is likely to increase by 60%. Further, the population aged between 75 and 84 years is likely to increase by 146%. The number of cases for surgery (for persons aged 65 years and over) will rise from 10150 in 1986 to 18550 in the year 2011. The number of surgical bed·days (days a patient remains hospitalized) for femoral neck fracture is expected to increase from 315000 to an estimated 579000. Based on these projections, the cost of providing acute hospital care for persons suffering from femoral fracture will increase from AUS$37.8 million to AUS$69.5 million [3].

Symptoms and Complications of Osteoporosis

Another complication of osteoporosis is vertebral fracture. Falls do not play a large part in causing these fractures. Generally they occur from the substantial loads placed on the spine during daily activities like bending forward, lifting objects, and climbing stairs.

As many as 20%–30% of ambulant women over the age of 60 show one or more asymptomatic vertebral fractures on routine X-ray, resulting in anatomical changes such as vertebral wedging and ballooning, as well as total vertebral collapse [5].

Osteoporosis has become a major community health problem affecting up to half of the elderly female population of industrialized countries. Research has suggested that the incidence of this skeletal disease is increasing in the population [2–5].

Women also appear to be presenting with the clinical manifestations of osteoporosis at a much earlier age than previously recorded. Generally, life expectancy rates for men and women have risen. The implications of a lower limit for the onset of the disease in a population that is increasingly aging suggests a problem of extreme magnitude for both health care systems and the people at risk.

Etiology

Peak bone mass occurs as a result of age, sex, genetically determined factors, and environmental influences [1, 6, 7]. Insufficient accumulation of skeletal mass in young adulthood predisposes a person to fracture later in life.

Factors contributing to low attainment of potential skeletal bone mass and subsequent bone loss are multifactorial. These influences, with the potential to decrease bone density and thus increase the risk of osteoporosis, include being a Caucasian or Asian woman, premature menopause or prolonged amenorrhea, a positive family history, short stature, and low muscle mass, low calcium intake or absorption, inactivity, nulliparity, and decreased breast-feeding.

Smoking, high levels of alcohol intake, and caffeine consumption are also important elements in the reduction of bone density [8–12].

The extent and significance of some of these factors on the development of osteoporosis remains controversial. However, the factors appear to play some role in the development of the disease state.

There also exist a number of secondary causes for osteoporosis. These include pharmaceutical agents used in steroid and anticonvulsant therapy and in management of various metabolic disorders, diabetes mellitus, Cushing's syndrome, skeletal metastases, and thyrotoxicosis [13].

Osteoporosis is therefore the end-state of many different processes. Application of risk factors can categorize people into those who are likely to develop the disease, and those who are less likely.

Mentally Disabled and Osteoporosis

Due to their disability and treatment, women with intellectual disabilities are exposed to many of the significant risk factors associated with osteoporosis. Some of these specific risk factors include having premature menopause, nulliparity and subsequent reduced breast-feeding, inactivity, low dietary calcium intake, anticonvulsant therapy, steroid therapy, and diabetes mellitus.

In addition to these factors, earlier onset of old age and a higher mortality rate have been observed in intellectually disabled persons. However, a marked increase in longevity has occurred among persons with intellectual disabilities during the past 30 years [14].

This has been due mainly to the introduction of new antibiotics and anticonvulsant drugs, as well as better diet, care, and environment. Longevity, however, has also brought with it the diseases and disorders associated with aging in the general population.

Studies have shown that the incidence of some diseases was, in fact, higher among persons with intellectual disabilities [15]. Results have indicated the existence of biological factors (physiological, genetic, and environmental) that placed intellectually disabled adults residing in a community setting at a higher risk of suffering from a range of health disorders [14]. These findings are very significant in a climate of increasing deinstitutionalization.

Beange [16], in a study of a randomly selected population of mildly and severely intellectually disabled persons, found each individual to have an average of four medical problems of significance, the majority of which were previously undiagnosed. There was also a range of lifestyle factors present (poor accommodation, low incomes, inadequate education, and low levels of marriage) which are associated with reduced health standards.

Beange also identified a variety of modifiable health risks such as physical inactivity and poor diet. Overall, people with intellectual disabilities suffered from more illnesses than the general population, had far more chronic diseases, and experienced much higher mortality levels.

A recent Australian study designed to permit comparisons with approximately matched nondisabled controls assessed the prevalence of osteopororsis and its risk factors among people with intellectual impairment and demonstrated a higher than normal degree of osteoporosis [17]. The data suggests that osteoporosis may be a common problem among the intellectually disabled.

Prevention of Osteoporosis

Currently, there are two approaches to the prevention of osteoporosis: increasing peak bone mass to optimum at skeletal maturity, and reducing the rate of bone loss after skeletal maturity. The successful treatment of osteoporosis is linked with the controversy over the particular significance of specific risk factors. Current studies are assessing the relationship between peak bone mass, nutrition, and physical activity.

Jancar [15], stated that to prevent osteoporosis and fractures within the intellectually disabled population, regular physical and mental examination was essential to detect early signs of disease and disorder. Drugs should be constantly monitored and adjusted according to their effects and side effects, and dietetic services made available to ensure that residents are receiving appropriate nutrients including minerals, vitamins, fiber, and trace elements. Regular exercise is essential to help maintain skeletal mass.

Increasing numbers of people with intellectual disabilities are being placed into the community and out of institutions. To ensure the well-being of these people, there exists a great need to meet all the requirements of this particular population, be they emotional, social, financial, or health-based. Concern about the increasing incidence of osteoporosis in industrialized countries and the need to implement preventive treatments are receiving growing medical attention. This attention must also be directed towards those with a higher risk of acquiring the disease but with a lesser means of dealing with such health issues: the intellectually disabled.

References

1. Riggs BL, Melton LJ (1986) Involutional osteoporosis. New Engl J Med 314:1676–1686
2. Avioli LV (1991) Significance of osteoporosis: A growing international health care problem. Calcif Tissue Int 49(Suppl):S5–S7
3. Lord SR, Sinnert PF (1986) Femoral neck fractures: admissions, bed use, outcome and projections. Med J Aust 145:493–496
4. Miller C (1978) Survival and ambulation following hip fracture. J Bone Joint Surg 60(A):930–933
5. Cooper C (1992) Vertebral fractures. How large is the silent epidemic? BMU 304:793–794
6. Matkovic V, Fontana D, Tominac C, Goel P, Chestnut C (1990) Factors that influence peak bone mass formation: a study of calcium balance and the inheritance of bone mass in adolescent females. Am J Clin Nutr 52:878–888
7. Pocock NA, Eisman JA, Hopper JL, Yeates MJ, Sambrook PN, Eberl S (1987) Genetic determinants of bone mass in adults. J Clin Invest 80:706–710
8. Stevenson JC, Lees B, Devenport M, Cust MP, Ganger KF (1989) Determinants of bone density in normal women: risk factors for future osteoporosis? Br Med J 198:924–928
9. Aloia JF, Cohn SH, Vaswani A, Yeh JK, Ellis K (1984) Risk factors of post-menopausal osteoporosis. Am J Med 78:95–100
10. Honkanen R, Alhava EM, Saarikoski S, Tuppurainen M (1991) Osteopororsis risk factors in perimenopausal women. Calcif Tissue Int 49(Suppl):S74–S75
11. Mazess R (1981) On aging bone loss. Clin Orthop 165:239–252
11. Slemenda CW, Miller JZ, Hui SL, Reister TK, Johnston CC (1991) Role of physical activity in the development of skeletal mass in children. J Bone Miner Res 6:1227–1233
12. Pocock NA, Eisman JA, Yeates MJ, Sambrook PN, Eberl S (1986) Physical fitness is a major determinant of femoral neck and lumbar spine bone mineral density. J Clin Invest 78:618–621
13. Francis RM Edt (1990) Osteoporosis, pathogenesis and management. Kluwer Academic Publishers, Dordrecht
14. Pitetti KH, Campbell KD (1990) Mentally retarded individuals—a population at risk? Med Sci Sports Exerc 23:586–593
15. Jancar J (1989) Fractures in older persons with mental handicap. Aust N Z J Develop Disab 12:329–335
16. Beange H (1991) The neglected health of the intellectually disabled. Paper presented at the National Conference of the Australian Society for the Study of Intellectual Disability. Geelong, Victoria, Australia
17. Centre J (1992) Osteoporosis may be a common problem in young people with an intellectual impairment. Presented at the 9th World Congress, International Association for the Scientific Study of Mental Deficiency, Broadbeach, Queensland, Australia

—Part VI—

Future Trends in APA

Adapted Physical Activity at the Dawn of the 21st Century

Jean-Claude de Potter

Abstract. During the last 20 years, professionals from different areas of expertise have implemented segregated, parallel, and integrated programs in the field of adapted physical activity (APA). Tremendous increases may be pointed out in the number of sports disciplines and performances, quality of investigations, exchange of information, and teacher training programs. Nevertheless only a small proportion of the population with a disability takes part in sports activities, for many reasons which may include limited access, the role of the media, and socialization factors. At the forefront of the present adapted sports movement is the inclusion of athletes in the Olympic Games. This trend requires closer attention to investigation and particularly to the criteria for recognition of an integrative sports event, such as autonomy, ability, and minimal disability. At the present time most scientific work has been done on elite sports for wheelchair users and amputees participating in adapted physical activities, but many issues still need to be investigated: the impact of training, the aging process, APA and misunderstood disabilities, future technology, and doping, among others. Among these fields, some involve the continued expansion of high-level competition, and others refer to the most adequate adapted sports disciplines. Elements that will certainly influence the future of APA include cultural elements in sport programs developed in Asia, Africa, and South America; the relationship between Olympic and Paralympic movements and criteria for the inclusion of athletes; sports relative to nature; and the participation of women athletes. But first of all, the prerequisite for progress is cooperation between administrative structures, authorities, scientists, and experts in order to increase the quality of research in the field of APA for the benefit of people with a disability.

Introduction

Modern sports, born in the last 20 years of the 19th century, received great momentum with the rebirth of the olympics in 1896. Since then, the sports world evolved quickly in terms of the number of areas of sports and in the involvement of governments. However, the emergence of the Sport for All Movement, the sports manifesto of 1964, and the International Charter on Physical Education and Sport enacted at the UNESCO General Conference in 1978, confirmed and enlarged the understanding that everybody had the right to participate in sports. From that time, disabled persons have had equal access to sports activities based on the sports equality policy which does not favor one group of the population above any other. This revised concept, combined with economic problems, gave sports a greater social meaning and redefined the roles of governments and sponsors.

Governments have traditionally limited their actions and invested in sports performances as an aspect of national sovereignty and supremacy. Some of the consequences are manifest in the form of violence, lack of respect of limitations, drug abuse, commercialization of sports, and so on.

Sports and Disability

Sports for disabled persons were originally introduced as an aid in remedial treatment and rehabilitation programs and not because of fitness, motivation, self-esteem, competitive spirit, or . . . fun.

With the evolution of the sports world, sports for the disabled moved from the realm of therapy to one of physical activities adapted to all kinds of disabilities and used for purposes of education, leisure, or fun.

Nevertheless, whereas 30% of the able-bodied population in Europe and 34% in the USA participate in sports on a regular basis, only 3% of the population with a disability participates in sports during leisure time.

This difference raises a few questions. Does it mean that:

— able-bodied people still have easier access to sports activities than disabled individuals?
— the Olympics Games have a direct impact on sports participation among the general population but that Paralympics have no impact?
— television coverage is insufficient and inadequate for Paralympics?
— socialization factors like medical personnel, the mass media, teachers, athletes, and sports administrators do not provide the relevant information, access, opportunity, and choice?
— there is a gap between the actual promoted sports level and the real aptitudes and motivations of disabled individuals?
— policy still favors one group of the population above any other?

However, within the last decade, there has been tremendous progress in numerous areas:

1. The number of sports disciplines has increased.
2. Access to sports for people with all kinds of disabilities has improved.
3. The number and quality of investigations is increasing.
4. More information and issues are being exchanged.

5. The concept of adapted physical activity is being introduced or emphasized in all teacher training programs.
6. More athletes are prepared to compete.
7. Performances are improving.
8. The best athletes are being included in physical activities on both the recreational and competitive levels.

However, the question still remains open as to whether attitude, classification, and regulations facilitate the participation of all disability groups according to their aptitudes and motivations. Everyone must have full opportunities in accordance with their national sports traditions to practice physical education and sports, develop physical fitness, and attain a level of achievement corresponding to their gifts and motivations. As Claudine Sherrill writes in her recent book, "The broad and inclusive concept of adapted physical activity (APA) emphasizes the needed adaptations for all persons not just labeled as disabled but with individual capabilities and interests" Therefore, APA refers to movement and sports for people of all ages in all settings. Progressively, society is shifting from the perception of limitations to the individual potential that persons with a disability have to maximize their abilities.

Unfortunately, what society identifies as a person with a disability sometimes becomes unclear. On the one hand, certain specific sports allow persons with minimal disability to compete for Paralympic medals; in sitting volleyball, for example, two-finger and two-toe amputees are eligible and become medal-winning athletes. To maintain their credibility, sports must define eligibility criteria for competition and these criteria must gradually be made more stringent. On the other hand, adapted physical activities emphasize the abilities of the most severely disabled and implement appropriately adapted sports disciplines.

Current trends have moved from educational, technical, or structural adaptations to the analysis of needed adaptations for mainstreaming, integration, and inclusion, but the obvious foundations—the educational and social implications—must be analyzed in greater detail.

Inclusion in Sports

At the forefront of the actual and future sports movement is the inclusion of selected athletes in the Olympic Games. There is indeed great pressure to give priority to this inclusion but the effects have to be weighed to make sure that it is beneficial for all the athletes. Inclusion means that events for athletes with disabilities will be equal to other events in the Olympic program and will have full medal status. The tremendous skill and athletic level exhibited by disabled athletes justifies their right to full and equal participation in all major international sports events. Persons with a disability have a rightful place within society; in the same way, disabled athletes have an equal place within the sports milieu. This inclusion in sports will hopefully be a prelude to greater inclusion in all aspects of society.

However, the following standards should be applied to the recognition of an integrative sports event:

1. Locomotor autonomy is one of the fundamental criteria of ability.
2. No athlete may be disadvantaged in competing: that means that the basic principle is grouping by ability.
3. The more similar the skill levels are among athletes on a team, the greater the chance that each one will play a meaningful role.
4. Sports disciplines must be widely practiced in member nations on a high level of competitive excellence.
5. Minimal disability for participation in normal competition must be defined.
6. Events must provide equal opportunity for men and women.

The question remains: will this concept of excellence in sports not limit the integration of severely disabled athletes into world-class competition? It is possible that able-bodied individuals and minimally disabled persons taking part together in competitions will set themselves apart from the most severely disabled individuals.

A system of open competition in which all who are classified as being handicapped compete without further subclassification has been adopted for the mentally handicapped by INAS-FMH. In addition, a second class of competition has been developed: the banded competition in which athletes are put into events according to their best performances.

The open system of classification reflects the principle of normalization and intergration. The banded system reflects the need to treat the person with a mental deficiency as "special".

This second system can be beneficial in extending participation, developing skills and sporting abilities, and addressing the needs of the profoundly and multi-disabled. This implies the need for technical and pedagogical adaptations which require the particular attention of researchers in this field.

Research Trends and Issues

At a glance, we can state that most work and investigation has been done in the two broad areas listed below.

Elite Sports for Wheelchair Users and Amputees

The number of sporting events available to disabled athletes has grown and competition has improved. There have been increases in the number and range of competitive sports that have mainly been the result of improved and more knowledgeable technical input and coaching from qualified sports teachers and technicians. It is clear that technology and scientific methods have parts to play.

Furthermore, because of improvements in prosthetics technology, performances of amputee athletes have also increased. Recent advances in wheelchair sports and research findings include the evolution of wheelchair design (track, road, field, and court chairs) and racing wheelchairs (propulsive and retarding forces, wheelchair geometry, and the effect on performance).

Adapted Physical Activity

Considering that more and more persons with disabilities will be integrated into regular settings, sports professionals will need to acquire the necessary skills for coping with a wide range of abilities.

The goal of adapted physical activity, by means of movement, physical activity, and sports, in which special emphasis is placed on the interest and capabilities of individuals, is to improve these abilities. Adaptations may be educational, technical, and/or structural. Movement experiences and participation may be motivated by therapy, rehabilitation, education, recreation, and/or competition. Such a cross-disciplinary and lifelong approach makes up the basic elements of pedagogical research.

Focusing on the current research in APA, the main areas are expected to be: matching the activity to ability, training methods, integration and social acceptance, methodological and pedagogical aspects, effects of fitness programs, physical activity and therapy, and human movement analysis and mathematical modeling. It is obvious that physical activities and sports for the disabled are changing and that this change will and must affect research objectives.

As the level of technical development becomes more sophisticated and complex, future growth in such a broad area will depend on emphasizing the relationship between the research domain and the field of practice on the one hand between scientists, and application of the results of research at universities.

Furthermore, many disabilities have virtually been ignored by scientists. Adapted physical activities and sports for individuals with cerebral plasy are an example: most work has been done with young children, the results on effectiveness of physiotherapy are unclear, and virtually no studies have been done on the effect of physical fitness training. Research is also limited by methodological factors like the heterogeneity of disability groups.

Perspectives in Adapted Physical Activity

When considering the future of APA, we must bear in mind some elements which could influence APA and sports.

Cultural Elements

The principal Olympic sports disciplines come from Western countries, and today the same holds true for Paralympics. It may be expected that Asian,

African, South American countries will emphasize the influence of different cultures on their disciplines. It is also obvious that a large concept like mainstreaming may be applied or rejected depending on local culture.

Discourses on Disability

Disability is no longer considered as an object of charity. More countries now have a vision of society where strategies are based on equity. More and more, sports for the disabled are considered as part of the sporting world, but it is disturbing to note that some disability groups are still being segregated or excluded. For example, 85% of national and international sports budgets go to elite sports to which severely disabled athletes have no access.

Olympic and Paralympic Movements

Today there are about 170 nations in the world and 169 National Olympic Committees in what can only be described as a prodigious success. From this perspective, most financial resources come from and go to elite sports. The "Sport for All" movement seems to have been implemented in only 50% of nations: structures, programs, and governmental services exist in only 79 countries. How many countries have a national policy promoting adapted physical activity? Very few have a national Paralympic committee which coordinates and promotes sports for all groups of disabled people. The responsibility of the Olympic and Paralympic movements, governments, community sports organizations, schools, and universities, is to offer the largest range of services to all categories of citizens.

Sports Relative to Nature

We are now facing a continuing emergence of sports areas relative to nature. This movement is already strong; sports are moving closer to the environment, and they include adventure sports like wheelchair competitions related to nature or simply orientation and endurance walks for mentally retarded individuals. Such rather new sports disciplines encourage the integration of disabled athletes into able-bodied sports associations on their own initiative.

Participation of Women Athletes

It is obvious that disabled women athletes have to be encouraged to participate in sports events and to become coaches, trainers, officials, and leaders. "As the barriers to participation in sport are eliminated, sport programs for disabled girls and women will become increasingly available and accessible." (K. DePauw—Vista 1993).

Perspectives in Research

Coaches and teachers need methods and techniques based on evidence and issues. Some scientific areas where such issues are needed may include: aerobic capacity, cardiorespiratory function, muscular strength and endurance, body composition, nutrition, flexibility, injury, impact of training, specific sports disciplines at different training levels, indicated and contraindicated activities, the aging process (youth and senior programs), APA and misunderstood disabilities, construction materials, future technology (within the present rules and with unrestricted development), doping, and marketing.

Among these many fields, some are related to the continued expansion of high-level evaluation and competition, and others are related to the most adequate and adapted sports disciplines for different training levels. Longitudinal training studies must focus on issues which pertain not only to immediate performance enhancement but also to individual quality of life.

It is generally agreed that the so-called sports sciences include: medicine, biomechanics, psychology, pedagogy, sociology, history of sports, and philosophy of sports, as well as other fields of human knowledge with scientific connections to physical activities or sports science.

In these scientific areas, there should be no discrimination between able-bodied and disabled persons because the science of human movement includes normalities and abnormalities. The distinction between these concepts of normalities and abnormalities is difficult to determine and scientists should analyze the movement of able-bodied and disabled persons with the same technology, scientific tools, and discipline.

Inclusion is not only an objective for athletes in sporting events but also for scientists who are focusing on new cross- and multidisciplinary perspectives.

Conclusion

During the last 20 years, the adapted physical activity movement has tried to extend the benefits of adapted sports to as many people as possible.

Future goals could be summarized in the following five points:

1. A coherent policy for disability groups on local, regional, national, and international levels
2. Cooperation between governing bodies, community sports organizations, schools, and universities
3. Cooperation between sports scientists, medical experts, and sports technicians, coaches, and athletes
4. Cooperation between sports scientists themselves in avoiding duplication of research and addressing the appropriate questions by coordinated research
5. Cooperation between university authorities in preparing teachers for adapted sports leadership

Men always build too many walls . . . and not enough bridges—Isaac Newton

Appendix

International Federation of Adapted Physical Activity (IFAPA)

The **International Federation of Adapted Physical Activity (IFAPA)** was founded in Quebec, Canada in 1973. Since then it has expanded rapidly to become a worldwide organization with an international charter.

The objective of IFAPA is to provide a global focus for professional using adapted physical activity for instruction, competition, recreation, education, remediation and research. Adapted physical activity means movement, physical activity, and sports in which special emphasis has been placed on the interests and capabilities of individuals with limiting conditions. A biennial symposium serves as an international forum to bring together people, programs and research findings to the benefits of disabled peoples all over the world.

Previous International Symposia on Adapted Physical Activity have been held:

1977 in Quebec, Canada
1979 in Brussels, Belgium
1981 in New Orleans, U.S.A.
1983 in London, Great Britain
1985 in Tronto, Canda
1987 in Brisbane, Australia
1989 in Berlin, Germany
1991 in Miami, U.S.A.

IFAPA Executive Board 1993–95

Gudrun Doll-Tepper	President	Germany
Karen P. DePauw	President-Elect	U.S.A.
Claudine Sherrill	Vice President	U.S.A.
Garry D. Wheeler	Secretary General	Canada
Claudia Emes	Treasurer	Canada
Jean-Claude De Potter	Past President	Belgium

IFAPA Office

Dr. Garry D. Wheeler
University of Alberta, Rick Hansen Center

W1-67 Van Vliet Complex, Edmonton, AB, Canada T6G2HA
Fax: 1-403-492-7161

Asian Society for Adapted Physical Education and Exercise (ASAPE)

The Asian Society for Adapted Physical Education and Exercise (ASAPE) was founded in Seoul, Korea in 1986. More than 250 professionals from 11 countries have been registered as ASAPE members.

The objectives of the ASAPE is to contribute to the development of research and study on adapted physical education and exercise for individuals with special needs and the elderly.

Previous International ASAPE conferences have been held:
1989 in Nagoya, Japan
1991 in Miyazaki, Japan
1994 in Taipei, Taiwan R.O.C.

ASAPE Executive Board

Kyonosuke Yabe	President	Japan
Yang Ja Hong	Vice President	Korea
Katsuhiko Kusano	Chairperson	Japan
Hideo Nakata	Secretary General	Japan

ASAPE Office

Prof. Hideo Nakata
Institute of Special Education
University of Tsukuba
Tsukuba-shi 305 Japan
Fax 81-298-53-6748

9th International Symposium on Adapted Physical Activity (9th ISAPA)

The 9th ISAPA was held in Yokohama 4–7 August 1993.

The theme was

Stepping Forward Beyond Barriers Through Physical Activity

The objectives of the symposium were:

— to promote research on health and fitness programs for persons with disabilities and the elderly,

— to present the results of basic and practical research to evaluate the role of physical activity in the rehabilitation of mental and physical functions of persons with disabilities and the elderly, and
— to promote understanding and awareness towards persons with disabilities and the elderly through sports, and to consider improvements in the environment and facilities provided for these activities.

Organizing Committee

Honorary Patron
His Imperial Highness Prince Tomohito of Mikasa

Honorary Presidents

Kazuji Nagasu	Governor of Kanagawa Prefecture
Hidenobu Takahide	Mayor of Yokohama City

Chairperson

Kyonosuke Yabe	ASAPE President, Nagoya University

Vice Chairperson

Katsuhiko Kusano	Miyazaki University

Secretary General

Hideo Nakata	University of Tsukuba

Committee Members

Tetsuo Fukunaga	University of Tokyo
Yasumasa Kaneda	National Rehabilitation Center for the Physically Disabled
Yoshifumi Kobayashi	Yokohama National University
Reijiro Shimo	Shimo Orthopedic Clinic
Hiroshi Uozumi	Hyogo Women's College

International Scientific Committee

Jean-Claude De Potter	Université Libre de Bruxelles, Belgium
Karen P. DePauw	Washington State University, U.S.A.
Yang Ja Hong	Ewha Womans University, Korea
Kyonosuke Yabe	ASAPE President, Nagoya University, Japan

Endorsement/Cooperation

— Ministry of Foreign Affairs
— Ministry of Education
— Ministry of Health and Welfare

— Kanagawa Prefecture
— Yokohama City
— Japanese Society of Physical Education
— Japanese Society of Physical Fitness and Sports Medicine
— Japanese Society of Special Education
— The Japanese Association of Rehabilitation Medicine
— Japanese Physical Therapy Association
— Japanese Sports Association for the Disabled
— National Strength and Conditioning Association Japan
— Foundation of Social Development for Senior Citizens
— Japan Broadcasting Corporation (NHK)
— The Asahi Shimbun
— International Council of Sport Science and Physical Education (ICSSPE)
— Foundation for Advancement of International Science

Acknowledgements

— Kashiwa Welfare Fellowship
— The Commemorative Association for the Japan World Exposition (1970)
— Keidanren
— IBM Japan, Ltd.
— Takashimaya Co., Ltd.
— Tokyo Gas Co., Ltd.
— Ishibashi Foundation
— Sony Corporation
— International Communications Foundation
— Chubu Ikeda Co., Ltd.
— The Federation of Pharmaceutical Manufacturers' Associations of Japan (FPMAJ)
— Toyota Motor Corporation
— Dr. Yutaka Nakamura Memorial Foundation for the Disabled
— Science Promotion Foundation of Nagoya University
— ASAPE Foundation

In addition, we thank all those who have contributed to the success of the symposium through their strong and constant efforts and support.

Subject Index

(Letter after page number: f = figure; t = table)

SPRINGER NATURE

GPSR Compliance

The European Union's (EU) General Product Safety Regulation (GPSR) is a set of rules that requires consumer products to be safe and our obligations to ensure this.

If you have any concerns about our products, you can contact us on ProductSafety@springernature.com

In case Publisher is established outside the EU, the EU authorized representative is:

Springer Nature Customer Service Center GmbH
Europaplatz 3
69115 Heidelberg, Germany

The manufacturer's authorised representative in the EU is Springer Nature Customer Service Centre GmbH, Europaplatz 3, 69115 Heidelberg, Germany. If you have any concerns regarding our products, please contact ProductSafety@springernature.com

Printed and bound by CPI Group (UK) Ltd, Croydon, CR0 4YY
25/09/2026
02222896-0008